TEXTBOOK *of* Naturopathic Integrative Oncology

TEXTBOOK *of*

Naturopathic Integrative Oncology

DR JODY E. NOÉ, MS, ND

Foreword by DR PETER J. D'ADAMO, ND

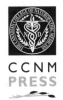

CCNM
PRESS

Canadä

Cataloging in publication data is available.
ISBN 897025-34-5

Edited by Bob Hilderley.
Indexed by Jo-Anne Pellisier.
Design and type by Sari Naworynski.
Illustrations courtesy of Susan Hannah, Teresa Winslow, and ASCO.
Cover photograph of *Camellia sinensis* by Henriette Kress.
Printed and bound in Canada.
Published by CCNM Press,
1255 Sheppard Avenue East,
Toronto, Ontario, M2K 1E2.
www.ccnmpress.com

CONTENTS

For various reasons, people often want to know my astrological sign. Having been born on July 17th, I've noticed over the years that the inquirer inevitably shudders a bit as I reply with the word 'cancer.' It seems that the word itself, originally derived from the Greek karkinos; meaning 'crab,' has the power to both awe and intimidate. Its medical meaning stems from the fact that the word can also be interpreted to mean 'hard' (like the shell of a crab) and the fact that from ancient times the diagnosis of cancer has been from the appearance of the hard, solid external lesion. The tumor, with its attendant swollen blood vessels, reminded Hippocrates of a crab dug into the sand. However, the karkinos of Hippocrates were the large superficial tumors readily seen on the skin, tongue, breast and neck.

We now know that cancer is not just a superficial illness, but also a systemic disease of widespread manifestation and mind-numbing complexity. Medicine has grown up with the cancer dilemma. It has taught us much, and much remains to be learnt. It has metaphorically evolved with each new and passing paradigm, from a humoral imbalance, to a chemical disruption, and finally to genomic instability; all the while tantalizingly fitting the exemplar of each new model, but remaining elusive of final accounting. We are now moving to a more complex, network-like, approximation of it inner workings. Only time will tell if these new systems-based models will suffice, but they at least allow for the possibility that the best models of the future will be non-reductionist, and that fact alone warrants a role for an integrative approach to its treatment and management.

Dr. Jody Noé has provided an important first step in the process of elucidating this integrative approach with the first edition of *The Textbook of Naturopathic Integrative Oncology*. I am impressed by the many facets of this work. Designed for naturopathic medical students, it exhibits wide explanatory scope, never neglecting that the active mind of the student requires contextualization, the relationship of information that throws light on their meaning, in addition to ostension, the act of teaching things by simply showing what they are about.

It's important and all well and good to know the molecular biology of genetic regulatory networks, and their influence on transcription factors, but the student must always remember that in practice everything boils down to that complex adaptive system in the examination room that we call a 'patient.'

June Goodfield, the British historian and scientist, wrote that 'Cancer begins and ends with people. In the midst of scientific abstraction, it is sometimes possible to forget this one basic fact. Doctors treat diseases, but they also treat people, and this precondition of their professional existence sometimes pulls them in two directions at once.'

Make no mistake, this is a highly nuanced and technical work and considerable effort on the part of the student will be required in order to master its precepts. It contains much new information on nutritional and botanical medicines, highlighting both their capabilities and risks of drug interaction. The sections dealing with specific common malignancies are authoritative, clearly organized and written. Important aspects of case management, including an excellent section on stress management, will allow naturopathic physicians to better integrate the workings of the mind-body into the therapeutic mix, a factor often given cursory attention by a harried and time-sensitive health care system.

Contrary to the prevailing stereotype that they are poorly educated, gullible, susceptible to wild promises and clutching at straws, research has shown that patients electing to incorporate integrative therapies in the cancer treatment are on average more informed and better educated than those who do not opt for such an approach. The naturopathic oncologist must be prepared to offer explanations and suggestions in an erudite, sagacious and perspicacious manner. This book will help them to do just that.

Every oncology patient, no matter how dire the prognosis, maintains the promise of being the 'exceptional patient.' Proper and rational integration of conventional treatment options with naturopathic modalities cannot but increase the odds of every patient's exceptionalness.

Most cancer patients have a pretty good idea of what their five-year survival odds are, and no doubt are prepared to hear just what survival rate my particular patients enjoy. I usually try to turn the dialectic around and offer instead an alternate interpretation: That even in cancers with low (5% to15%) odds of five year survival, the fact is that someone will have to be in that percentile, and I will try to do everything in my power to get them into that group.

Cancer treatment is just that personal.

Dr Peter J. D'Adamo

Integrative Medical Model

By definition, the word integrative means to unify, to make a whole by bringing all parts together. On the one hand, integrative medicine treats the person as a whole, integrating body, mind, and spirit. The patient is respected as a whole being, not just managed as a disease condition, and becomes empowered as a result to participate consciously in the healing process. On the other hand, integrative medicine calls on many different healing traditions and modalities to treat the whole person, ranging from conventional Western chemotherapy, radiation, and surgery to Traditional Chinese Medicine (TCM) and other complementary and alternative medicines (CAM). Naturopathic medicine straddles these extremes, playing an adjunctive role at the center of cancer patient care. Naturopathic medicine is particularly well-suited for this role because of the modalities encompassed in this practice of medicine.

ROLE OF NATUROPATHIC MEDICINE IN CANCER CARE

Chemotherapy   Radiation

Naturopathic
Medicine

Surgery   Palliative Care

Naturopathic Medical Modalities
- Lifestyle counseling
- Clinical nutrition
- Botanical medicine
- Homeopathic medicine
- Traditional medicines (Chinese, Ayurvedic, Native)
- Mind-Body therapies

PATIENT-CENTERED CARE

Integrative partnerships between conventional medical doctors (MDs) and licensed naturopathic doctors (NDs) are becoming quite common. This collaboration makes many more effective therapies available to patients and allows the physician to better customize management programs for individual patients. Gone are the days of treating all cancers and all patients with one modality, such as chemotherapy. In this collaborative model, naturopathic physicians are integral to the full patient care continuum, following the patient from diagnosis through treatment to recovery or palliative care if treatment fails. They also play the central role in prevention education.

CANCER PATIENT CARE CONTINUUM

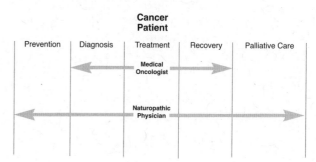

The medical oncologist specializes in immediate diagnosis, treatment, and recovery care, while the naturopathic physician also manages prevention and palliative care.

CIRCLES OF CARE

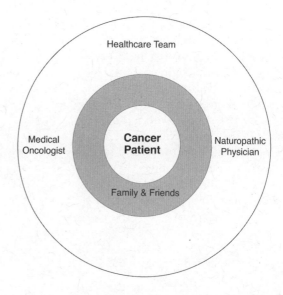

INTEGRATIVE EDUCATIONAL PROGRAMS

In recent years, integrative approaches to patient care have been instituted as part of residency training programs at many schools of medicine in North America, and several comprehensive textbooks have been published to support these educational initiatives. Celebrated physicians and professors Andrew Weil, Tierona LowDog, and their colleagues have founded the Program in Integrative Medicine at the University of Arizona. Dr David Rakel at the University of Wisconsin Integrative Medicine Program has written the authoritative textbook, *Integrative Medicine*, while Dr Marc S. Micozzi at the Thomas Jefferson University Center for Complementary and Integrative Medicine has compiled a textbook on the *Fundamentals of Complementary and Integrative Medicine* to introduce medical professionals to the principles and practices of this approach. Dr. Donald Abrams at the University of California, San Francisco, has developed the highly respected Osher Center for Integrative Medicine.

Other integrative medicine programs can be found at the five naturopathic medicine colleges in North America – National College of Natural Medicine, Bastyr University, Canadian College of Natural Medicine, Southwest College of Naturopathic Medicine, University of Bridgeport College of Naturopathic Medicine, Boucher Institute, and National University of Health Sciences.

Beyond these introductory textbooks, however, few academic books on integrative approaches to specific disease conditions have been published for use in the classroom and clinic. In the field of cancer care, this *Textbook of Naturopathic Integrative Oncology* is a fundamental work.

Learning Objectives

This textbook is designed to teach health science and medical college students fundamental cancer cell biology and inflammatory pathway biochemistry in preparation for managing patients with various forms of cancer, integratively. Integrative cancer treatment combines conventional allopathic chemotherapy, radiation, and surgery with naturopathic modalities, chiefly lifestyle counseling, clinical nutrition (dietary and nutraceutical therapy), and botanical medicine. These integrated modalities can be applied not only to cancer treatment but also to cancer prevention and palliative care.

Contents

Part 1 of this book reviews basic cell division and introduces abnormal cell biology leading to development of a cancer cell. Various theories of cell mutation are examined with the focus on inflammatory pathway biochemistry. In Part 2 stress management, clinical nutrition, and botanical medicines are presented as the chief naturopathic preventive and therapeutic modalities for cancer. In Part 3, these naturopathic modalities are integrated with conventional chemotherapy, radiation, and surgery, showing how naturopathic approaches can enhance these conventional treatments while decreasing side effects.

In Part 4, common types of cancer are discussed chapter by chapter in terms of their epidemiology and pathophysiology, leading to a discussion of their possible etiology, diagnosis, staging, and conventional treatment protocols. Naturopathic recommendations for each cancer are included with integrative applications.

Not all cancers are discussed, providing an opportunity for students to apply naturopathic integrative protocols to cancers of the bladder, bone, brain, kidney, liver, and soft tissue (sarcoma), as well as cervical, skin (melanoma), testicular, thyroid, and uterine cancers, for example. In group projects, students could work up a chapter on one of these cancers, following the clinical reasoning pattern established in this textbook, moving from pathophysiology and epidemiology through assessment and diagnosis to conventional and naturopathic integrative therapeutic protocols.

Evidence-Based Guidelines

The body of literature on integrative practices is growing rapidly, with studies supported by key government bodies, university research centers, and cancer institutes. Throughout this book, medical information and clinical guidelines are grounded in the most current research and best practice standards established by medical associations. The extensive references at the end of each chapter are augmented with a special chapter listing the most important integrative medicine publications on in the field. Taken together, this book is the most complete and current list of integrative and naturopathic research on cancer in the medical literature.

Pedagogical Tools

Within the individual chapters on cancer types, clinical reasoning and case management skills are developed by presenting information in recurring SOAP order and by presenting case histories of patients who have been managed integratively. Open-ended case management studies are provided at the back of the book for instructors to use in directing classroom discussions and for students to use in preparing for board examination questions. Students should also find the extensive references to be an excellent springboard for new laboratory research and independent study. To assist instructors adopting or recommending this book for course use, a basic syllabus for a quarter, semester and full-year course is available. For an instructor's manual and a complementary book of case studies, contact the publisher at ccnmpress.com.

GLOSSARY

This glossary is adapted from the National Cancer Institute, by permission, available at http://www.nci.nih.gov.

Acute lymphocytic leukemia: Type of blood cancer that originates in lymphatic cells of the bone marrow.

Acute myelogenous leukemia: Type of blood cancer that involves accumulation of myeloid cells in the bone marrow and bloodstream.

Adenocarcinoma: Cancer that begins in cells that line certain internal organs.

Adenoma: Noncancerous tumor.

Alpha-fetoprotein: Protein often found in abnormal amounts in the blood of patients with liver cancer.

Ames test: Mutagenesis assay (a measure of mutagenic ability) that involves specially engineered strains of bacteria. Because of the relationship between mutagenicity and carcinogenicity, the test is used as a rapid and relatively inexpensive first screening of untested chemicals that are suspected to be carcinogens.

Anaplastic: Term used to describe cancer cells that divide rapidly and bear little or no resemblance to normal cells.

Angiogenesis: Blood vessel formation, which usually accompanies the growth of malignant tissue.

Angiosarcoma: Type of cancer that begins in the lining of blood vessels.

Apoptosis: Normal cellular process involving a genetically programmed series of events leading to the death of a cell.

Asymptomatic: Presenting no signs or symptoms of disease.

Ataxia telangiectasia: Hereditary disorder characterized by problems with muscle coordination, immunodeficiency, inadequate DNA repair, and an increased risk of developing cancer.

Atypical hyperplasia: Benign (noncancerous) condition in which tissue has certain abnormal features.

Basal cell: Small, round cell found in the lower part, or base, of the epidermis, the outer layer of the skin.

Basal cell carcinoma: Type of skin cancer that arises from the basal cells.

Benign: Not cancerous; does not invade nearby tissue or spread to other parts of the body.

Benign tumor: A noncancerous growth that does not spread to other parts of the body.

Biological therapy: Use of the body's immune system, either directly or indirectly, to fight cancer or to lessen side effects that may be caused by some cancer treatments. Also known as immunotherapy, biotherapy, or biological response modifier therapy.

Biopsy: Removal of a sample of tissue, which is then examined under a microscope to check for cancer cells.

Bone marrow: Soft, spongy tissue in the center of large bones that produces white blood cells, red blood cells, and platelets.

Bone marrow aspiration: Removal of a small sample of bone marrow (usually from the hip) through a needle for examination under a microscope to see whether cancer cells are present.

Bone marrow biopsy: Removal of a sample of tissue from the bone marrow with a large needle. The cells are checked to see whether they are cancerous. If cancerous plasma cells are found, the pathologist estimates how much of the bone marrow is affected. Bone marrow biopsy is usually done at the same time as bone marrow aspiration.

Bone marrow transplantation: Procedure in which doctors replace marrow destroyed by treatment with high doses of anticancer drugs or radiation. The replacement marrow may be taken from the patient before treatment or may be donated by another person.

Bone scan: Technique to create images of bones on a computer screen or on film. A small amount of radioactive material is injected and travels through the bloodstream. It collects in the bones, especially in abnormal areas of the bones, and is detected by a scanner.

Brachytherapy: Internal radiation therapy using an implant of radioactive material placed directly into or near the tumor.

BRCA1: Gene located on chromosome 17 that normally helps restrain cell growth. Inheriting an altered version of *BRCA1* predisposes an individual to breast, ovarian, or prostate cancer.

BRCA2: Gene located on chromosome 13 that scientists believe may account for 30% to 40% of all inherited breast cancer.

Breast reconstruction: Surgery to rebuild the shape of a breast after a mastectomy.

Burkitt lymphoma: Type of non-Hodgkin lymphoma that most often occurs in young people between the ages of 12 and 30. The disease usually causes a rapidly growing tumor in the abdomen.

Cancer: Term for a group of more than 100 diseases in which abnormal cells divide without control. Cancer cells can invade nearby tissues and can spread through the bloodstream and lymphocytic system to other parts of the body.

Carcinogen: Any substance that is known to cause cancer.

Carcinogenesis: Process by which normal cells are transformed into cancer cells.

Carcinoma: Cancer that begins in the lining or covering of an organ.

Carcinoma in situ: Cancer that involves only the cells in which it began and has not spread to other tissues.

CEA assay: Laboratory test to measure the level of carcinoembryonic antigen (CEA), a substance that is sometimes found in an increased amount in the blood of patients with certain cancers.

Cell cycle: Sequence of events by which cells enlarge and divide. Includes stages typically named G1, S, G2, and M.

Chemoprevention: Use of natural or laboratory-made substances to prevent cancer.

Chemotherapy: Treatment with anticancer drugs.

Chronic lymphocytic leukemia: Type of blood cancer that involves overproduction of mature lymphocytes.

Chronic myelogenous leukemia: Type of blood cancer that involves accumulation of granulocytes (a type of white blood cell) in the bone marrow and bloodstream.

Clinical trial: Research study that involves patients. Each study is designed to find better ways to prevent, detect, diagnose, or treat cancer and to answer scientific questions.

Colonoscopy: Procedure that uses a flexible fiber optic endoscope to examine the internal surface of the colon along its entire length.

Combination chemotherapy: Treatment in which two or more chemicals are used to obtain more effective results.

Computed tomography: X-ray procedure that uses a computer to produce a detailed picture of a cross section of the body; also called CAT or CT scan.

Contact inhibition: Inhibition of cell division in normal (noncancerous) cells when they contact a neighboring cell.

CT (or CAT) scan: *See* computed tomography.

Cytotoxic: Poisonous to cells. In chemotherapy, used to describe an agent that is poisonous to cancer cells.

Diagnosis: Process of identifying a disease by the signs and symptoms.

Dysplasia: Abnormal cells that are not cancer.

Dysplastic nevi: Atypical moles; moles whose appearance is different from that of common moles. Dysplastic nevi are generally larger than ordinary moles and have irregular and indistinct borders. Their color often is not uniform and ranges from pink or even white to dark brown or black; they usually are flat, but parts may be raised above the skin surface.

Encapsulated: Confined to a specific area; an encapsulated tumor remains in a compact form.

Endometrial: Having to do with the mucous membrane that lines the cavity of the uterus.

Environmental tobacco smoke: Smoke that comes from the burning end of a cigarette and smoke that is exhaled by smokers. Also called ETS or secondhand smoke. Inhaling ETS is called involuntary or passive smoking.

Epidemiology: Study of the factors that affect the prevalence, distribution, and control of disease.

Epidermis: Upper or outer layer of the two main layers of cells that make up the skin.

Epstein-Barr virus: Virus that has been associated with the development of infectious mononucleosis and also with Burkitt's lymphoma.

Estrogen: Female hormone produced by the ovary. Responsible for secondary sex characteristics and cyclic changes in the lining of the uterus and vagina.

Etiology: Study of the causes of abnormal condition or disease.

Familial polyposis: Inherited condition in which several hundred polyps develop in the colon and rectum. These polyps have a high potential to become malignant.

Fecal occult blood test: Test to reveal blood hidden in the feces, which may be a sign of colon cancer.

Fiber: Parts of fruits and vegetables that cannot be digested. Also called bulk or roughage.

Fibroid: Benign uterine tumor made up of fibrous and muscular tissue.

Gene therapy: Treatment that alters genes (the basic units of heredity found in all cells in the body). In studies of gene therapy for cancer, researchers are trying to improve the body's natural ability to fight the disease or to make the tumor more sensitive to other kinds of therapy.

Genetic: Inherited; having to do with information that is passed from parents to children through DNA in the genes.

Glandular: medicine derived from the glands of other animals, such as porcine insulin and adrenal tissue.

Grade: Describes how closely a cancer resembles normal tissue of its same type, along with the cancer's probable rate of growth.

Grading: System for classifying cancer cells in terms of how malignant or aggressive they appear microscopically. The grading of a tumor indicates how quickly cancer cells are likely to spread and plays a role in treatment decisions.

Herpes virus: Member of the herpes family of viruses. One type of herpes virus is sexually transmitted and causes sores on the genitals.

Hormonal therapy: Treatment of cancer by removing, blocking, or adding hormones.

Human papillomaviruses: Viruses that generally cause warts. Some papillomaviruses are sexually transmitted. Some of these sexually transmitted viruses cause wartlike growths on the genitals, and some are thought to cause abnormal changes in cells of the cervix.

Hyperplasia: Precancerous condition in which there is an increase in the number of normal cells lining an organ.

Imaging: Tests that produce pictures of areas inside the body.

Immunotherapy: Treatment that uses the body's natural defenses to fight cancer. Also called biotherapy or biological modifier response therapy.

Incidence: Number of new cases of a disease diagnosed each year.

Incidence rate: Number of new cases per year per 100,000 persons.

Initiation: Preneoplastic change in the genetic material of cells caused by a chemical carcinogen. Cancer develops when initiated cells are subsequently exposed to the same or another carcinogen.

In situ cancer: Cancer that has remained within the tissue in which it originated.

Invasion: As related to cancer, the spread of cancer cells into healthy tissue adjacent to the tumor.

Invasive cancer: Cancer that has spread beyond the layer of tissue in which it developed.

Keratin: Insoluble protein that is the major constituent of the outer layer of the skin, nails, and hair.

Lesion: Area of abnormal tissue change.

Leukemia: Cancer of the blood cells.

Lifetime risk: Probability that a person, over the course of a lifetime, will develop cancer.

Li-Fraumeni syndrome: Rare family predisposition to multiple cancers, caused by an alteration in the *p53* tumor suppressor gene.

Lumen: An enclosed space bounded by an epithelial membrane; for example, the lumen of the gut.

Malignant: Cancerous; can invade nearby tissue and spread to other parts of the body.

Melanin: Skin pigment (substance that gives the skin its color). Dark-skinned people have more melanin than light-skinned people.

Melanocyte: Cell in the skin that produces and contains the pigment called melanin.

Melanoma: Cancer of the cells that produce pigment in the skin. Melanoma usually begins in a mole.

Metastasis: Cancer growth (secondary tumors) that is anatomically separated from the site at which the original cancer developed.

Metastasize: To spread from one part of the body to another. When cancer cells metastasize and form secondary tumors, the cells in the metastatic tumor are like those in the original (primary) tumor.

Mole: Area on the skin (usually dark in color) that contains a cluster of melanocytes. *See also* nevus.

Monoclonal: Population of cells that was derived by cell division from a single ancestral cell.

Morbidity: Disease.

Mortality: Death.

Mortality rate: Number of deaths per 100,000 persons per year.

Mutagen: Any substance that is known to cause mutations.

Mutagenesis: Process by which mutations occur.

Mutation: Change in the way cells function or develop, caused by an inherited genetic defect or an environmental exposure. Such changes may lead to cancer.

National Cancer Institute (NCI): The largest of the 24 separate institutes, centers, and divisions of the National Institutes of Health. The NCI coordinates the federal government's cancer research program.

National Institutes of Health (NIH): One of eight health agencies of the Public Health Service (the Public Health Service is part of the U.S. Department of Health and Human Services). Composed of 24 separate institutes, centers, and divisions, NIH is the largest biomedical research facility in the world.

Necrosis: Cell death.

Neoplasia: Abnormal new growth of cells.

Neoplasm: New growth of tissue. Can be referred to as benign or malignant.

Nevus: Medical term for a spot on the skin, such as a mole. A mole is a cluster of melanocytes that usually appears as a dark spot on the skin.

Non-Hodgkin lymphoma: One of the several types of lymphoma (cancer that develops in the lymphocytic system) that are not Hodgkin lymphoma. Hodgkin lymphoma is rare and occurs most often in people age 15 to 34 and in people over 55. All other lymphomas are grouped together and called non-Hodgkin lymphoma.

Nutraceutical: Term for a nutritional supplement, such as a vitamin, mineral, or amino acid, used medicinally.

Rous sarcoma virus: Chicken retrovirus that was the first virus shown to cause a malignancy.

Sarcoma: Malignant tumor that begins in connective and supportive tissue.

Screening: Checking for disease when there are no symptoms.

Secondary tumor: Metastasis.

SEER Program: Surveillance, Epidemiology, and End Results Program of the National Cancer Institute. Started in 1973, SEER collects cancer incidence data in nine geographic areas with a combined population of approximately 9.6% of the total population of the United States.

Side effect: Problem that occurs when treatment affects healthy cells. Common side effects of cancer treatment are fatigue, nausea, vomiting, decreased blood cell counts, hair loss, and mouth sores.

Somatic cell: Any of the body cells except the reproductive cells.

SPF (sun protection factor): Scale for rating sunscreens. Sunscreens with an SPF of 15 or higher provide the best protection from the potentially harmful rays of the sun.

Squamous cell cancer: Type of skin cancer that arises from the squamous cells.

Stage: Extent of a cancer, especially whether the disease has spread from the original site to other parts of the body.

Staging: Doing exams and tests to learn the extent of the cancer, especially whether it has spread from its original site to other parts of the body.

Stem cells: Cells from which all blood cells develop.

Sun protection factor: *See* SPF.

Sunscreen: Substance that blocks the potentially harmful effect of overexposure to the rays of the sun. Using lotions or creams that contain sunscreens can protect the skin from damage that may lead to cancer. *See also* SPF.

Survival rate: Proportion of patients alive at some point after their diagnosis of a disease.

Telomerase: Enzyme that is present and active in cells that can divide without apparent limit (for example, cancer cells and cells of the germ line). Telomerase replaces the missing repeated sequences of each telomere.

Telomere: End of a chromosome. In vertebrate cells, each telomere consists of thousands of copies of the same DNA sequence, repeated again and again. Telomeres become shorter each time a cell divides; when one or more telomeres reaches a minimum length, cell division stops. This mechanism limits the number of times a cell can divide.

Testosterone: Male sex hormone.

Transformation: Change that a normal cell undergoes as it becomes malignant.

Tumor: Abnormal mass of tissue that results from excessive cell division. Tumors perform no useful body function. They may be either benign (not cancerous) or malignant (cancerous).

Tumor marker: Substance in blood or other body fluids that may suggest that a person has cancer.

Tumor suppressor gene: Gene in the body that can suppress or block the development of cancer.

Ultraviolet (UV) radiation: Invisible rays that are part of the energy that comes from the sun. UV radiation can burn the skin and cause melanoma and other types of skin cancer.

X-chromosome inactivation: Process by which one of the two X chromosomes in each cell from a female mammal becomes condensed and inactive. This process ensures that most genes on the X chromosome are expressed to the same extent in both males and females.

X-ray: High-energy radiation used in low doses to diagnose diseases and in high doses to treat cancer.

Xeroderma pigmentosum: Hereditary disease characterized by extreme sensitivity to the sun and a tendency to develop skin cancers. Caused by inadequate DNA repair.

ONCOLOGY ACRONYMS
AND ABBREVIATIONS

DISEASES
ALL: Acute Lymphoblastic Leukemia
AML: Acute Myelooid Leukemia
ANLL: Acute Non-Lymphocytic Leukemia
APL: Acute Promyelocytic Leukemia
APML: Acute Promyelocytic Leukemia
BCP-ALL: B-cell Precursor Acute Lymphoblastic Leukemia
CLL: Chronic Lymphocytic Leukemia
CML: Chronic Myelogenous Leukemia
CNSL: Central Nervous System Lymphoma
HCL: Hairy Cell Leukemia
HD: Hodgkin Lymphoma
MCL: Mantle Cell Lymphoma
MDS: Myelodysplastic Syndrome
MF: Mycosis Fungoides
MM: Multiple Myeloma
MPD: Myeloproliferative Disorders
NHL: Non-Hodgkin Lymphoma
PV: Polycythemia Vera
WM: Waldenstrom's Macroglobulinemia

TREATMENT OPTIONS
ABMT: Autologous Bone Marrow Transplantation (your own marrow)
BMT: Allogeneic Bone Marrow Transplantation (someone else's marrow)
SBMT: Syngeneic Bone Marrow Transplantation (identical twin's marrow)
PBPC: Peripheral Blood Progenitor Cell Transplant
PBSCT: Peripheral Blood Stem Cell Transplant
PBSCR: Peripheral Blood Stem Cell Rescue
PSCT or PSCR: Peripheral Stem Cell Transplant or Peripheral Stem Cell Rescue; same as PBSCT or PBSCR without the word "blood"

CHEMOTHERAPIES
ABVD: doxorubicin, vinblastine, bleomycin, DTIC
ACOB: doxorubicin, cyclophosphamide, vincristine, bleomycin
ARA-C: cytarabine
ATRA: all-trans retinoic acid, or Vesanoid

BACOP: bleomycin, doxorubicin, cyclophosphamide, vincristine, prednisone
BEAM: busulfan, etoposid, ara-c, melphalan
BLEO: bleomycin 2CdA - 2-chlorodeoxyadenosine (generic name = cladribine)
CCNU: (1-2-chloroethyl)-3-cyclohexyl-1-nitrosourea)
CHOD: cyclophosphamide, doxorubicin, vincristine, dexamethasone
CHOP: cyclophosphamide, adriamycin, vincristine, prednisone
CHOP-BLEO: cyclophosphamide, doxorubicin, vincristine, prednisone and bleomycin
CMF: cyclophosphamide, methotrexate, fluorouracil
C-MOPP: cyclophosphamide, oncovin, procarbazine, prednisone
COP: cyclophosphamide, vincristine, prednisone
COPP-CCNU: vincristine, procarbazine, prednisone
CyA: cyclosporin A
DCF: 2-deoxycoformycin (pentostatin)
DTIC: dacarbazine, 5-(3, 3-dimethyl-1-triazino) imidazole-4- carboxamide
EPOCH: etopside, prednisone, vincristine, cyclophosphamide (cytoxan), Adriamycin
FAC: fluorouacil, adriamycin, cyclophosphamide
Fludara: fludarabine
IFN: Interferon (comes in alpha2a, alpha 2b, human leukocyte, and beta; another one, "concensus, " is still in trials)
MOPP: Nitrogen mustard, vincristine, procarbazine, prednisone

BLOOD STIMULATING FACTORS
EPOIETIN: erythropoietin (Epogen); stimulates red cell growth
G-CSF: granulocyte colony stimulating factor (Neupogen); stimulates growth of white cells
GM-CSF: granulocyte macrophage; colony-stimulating factor (sargramostim)
NEUMEGA: platelet-stimulating factor

TPOIETIN: thrombopoietin; platelet-stimulating factor that is still in clinical trials

GENERAL TERMINOLOGY

B/P: Blood Pressure
B2M: beta 2 microglobulin test. Beta-2-microglobulin is a protein found on all the surface of all cells and small amounts are shed into the serum. People diagnosed with blood diseases and who have levels of beta-2-microglobulin below 3. 0 seem to have a longer survival rate.
BMB: Bone Marrow Biopsy
BMT: Bone Marrow Transplant
Bx: Biopsy
CBC: Complete Blood Count
CDRT: Cell culture drug resistance testing
CR: Complete Remission
CRN: Complete Remission with Nodular Pattern in Marrow
CS: Clinical Stage
Dx: Diagnosis
FISH: Fluorescence In Situ Hybridization. This is a test used to detect chromosome abnormalities in cells. The results help predict prognosis.
GVHD: Graft vs. host disease
GVL: Graft vs. leukemia or graft vs. lymphoma

HCT: Hematocrit; the percentage of red blood cells in the blood. A low hematocrit measurement indicates anemia.
HDC: High-dose chemotherapy, often used before a BMT or PBSCT
Hem/Onc: Hematologist/Oncologist
HGB: Hemoglobin
HLA: Human Leukocyte Antigen Test; a special blood test used to match a blood or bone marrow donor to a recipient for transfusion or transplant
Ig: Immunoglobulin (IgA, IgD, IgE, IgG, IgM)
IV: Intravenous (placed directly into a vein)
Mab or MoAb: monoclonal antibodies (for example, Campath-1H, Rituxan, Bexxar)
Matched Unrelated Donor of bone marrow
NR: Nodular remission (nodules of cancer cells remain in the marrow, but there are less than 10% cancer cells throughout)
OR: Overall Remission
PR: Partial Remission
RBC: Red Blood Count
Rx: Prescribed medication
WBC: White Blood Count
WBC/HPF: White Blood Cells Counted Per High Powered Field
WD: Well Differentiated
XRT: External Radiation Therapy

PART 1:
CANCER BASICS

CANCER CELL BIOLOGY AND INFLAMMATORY PATHWAYS

Dedicated cancer research during the past few decades has revolutionized our understanding of cancer. This success was made possible by molecular biologic techniques that have enabled researchers to probe features of individual cells. We now know that cancer is a disease of molecular genetics, and we are identifying these molecules and genes in order to create new strategies for treating cancer. As our understanding of the molecular genetics of the different types of cancers grows, we are developing new strategies aimed at avoiding, forestalling, and even changing genetic mutations that can lead to the development of that one aberrant cell that becomes cancer. This has become the study of epigenetics and genome expression.

Cancer Prefixes

Cancers are often referred to by terms that contain a prefix related to the cell type in which the cancer originated and a suffix, such as -sarcoma, -carcinoma, or just -oma. Common prefixes include:

- Adeno = gland
- Chondro = cartilage
- Erythro = red blood cell
- Hemangio = blood vessels
- Hepato = liver
- Lipo = fat
- Lympho = white blood cell
- Melano = pigment cell
- Myelo = bone marrow
- Myo = muscle
- Neuro = brain
- Osteo = bone
- Retino = eye
- Uro = bladder

Cell Review

The fundamental unit of life is the cell. In its small structure, the cell is capable of performing all of the functions that define life. Each of the organs in the body, including the heart, lungs, breasts, gonads, pancreas, colon, and brain, consists of specialized cells that carry out that organ's functions. Injured cells must be replaced to assure proper function of the organ. To reproduce a cell that is the replacement for an injured cell is a process of normal cell division. It is a highly regulated process.

DNA

DNA Cell growth, inheritance, and containment are regulated by its DNA (deoxyribonucleic acid). DNA is a highly complex molecule manufactured in the cell nucleus, which serves as the "brain" of the cell. DNA is the blueprint for cell functions. In a human cell, the DNA is arranged in 46 distinct sections called chromosomes. They are arranged in pairs, 23 chromosomes from each biological parent. The 46 chromosomes contain more than 100,000 genes.[1]

GENES

A gene is a segment of DNA that determines the structure of a protein, which is needed for growth and development, as well as carrying out vital chemical functions in the body. Genes are arranged in pairs - one gene from the progenitor female and one from the male.[1]

Each gene occupies a specific place on the chromosome, and through a series of biochemical steps, it tells the cell to make specific proteins. Some proteins are structural and some are regulatory. They tell the genes when to "turn on or off." Genes can also tell the cell to produce hormones, cytokines, and growth factors, which, in turn, exit the cell to communicate with other cells.[1]

When a gene is turned on, it manufactures a molecule called ribonucleic acid (RNA), which contains all the information the cell needs to make new proteins. Cells divide only when they receive the proper signals from growth factors that circulate in the bloodstream or from a cell in direct contact. Once that message is received by the cell, a normal cell reproduction is initiated involving several phases of division. Checkpoints along the way assures that the cell is undergoing normal cell division.[1]

FOUR PHASES OF MITOSIS[2]

1. Prophase
- Centrosomes separate and migrate to opposite poles.
- Centrioles separate.
- Chromatin is transformed into chromosomes composed of pairs of filaments called chromatids (each is a complete genetic copy of its chromosome).
- Nuclear membrane disappears.

2. Metaphase
- Paired chromosomes become lined up between the centrioles.

3. Anaphase
- Chromatids are pulled toward the centrioles. One chromatid from each pair goes to each daughter cell.

4. Telophase
Telophase I
- Chromosomes become more polarized and transformed into thread-like structures.
- A nuclear membrane forms around each set of chromosomes forming a new nucleus with a nucleolus.
- The centrioles duplicate.

Telophase II
- Actual dividing of the cell occurs (cytokinesis).
- Cytoplasm splits and two daughter cells are formed.

CELL CYCLE: MUTATIONS CREATE ABBERANT GENE
(www.nei.nih.gov[2])

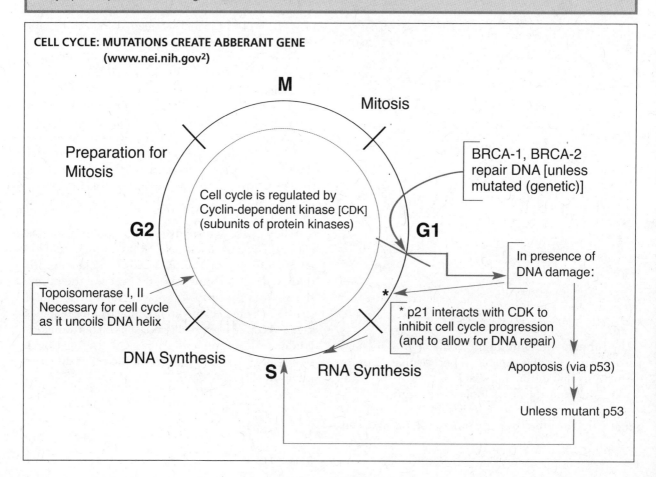

NORMAL CELL DIVISION

Cells reproduce by division. Cell division starts and ends with the mitosis phase, which forms two daughter cells. Normal cell division follows a cycle, starting and ending at mitosis or "M" while passing through G-1, S, and G-2 phases. The gap or G1-phase produces the RNA, proteins, and enzymes that direct DNA synthesis. The time it takes to complete this transcription varies, determined by the length of the individual cell cycle. In the S-phase, DNA synthesis occurs. Cells are thought to prepare for mitosis in the G-2 phase when specialized proteins and RNA are produced. G-0 designates a dormant phase of the cell cycle. The duration of S, M, and G-2 is considered relatively constant in different tissues.

ABNORMAL CELL DIVISION

Throughout the process of cell division each phase must take place correctly for proper cell reproduction. If one step is aberrant, then the whole process of cell division is askew.

A cancer cell grows rapidly out of control, ignoring normal cell signals and boundaries. Unlike normal cells, cancer cells ignore these signals to stop reproduction, to specialize highly, or to undergo apoptosis (normal cell death). As a cell able to grow in an uncontrollable manner, unable to recognize its own natural boundary signals, the cancer cell has the ability to evade the body's own immune system response and spread to distant areas of the body, a process called metastasis.

Cell Mutations

For a normal cell to become an aberrant cell, several genes must become mutated in the coding for cell reproduction. Generally there are two types of gene mutations: dominant and recessive.[3]

Dominant Gene

Dominant gene mutation is caused by an abnormality in one gene from a pair. This results in messages that create an aberration in the normal cell, such as a defective protein, that in turn signals for epithelial growth factor to constantly be "on." This results in the constant message to divide. The dominant gene mutated is called an oncogene.[3]

Recessive Gene

Both genes in the pair are damaged in the recessive mutation type of cell aberration. In cancer, one of the worst recessive mutations is the p53 tumor suppressor gene. The normal function of this gene is to produce a protein that turns off the cell cycle and helps to control normal cell reproduction. The p53 also is coded to repair or destroy defective cells, which is one of the normal gene functions that become aberrant in cancer cell division. The failure of this gene to repair or destroy defective cells takes away the potential to control precancerous and cancerous cells. The ability for the tumor suppressor activity of the p53 is only lost when both genes in the pair are mutated. One of the pair of p53 gene will still function to control the cell cycle.[3]

Cancer Cell Growth

Cancer is not a single disease. It is a group of many diseases characterized by uncontrolled growth and spread of abnormal cells. Aberrant cell division can occur either when active oncogenes are expressed or when tumor suppressor genes are lost. For this aberrant cell to become malignant, multiple mutations must occur. Both dominant and recessive mutations may occur within the same aberrant cell. These gene mutations allow for the aberrant cell then to act in unnatural ways within the system. It may invade normal tissue, where the original hyperplastic activity began, or can travel unchecked through the bloodstream to metastasize at a distant site in the body. There, the aberrant cell can continue its mutated hyperplastic division successfully.[4]

Aberrant Cell Actions

Multiple mutations of various kinds over time can result in cancer in the cell:
1. Rapid reproduction (hyperplasia)
2. Abnormal architecture (dysplasia)
3. Changes within the cell (in situ)
4. Loss of intracellular communication (invasive cancer)
5. Loss of cell adhesion (metastasis)

Cancer Cell Characteristics
1. Self sufficient growth signals
2. Insensitive to anti-growth signals
3. Evade apoptosis
4. Limitless replicative potential
5. Sustained angiogenesis
6. Tissue invasion and metastasis

CANCER CELL BEHAVIOR

What causes the damage to the normal cell can vary. First, if a cell becomes abnormal either by deletion of a part of a gene, a translocation in a chromosome, or a deficit in the DNA blueprint for the production of a defective protein, the normal cell becomes damaged.

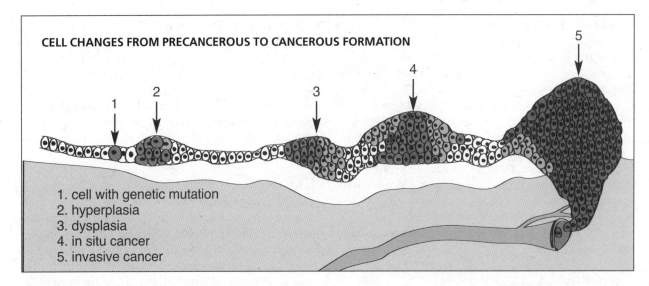

CELL CHANGES FROM PRECANCEROUS TO CANCEROUS FORMATION

1. cell with genetic mutation
2. hyperplasia
3. dysplasia
4. in situ cancer
5. invasive cancer

Second, viral infections can also cause an aberration in the cell cycle by imposing a viral reproductive life cycle. Depending on the virus and sometimes the viral strain, when a virus codes (either DNA or RNA) in the host genome, it can cause an aberration in the sequence, causing the protein function not to work because of the viral genomic code left behind.

How the aberrant cancer cell then behaves in the body is dependant on the mutations that have occurred. These mutations turn "on" or turn "off" functions of the cell's behavior and therein the virility of the cancer growth and behavior is determined. Some cancer cells simply divide and produce a hyperplastic lesion that remains localized. Other cancer cells are able to evade the body's immune function and successfully invade local tissue as well as enter the bloodstream, lymph system, or central spinal fluid and metastasize to a distant site of the body. These defects in the cancer cell are a direct result of gene mutation that can be caused by exogenous stimuli, such as an infectious virus.[5]

Aberrant Chromosomes

Chromosomal aberrations, according to the *CURRENT Medical Diagnosis and Treatment (2010)*,[6] include:

- In Burkitt's lymphoma, the c-*myc* oncogene is activated by translocation of genetic material from chromosome 8 to chromosome 14.
- In chronic myelogenous leukemia (CML) by definition a reciprocal translocation of the long arms of chromosomes 9 and 22, resulting in the generation of a fusion protein (BCR-ABL) with tyrosine kinase activity.
- In colon cancer, loss of the long arm of chromosome 18 (18q) predicts a poor outcome, whereas mutations in the gene for the type II receptor for

transforming growth factor-1 (TGF-1) with microsatellite instability predict a favorable outcome.
- In chronic lymphocytic leukemia (CLL), genetic mutations have been shown to occur in up to 82% of cases and strongly predict outcomes.
- Amplification of the HER-2/*neu* oncogene in breast cancer has been associated with more aggressive tumors, a higher stage at diagnosis, and a shorter survival. However, this gene has also been associated with marked chemotherapy responsiveness to specific agents, and has provided a successful target for a targeted biologic agent (trastuzumab) in the treatment of breast cancer. Treatment of HER-2/*neu*-positive early-stage breast cancer with the combination of chemotherapy and the targeted agent trastuzumab has resulted in striking improvements in outcome—so much so that finding this gene not only predicts response to treatment but also a lower risk of recurrence.

Tumor Development

Most tumors exhibit chromosomal abnormalities, and, although usually nonspecific, certain genetic alterations are strongly associated with specific malignancies, and in some cases can be used to direct therapy or act as a prognostic factor.[7]

HYPERPLASIA

This is the first aberration in the development of cancer. The cell is not restrained by normal signaling, and cell division begins a rapid proliferation. The first aberrant cell that causes the proliferation is called the ancestral cell or the progenitor cell. All of the cells that divide off this ancestral cell line, the progeny, will

Differences between cancer cell and normal cell behavior[7]

- Increased cGMP activity in cancer cells
- Increased uptake of sugars and iron in cancer cells
- Increased receptors for growth factors in cancer cells
- Increased production of TGF (both alpha and beta) in cancer cells
- Increased production of prostaglandin 2 series (pro-inflammatory) in cancer cells

Genetic differences between cancer cells and normal cells

- Cancer occurs through a series of mutations
- Cancer cells have developed through clonal selection
- Most cancer cells develop genetic instability, allowing multiple mutations
- Genetic variation can affect somatic cells or germ cells

Cell differentiation

- Cancer cells tend to be less highly differentiated
- The less differentiated a cell, the harder to control

system must endure, the more likely the threat on the individual's life. The disruption of normal tissue and organ function by the cancer growth decreases the survival rate for the patient.

Stages of Tumor Development[7]

Hyperplastic cells develop over time due to genetic mutations: a normal cell can become fully malignant with less than ten mutations!

- Tumor development is successful when the aberrant cell begins hyperplasia.
- The altered ancestral cell and its progeny rapidly divide, creating hyperplastic changes.
- The cell's progeny create dysplasia, and the increased risk of continual cellular mutations
- If the aberrant cell growth is contained in the tissue of origin (in situ), it may remain contained indefinitely.
- If additional mutations exist, the risk of increased tumor invasion and shed is likely and metastases may occur.

display aberrant cellular proliferation. A tumor, or mass of cells formed by this hyperplastic cell line, may remain local where it originated (carcinoma in situ) or it may invade local surrounding healthy tissue (invasive carcinoma). When a tumor becomes invasive, it is then considered malignant. Malignancy may be shed into the lymphatic, hematologic, or central spinal fluid, which, in turn, may establish new tumor growth sites, or metastatic sites. The more tumor burden a

Proteomics

This new science studies how genes encode proteins, which are easier to evaluate than genes. Proteomics seeks to find specific patterns of protein expression with specific disease states, prognosis, and response to treatment. By utilizing proteins, evaluation can be assayed in both tissue and serum analysis. Proteomics has already been successful in early detection of cancer; a good example of this is prostate-specific antigen used for the early detection of prostate cancer.[8]

Profile of Carcinogens

Pro-carcinogens	**Co-carcinogens**
↓	↓
Require cP450 metabolic activation to become carcinogens capable of binding to cells	Enhance the action of carcinogens and promote tumors
↓	↓
Carcinogens bind to proteins, RNA, and DNA	Tumor promoters increase genetically determined inflammation, hyperproliferation, and tissue remodeling
↓	↓
Cells mutated via DNA damage = initiated cells	Neoplasm
↓	
Neoplasm	

Carcinogens	*Co-carcinogens*
Physical: radiation exposure, chronic irritations	Behavior • Stress • Occupation •
Biological: infections, hormone inbalance	Alcohol or drug abuse • Geophysical factors
Chemical: diet, tobacco smoke, pollution, heavy metals	Tumor promotes genetically determined damage: inflammation • hyperroliferation • tissue remodeling

> Oncogene Categories[9]
> Oncogenes fall into six categories (all of which are involved in signal transduction):
> 1. Growth factors – ras, myc family of genes
> 2. Growth factor receptors
> 3. Nonreceptor tyrosine kinases
> 4. Serine-threonine kinases
> 5. G proteins/GTPases
> 6. Nuclear proteins

ONCOGENES

Normal expression in healthy cells of oncogenes assist the normal cell in activities such as proliferation; it is only when the oncogene is over expressed that oncogenes transform healthy cells into cancer cells. Oncogenes are an overexpression of their normal function involving over proliferation of their proteins that stimulate growth. This can be caused by procarcinogens, such as radiation, viruses, and free radical damage produced by chronic inflammation.

The major cause of oncogene overexpression is mutations that can lead to abnormal production or activity of transcription and transduction and create progenetic aberrant cell lines. This is considered both a direct and indirect effect in the promotion of carcinogenesis. Proto-oncogenes are specific genes in normal cells that are target sites for chemical carcinogens. Once damaged, these become oncogenes.[9]

TUMOR SUPPRESSOR GENES

Tumor suppressor genes are normal genes that when expressed inhibit carcinogenesis. When these genes are under expressed or when they become mutated, their lack of activity enables carcinogenesis to develop, progress, and proliferate.

Genes that code for proteins block the action of growth promoting proteins. The Bcl-2 family of proteins acts as "arbiters of cell death" with a balance of both "antideath" and "prodeath" activity. Bcl-2 and Bcl-X_L appear to function as "antideath" proteins to prevent programmed cell death of cancer cells; overexpression of these proteins in cancer confers resistance to chemotherapy and radiation therapy. Bcl-2 and Bcl-X_L are overexpressed at a high level (50% to 100%) on common cancers, including cancers of the breast, colon, prostate, head and neck, and ovary.[5,7,10]

Anti-oncogene

The p53 tumor suppressor gene, when mutated, becomes inactivated, contributing to unregulated tumor growth. Inherited mutant p53 gene is the most

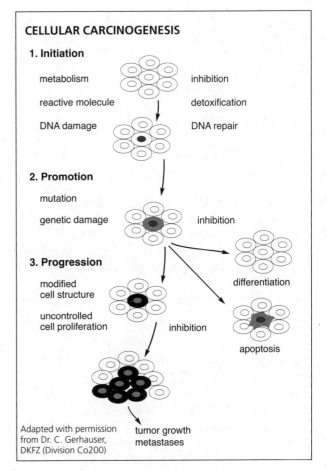

CELLULAR CARCINOGENESIS

1. **Initiation**

metabolism   inhibition

reactive molecule   detoxification

DNA damage   DNA repair

2. **Promotion**

mutation

genetic damage   inhibition

3. **Progression**

modified
cell structure   differentiation

uncontrolled
cell proliferation   inhibition

                                                  apoptosis

Adapted with permission from Dr. C. Gerhauser, DKFZ (Division Co200)   tumor growth
                                                    metastases

common genetic abnormality seen in human cancer. p53 is required for apoptosis (programmed cell death in response to genetic damage) .

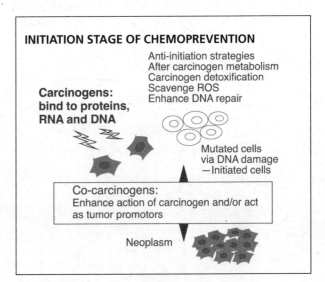

INITIATION STAGE OF CHEMOPREVENTION

Anti-initiation strategies
After carcinogen metabolism
Carcinogen detoxification
Scavenge ROS
Enhance DNA repair

**Carcinogens:
bind to proteins,
RNA and DNA**

Mutated cells
via DNA damage
—Initiated cells

Co-carcinogens:
Enhance action of carcinogen and/or act
as tumor promotors

Neoplasm

CARCINOGENESIS STAGES[5,7,10]

Carcinogenesis involves three stages or phases, first binding to DNA and finally showing malignancy:

Initiation

- Carcinogen binds to DNA (procarcinogen can be chemical, viral, radiation induced).
- Phenotypically normal tissue otherwise is initiated into aberrant cellular division, creating a mutation in the genomic information.

Promotion

- Expansion of the mutated cell line by unchecked rapid cellular division from the ancestral cell to the progeny promotes multiple genomic errors and hyperplastic cellular growth.
- Benign or early stage growths start in this fashion.

Progression

- Additional genetic changes cause an increase in mutations, which create a stronger virulence to the aberrant cell line.
- The cell line gains malignant characteristics:
  - Hyperplasia has greater success in invading surrounding tissues
  - Cellular shed of aberrant progenitor cells via blood, lymph, or CSF creates metastatic distant sites in the body of cancer growth
  - Loss of p53 tumor suppression normal function creates a highly aggressive growth pattern to the cancer cell line

---

Typical Sites of Metastasis[12]

- Breast: bone, liver, lung
- Prostate: bone
- Colorectal: liver, lung, brain
- Esophageal: lung, liver
- Lung: bone, liver, brain, adrenal
- Ovary: entire abdomen, brain
- Pancreas: liver, lung
- Thyroid: lung, bone
- Uterine: lung

TUMOR MARKERS

These marker molecules represent biological alterations in normal cellular function and may be found within the tumor or circulating in the serum. Most often they are made of proteins or glycoproteins, phospholipids, DNA or RNA, but they can also be produced by a tumor or by the body in an immunologic response to the tumor. Tumor markers are not generally used as routine screening devices due to their lack of sensitivity and specificity. Some cancers do not even shed tumor markers, while some non-cancerous lesions can raise certain tumor markers (like endometriosis and CA 125).

Tumor-specific antigens are a genetic response that produces specific proteins uniquely expressed in tumors as a result of genetic alterations or viral transformation. Tumor-associated proteins are an over expression by the tumor of normal gene proteins.

Diagnostic Markers[13]

Some tumor markers are sensitive and specific enough to be considered diagnostic markers. The gold standard for cancer diagnosis is the histopathologic exam. Tumor markers are used with histopathology to aid in differential diagnoses, characterization of metastatic lesions with an unknown primary lesion, and clarification of inconclusive histopathology.

Nearly all tumor markers lack complete organ specificity so that they do not make accurate diagnostic markers for the most part, with the exception of PSA (prostate specific antigen) and prostate cancer. The PSA marker also allows detection of possible cancer growth with sensitivity to changes within normal ranges, although there are several benign disease processes that can also elevate PSA.

CHARACTERISTICS THAT MAKE CANCER CELLS SUCCESSFUL[11]

Apoptosis

- Programmed cell death is inhibited in cancer cells.
- p53 mediates apoptosis (50% of cancers have abnormal p53).
- p53 gene mutation is an independent prognostic marker of early relapse and death in breast cancer.
- Measure p53 mutations to treat more effectively.

Angiogenesis

- Cancer cells promote growth of new blood vessels.
- Tumors cannot grow without a blood supply.

Metastasis

- Tumor cells from original tumor can spread to other sites in the body be via the lymphatic or hematologic or local extension systems.
- Cellular adhesion molecules are lost in cancer cells. Normal cells have contact inhibition and require attachment to basement membrane or other cells, but cancer cells loose one or both of these qualities.
- Once metastasized cancer is much less curable

ANTIGENIC TUMOR MARKERS

- Carcinoembryonic antigen (CEA): an elevated antigen that can be found in the serum of patients with gastrointestinal, colorectal, stomach, pancreatic, liver, kidney, and lung cancers.
- Prostate specific antigen (PSA): an elevated antigen that also can be found in the serum of patients with prostate cancer.
- Carbohydrate antigen 125 (CA 125): an antigen, found in the serum, primarily elevated in ovarian cancer but can be elevated in cancers of other organ systems — pancreatic, stomach, endometrium, and colon. CA 125 also can be insensitive to growing ovarian cancer and produce a false negative result.
- Carbohydrate antigen 15.3 (CA 15.3): an antigen found in the serum that can be elevated in breast cancer that usually has metastasized.
- Carbohydrate antigen 19.9 (CA 19.9): another antigen found in the serum that can be elevated in pancreatic cancer and other gastrointestinal and digestive tract cancers.
- HER2: a specific antigen that lies on the surface of some types of cancer cells. It is estimated that 30% of breast cancers have multiple copies of this gene in a single cell. This HER2 gene produces a growth factor cell surface receptor that aids in the rapid growth and division of cells. Breast cancer with an over expression of HER2 tends to be a more aggressive cell type with a tendency toward resistance to treatment.

OTHER TUMOR MARKERS: HORMONES, ONCOGENES, AND TUMOR SUPPRESSOR GENES

- Estrogen receptors (ER): can be expressed on a growing cancer cell, meaning that the cancer cells themselves have hormone receptor sites used to couple the hormone and stimulate tumor growth. ER positivity (ER+) has been seen in breast, ovarian, pancreatic, and colorectal cancers. Breast cancer estimates are about 75% ER+, with an estimated 65% of ER+ breast cancers having also positive progesterone receptors (PR+). These markers can be used both as prognostic markers and therapeutic markers.
- Hcg: human chorionic growth hormone can be used in some cancers as a diagnostic as well as prognostic marker.
- Bcl-2: an oncogene that protects cancer cells by inhibiting apoptosis (programmed cell death) and reduces damage from free radical.
- C-myc: a gene that with normal expression is needed to initiate cell division as well as to prevent differentiation. With over expression (as an oncogene) it affects cancer cell proliferation, differentiation, and apoptosis. Members of this gene family include n-myc and l-myc.
- Ki-ras: an oncogene that codes for a protein involved in a stimulatory signaling pathway (involved in lung, ovarian, colon, and pancreatic cancer).
- Ras: an oncogene induces several changes in tumor cells that range from structural to changes in the gene expression itself. This results in an excessive DNA synthesis with an increase in chromosomal abnormalities. Ras oncogenes increase tumor invasion, inhibit apoptosis, and protect cancer cells by increasing the expression of MDM2.
- MDM2: main function is to inhibit p53 activity in normal cells by degradation. In cancer cells, this oncogene is over expressed (as an oncogene) and causes chronically low p53 levels protecting the cancer cell from apoptosis.
- Fos and jun: proteins encoded to act as transcription factors that facilitate proliferation. These can be over expressed (as an oncogene) in certain cancer cell growth and create uncontrolled proliferation.
- P53: tumor suppressor gene that is the guardian of DNA when it functions normally (wild type) as a gene suppressor that initiates DNA repair and apoptosis of damaged cells. When p53 is mutated, it acts as an oncogen allowing rapid proliferation of cells with damaged DNA. Change in p53 is one of the most common mutations found in cancer cell growth and can happen in the course of a cancers progression, giving a poor prognosis.
- NF-1: tumor suppressor gene that codes for a protein and inhibits a stimulatory protein (involved in myeloid leukemia).
- RB: tumor suppressor gene that codes for the pRB protein, a key inhibitor of the cell cycle (involved in retinoblastoma and bone, bladder, and breast cancer).
- BRCA1 and BRCA2: tumor suppressor genes that code for a protein whose function is still unknown (involved in breast and ovarian cancers).
- Bax: promotes cell death by competing with Bcl-2 and acts as an inducer of apoptosis. When Bcl-2/Bax conjugate, a survival signal for the cells is created. The p53 is in part in control of the expression of Bcl-2 and Bax genes.
- Connexin Proteins (Cx32, Cx43): genes that produce the connexin proteins and form gap junctions between adjacent cells. Communication between the cells gap junction inhibits carcinogenesis while also normalizing malignant behavior of cells.
- EGFR (epidermal growth factor receptor): a tyrosine kinase mutation from oncogenes that can stimulate more of these receptor sites and promote cancer cell growth.
- PDGF: oncogene that codes for a protein called platelet-derived growth factor (involved in some forms of brain cancer).
- ADP-ribosylation factor-like tumor suppressor 1 (ARLTS1): a new gene that has been identified appears to be linked to a significant percentage of familial as well as sporadic cancers. Mutations in this tumor suppressor gene increase the risk of cancer only a little, but may represent the first in a set of genes that are important in cancer risk for large populations.

Prognostic Markers

Some tumor markers may be used in an additional classification and identification of subgroups and therefore can be considered prognostic markers (e.g., HER-2/neu).[13]

Response Markers

When tumor markers are used to predict if a patient will respond to specific treatments, these then are considered response markers. Response markers can be utilized to direct a specific treatment regimen and tailor the chemotherapy strategies toward those response markers. For example, determination of estrogen/progesterone receptors of a breast cancer tumor can direct what chemotherapy strategies are used, as well as determine whether hormone therapy will be appropriate.[13]

Therapeutic Response Markers

Tumor markers that can monitor the progress of the chemo/radio therapeutics during treatment are called therapeutic response markers. These tumor response markers can be drawn at regular intervals during active treatment to determine immediate efficacy and continued efficacy of the treatment protocol. A favorable response of the tumor to the treatment is a decrease in the tumor marker, therefore a measurable outcome for the treatment protocol.[13]

Recurrence Markers

Tumor markers that can be drawn at regular intervals after treatment to monitor for cancer recurrence are called recurrence markers. Minor fluctuations in tumor markers may normally occur, but a sudden significant increase or even a slower trend of increase suggests a recurrence. This allows correlation with imaging and other diagnostic studies to find the recurrent cancer growth.[13]

Risk Factors

The single most important risk factor for cancer is age, with more than 75% of cancers diagnosed in people who are over the age of 55. Based on the SEER database from 2002 to 2004, the lifetime probability of developing cancer is about 45% for men and 38% for women with variance by race and age.[14] In the United States, this accounts for almost one-third of deaths in men and women. In America, a decrease of cancer-related deaths by 2.1% per year from 2002-2004 has been attributed to changes in lifestyle as well as improved prevention and early detection. It is estimated that certain lifestyle factors, such as obesity, inactivity, and poor nutrition, could be prevented and that over one-third of the over 565,000

Cancer Risk Factors[12]
- Family history of cancer, genetic factors
- Lifestyle habits: smoking, alcohol, sunbathing, obesity, diet
- Exogenous factors: xenobiotics, hormones, pollution, customs, occupational, iatrogenic, habitat
- History of immunosuppressive drugs
- History of HPV
- History of chronic GERD
- History of insulin resistance or diabetes

Risk Factors for Specific Cancers
- Breast: female, Jewish, single, nullip, early menarche, alcohol, obesity, HRT exposures
- Lung: smoking, family history, Hx, radon, asbestos, welders, smelters, chem workers
- Prostate: male, black, American, high saturated fat, high IGF-1, low vit D, high calcium
- Colon: low calcium, red meats (charred), insulin, simple carbs, colitis, low veg diet, age, family history.
- Ovarian: white, history of breast cancer, family history, BRCA ½, radiation exposure, HRT, nullip, asbestos

Immunity Associated Risks
- People on immune suppressive medications have increased rates of certain cancers.
- Chronic viral infections are associated with increased incidences of cancer.
- Tumor recognition is often a problem; need to express tumor antigens on surface of cell to be recognized as abnormal/not self, by the immune system.

---

annual cancer deaths are related to these cofactors. These cofactors do not include tobacco smoking, which causes 170,000 cancer deaths annually in America.[14]

Cancer Theories

Our current molecular understanding of cancer began in the mid 1970s as scientists worked on developing a unified theory of cancer. The work done on the relationship between mutagenicity and carcinogenicity provided the support for the idea that carcinogens had chemical activities that acted directly to damage cellular genes. This idea led to the model for cancer initiation were carcinogens create mutations in genes that are critical for normal cell function and these mutations direct the cell (as well as all of its progeny) to grow abnormally. This abnormal growth and aberrant cellular behavior leads to the development of a cancer tumor. This model was now able to explain how cancers could run in families if the mutation was in a critical gene that could be inherited, thereby making the patient more susceptible to cancer developing.[15]

The primary flaw in this theory was that the nature of these cancer-causing mutations was unknown. Evidence with work from cancer causing viruses suggested which genes may be involved, and these were the key genes that controlled normal cell division and activity. It would take another 20 years, the deciphering of the human genome, and a revolution of biological research to find the information needed to bring the science and theory together.[16] Today, the picture of causes and development of cancer is so detailed that we now know many of the genes involved and are able to target strategies for prevention, detection, and treatment directly at these genes. With the emergence of epigenetics we can also target strategies at prevention directly by identifying SNPs on chromosomes that tells us of certain inborn errors of metabolism (like folic acid methylation errors) and possibly prevent the expression of cancer.

Cancer has specialized characteristics that enable the cell to successfully infiltrate the healthy tissue while evading immunosurveillance, avoiding programmed cell apoptosis, and, after adhering to host tissue, creating its own blood supply to feed the rapidly dividing neoplasia.

BOIK'S THEORY

It has been postulated by John Boik, PhD, that there are seven mechanisms of action for cancer cell development and success in the host system.[17] These mechanisms make the aberrant cell line successful not only in continuing its cellular division, but also in increasing it lethal ability to invade and destroy the host while evading the natural function of the immune system to scavenge these aberrant cells. The cancer cell line becomes more successful and more lethal as it exhibits more of these mechanisms successfully.

1. Induced genetic instability: Mutation of the normal cell into an aberrant cell is one of the first precursors of cancer cell development. The cell is able to pass on this genetic mutation to its progeny, thus enhancing its ability to mutate as needed in the body's unfavorable environment and be successful in its strategy to pro-generate cancerous cells.

2. Abnormal expression of genes: In the normal process of gene expression, it is the fundamental purpose of the gene to make proteins. Normal expression of these genes allows for the cell to function in a normal capacity and eventually die off when its life cycle is complete. In a cancerous cell, there is abnormal expression of genes and results in an abnormal function in relation to these protein formations. This results in not enough proteins being formed and therefore cannot inhibit the cancerous cell growth, and may even enhance it.

3. Abnormal signal transduction: Signaling is the way of cellular communication (*ras* proteins, kinases). A signal must be moved from outside of the cell to the internal environment of a cell. This is called signal transduction. Once a signal has reached its target, the normal function of various activities continues, keeping the cell healthy and effective. Growth factors are important soluble molecules that work in this way, binding to specific receptor sites to ensure healthy, normal cell function. Another important external cell signal is cell adhesion molecules. These cells are proteins that act like fingers regulating the amount of contact the cell will have with other cells and surrounding tissues. Its signal informs the cell of its surrounding environment. These proteins function to keep a normal cell within its boundaries and within its life cycle. When a cancerous cell line has mutated and reproduced successfully, it can create its own aberrant proteins that ensure its success in invading the host system.

   Cancer cells produce their own growth factors that allows them to reproduce and initiate their life cycle through the aberrant progenetic cell line. This self stimulation also allows for the cancer cell line to stimulate extra growth factor receptors and free radicals, which can make the growth factor receptors more responsive.

4. Abnormal cell to cell communication: Cancer cells are free to act independently once they have mutated to the point of initiating their own reproductive capacity and lose their contact with normal cells. Loss of this cell adhesion to normal cells effectively decreases the cell to cell communication. Normal cell to cell communication is important in maintaining healthy cell life cycles and inhibiting cancerous cell behavior. Now, with the aberrant cell line able to initiate its own reproductive capacity and evade normal cellular communication, it has begun its strategy to evade the defense system of the host and create more progeny.

5. Angiogenesis: The cancer cell proliferation has now created a mass of cells or tumor. The tumor is dependent on blood to supply its nutritional needs for rapid cellular division. Angiogenesis is how the tumor meets these needs. To stimulate the growth of new blood vessels toward the cancer-

ous tumor and within the tumor itself, the cancer cell produces protein growth factors. These growth factors stimulate the creation of new blood vessels that not only deliver the nutrition required to keep the tumor mass supplied, but also provide a route of escape in which the tumor cell line can metastasize to distant sites in the hosts' system.

6. Invasion and metastasis: A tumor seeks to spread its aberrant cell line. Invasion can be both local and distant. If there is local spread, the cancerous cell line has invaded the surrounding tissues and successfully implanted its reproductive strategy. This spread of local invasion, uncontrolled aberrant cell reproduction, and proliferation is a hallmark of cancer malignancy. Distant site invasion through the lymph, blood, or spinal fluid (to a lesser extent) is a metastatic event. Again, once the aberrant cell has reached the favorable distant site, it can successfully implant itself and proliferate uncontrollably.

7. Evading the immune system: Cancer cells create the ability to evade the natural surveillance function of the immune system and its ability to remove aberrant cells. The cancer cells can do this via several strategies by either disguising themselves or producing immunosuppressive compounds that impair the immune system from its normal function.

FREE RADICAL DAMAGE

Gene mutation is the cause of the oncogene "turn on" and overexpression as well as the "turn off" of natural tumor suppressor gene function. Genetic mutation also can affect any of Boik's seven mechanisms, creating a more virulent and aggressive aberrant cell line. When a gene is coded off the initiator DNA strand, there can be normal base sequence changes. If a sequence is aberrant, the normal function of the cell is to repair it; if it is not repaired, the cell survives and the changes are passed on through the following cell reproductive line through generations of progeny.[3] When the cell does not make these needed repairs, we call this "damage," and if the damage is found in a pro-oncogenic cell line, an oncogene is formed or a tumor suppressor gene is turned off and a cancer growth can be initiated. These genetic point mutations can be a part of the normal evolutionary growth of a species, if they are just aberrant and not toxic.[5]

Toxic sequence changes create mutations, and these mutations are the inherent cause of normal cells being transformed into cancer cells and developing into a mass of cells forming a tumor. External factors can transform, replace, or destroy sequence bases because of their similarity in structure to the external carcinogens. Some these external carcinogens have been identified, such as overexposure to ultraviolet light/radiation exposure, alkylating chemicals, or free radical damage.[11] Other sequence changes can be caused by additions or deletions of the DNA sequence, which can be caused by a toxic viral infection or a misplaced endogenous enzyme, both leading to errors in DNA synthesis.[11]

Free radicals are unstable molecules that have unpaired electron valences, which makes them highly reactive. This is explained by a free radical molecule either gaining or loosing electrons when in contact with a stable molecule. Biology not only wants to beget progeny, but is always looking for balance, so these free radicals are looking for balance by sharing electron stability with a stable molecule. However, the balance of the stable molecule is now disrupted because of the free radical, and therefore becomes a free radical molecule itself. This is coined as free radical damage to a cell. Free radicals damage DNA — proteins and fats and are one of the main causative factors in a cancerous cell mutated line formation.[18]

Antioxidants

The natural human body's own defense system uses a variety of antioxidants against free radical damage. These antioxidants are endogenous as well as exogenous. Endogenous antioxidants, such as glutathione, uric acid, and proteins, are synthesized by the host system to scavenge free radicals. Naturally produced biochemicals, such as superoxide dismutase (SOD), coenzyme Q10 (ubiquinone), alpha lipoic acid, catalase, and glutathione peroxidase function in the same way for free radical scavenging. Exogenous antioxidants, such as vitamins A, C, E, D, retinoids, carotenoids, betacarotene, bioflavonoids, and omega-3 fatty acids (especially EPA), have been shown to scavenge free radicals.[19]

Antioxidants[19]

Endogenous
- Glutathione, uric acid, and proteins

Exogenous
- Vitamins A, C, E, D, retinoids, carotenoids, betacarotene, bioflavonoids, and omega-3 fatty acids (especially EPA)

Naturally produced biochemicals
- Superoxide dismutase (SOD), coenzyme Q10 (ubiquinone), alpha lipoic acid, catalase, and glutathione peroxidase

The issues of cancer cell line progenitor comes into play when the free radicals are overproduced by the body or the endogenous antioxidant system becomes overwhelmed and cannot repair free radical damage or scavenging.

EPIGENETICS

Epigenetics is the study of inheritable changes in gene function that occur without a change in the DNA sequence.[20] These functional changes, which are inherited and affect the normal DNA, have shown that some inherited mutations lead to cancer cell growth. Mechanisms that affect the DNA without denaturing the sequencing, such as DNA methylation function, histone acetylation, and RNA interference, can effect a genes activation or deactivation. In turn, this effects the phenotypic expression of the progeny cell line and can lead to the aberrant cell development needed to create a cancer cell line.

Because these epigenetic changes are not true mutations, they are considered reversible and can be "normalized" back to proper functional status. Integrative naturopathic strategies are targeting this ability to normalize proper functional status as well as prevention of the epigenetic expression altogether.

According to one study, methylation of cytosine is a non-aberrant modification to DNA and determines which gene is activated for transcription in the replication process. Epigenetic changes are characterized by changes in the DNA, primarily by the attachment of a methyl group to a specific cytosine base: "Mammals appear to have taken advantage of the possibilities afforded by cytosine methylation to provide a heritable mechanism for altering DNA-protein interactions to assist in such silencing. Genes can be transcribed from methylation-free promoters even though adjacent transcribed and non-transcribed regions are extensively methylated. Gene promoters can be used and regulated while keeping noncoding DNA, including transposable elements, suppressed. Methylation is also used for long-term epigenetic silencing of X-linked and imprinted genes and can either increase or decrease the level of transcription, depending on whether the methylation inactivates a positive or negative regulatory element.

Abnormalities in cytosine methylation are common in the aberrant cancer cell line. In most cancer cell's genetics they are hypomethylated and overexpressed, which is especially true for oncogene expression. Tumor suppressor genes tend to be hypermethylated in cancer genesis and therefore are underexpressed, such is the case of the p53 tumor suppressor gene and cancer growth. This is called silencing a genetic expression. When hypermethylation occurs it can not only silence a genetic expression of a gene, but can also silence the production of controlling proteins that signal for specific cellular activities to occur.

Epigenetic changes in cancer cells are considered to be reversible thus invite strategies for prevention that can target these changes. These strategies are aimed at the possible reduction in the rate of mutations, thus inhibiting the tumors formation and progression.

MUTATOR PHENOTYPE THEORY

In the phenotype mutation theory, cancer cell survival is dependent on ongoing genetic alterations.[21] Whether these genetic mutations are classical point mutations or epigenetic changes doesn't matter. It is the goal of the cancer cell to survive the hostile environment of the host's system. The natural host's immune defense will attempt to inhibit the cancer cell activity as well as react to the cancer treatment strategies targeted to destroy the cancer cell. All of these strategies in concert create a hostile environment the cancer cell must overcome.

The cancer cell also competes with itself. Because of its hyperplastic proliferation, it overcrowds itself and must compete with its own progeny for oxygen and nutrients. These strong cancer cells that survive this environment from specific mutations also contain mutations that enhance their mutability, making them more changeable and toxic. This gives the phenotypic characteristic of genetic instability to the cancer cell line, which, in turn, makes that aberrant cell line more successful.

Mutations in the genes that code for stability are early events in the phenotype mutation theory. This would include the p53 tumor suppressor gene mutation causing the inactivity of this important anti-oncogene, DNA mutations that would affect genes that act as DNA repair enzymes, genes that control cell growth and replication, and enzymes (proteins) responsible for helping in DNA replication. Once these genetic mutations have occurred, it allows for a higher rate of continual mutation that can lead to the over expression of oncogenes and under expression of tumor suppressor genes (p53).

PERSISTENT OXIDATIVE STRESS THEORY

Mutations require both DNA damage and lack of DNA repair in order to occur.[22] Inflammation can be the environment in which these mutations can occur due to ROS (reactive oxygen species) enrichment associated with inflammation. Statistically, chronic inflammatory diseases producing a large amount of ROS are associated with higher incidence of cancers.

Not only is there an increase in the incidence of cancer, but also a marked increase in their recurrence and resistance. This is the postulate of the oxidative stress theory: the more ROS the cancer cells are exposed to, the better their survival and progression. It has been found that in extremely high levels of ROS cancer cells can be killed, but it is the mild chronic elevation that has been found to stimulate cancer cell proliferation and progression. This chronically elevated oxidative environment facilitates cancer cell growth by increasing the rate of mutation and proliferation. Proliferation is enhanced by the oxidative stress causing an increase to the sensitivity of growth factor receptors.

Cytokines and Inflammation

Inflammation is the milieu in which cancer exists, creating oxidative damage to the environment of the cell.[23] Chronic inflammation can be co-factorial in the mutation of the aberrant cell that leads to the development of the cancer growth. While some cells will die in the oxidative environment, others will survive and mutate. Inflammation is a known "promoting" agent that causes aberrant cell proliferation, with an increased capacity to mutate and successfully survive in the unfavorable climate. Over time, this promotion leads to a precancerous cell formation that, in turn, creates a genetically mutated aberrant progeny cell line that has become self capable of promoting and self stimulating. This is the creation of the autonomous cancer cell, which is now capable of making proteins (like tumor growth factor) and stimulates the cell line proliferation without interference. Inflammatory white blood cell lines, like macrophages and neutrophils, are attracted to the tumor site by tumor producing chemokines. MCP-1 and IL-8 are good examples of these chemotactic factors that attract white blood cell lines to the tumor site.

The growth of the cancerous cell line creates hypoxia in the tumor as the cells necrose, beginning centrally, causing an increase in tumor burden. Hypoxia induces these cells to secrete cytokines, such as TNF-alpha, IL-1 and IL-6, which, in turn, are pro-inflammatory in function. Vascular endothelial cells proliferate and migrate toward this hypoxic environment, which is also considered an angiogenic environment. This enables the cancerous lesion to connect these proliferative vascular endothelial cells and create a new capillary vessel, thus creating an oxygen and nutrient supply the rapidly growing cellular lesion, thereby creating tumor angiogenesis. Cancerous cells themselves secrete various growth factors, such as TGF (tumor growth factor). Platelets also secrete growth factors, and often with cancer cell progression, platelet factors are affected in cell growth and associated blood clots may form with some cancer progression.

Vascular Endothelial Growth Factor

As these cytokines and growth factors increase in concentration, an increase is noted in the expression of a substance called VEGF (vascular endothelial growth factor).[24,25,26] VEGF is a protein that is 50,000 times more active than histamine in enhancing vascular permeability. This increase in VEGF promotes the growth of blood vessels from the tumor into surrounding host tissue, creating angiogenesis. This strategy of tumor growth not only nourishes the cancerous growth, but also helps the lesion expand beyond its boundaries into healthy surrounding host tissues. The expanding cancer cell lesion activates the extrinsic coagulation cascade to protect VEGF and other tumor growth factors from degradation from the host immune system. Once this coagulation cascade is activated, thrombin and a fibrin-gel matrix are produced. VEGF and bFGF (basic fibroblast growth factor) are the primary angiogenic compounds, while all others are considered secondary.

Thrombin then encourages blood platelets to produce more VEGF, and the fibrin-gel matrix helps to concentrate the growth factors at the tumor site and provide a lattice work for the migrating endothelial and tumor cells to follow. Platelet activation factor (PAF) and epidermal growth factor (EGF) and Platelet derived growth factor (PDGF) are included in the secondary factors that stimulate angiogenesis at this point. These activation processes include the activation of fibrin and other products of coagulation to activate proteases. These proteases, such as matrix metalloproteinases (MMPs), are what promote metastasis as well as the ability to evade the immunosurveillance of the host's system. Monitoring these cytokines, VEGF levels, and coagulation markers can help to determine the activity of cancer growth as well as metastasis. VEGF has even been found to be a fairly good recurrence marker for colorectal cancers.

Prostaglandin and Leukotriene Synthesis

Prostanoids, such as prostaglandins and thromboxanes, are the biochemical shunts in the eicosanoid pathway that promotes inflammation.[27] Prostaglandins from the E2 series (PGE2) can increase vascular permeability while also suppressing normal immune cell activity. Some solid tumors are known to secrete PGE2 in excess. This is thought to enhance angiogenesis, proliferation, and immuno-evasion of the growing cancer. Thromboxanes, which function normally in blood clotting by platelet aggregation, are also considered proinflammatory. Leukotrienes are also responsible for the induction of inflammation and can be independently produced by tumor cells.

Through either the conversion of the enzymes cyclooxygenase or lipoxygenase either a prostanoid or a leukotriene is formed. There are two types of cyclooxygenase (COX), either COX-1 or COX-2. COX-2 is the series that produces an inflammatory event, while COX-1 acts to regulate normal tissue homeostasis. Some of our chemotherapeutic strategies are targeted at inhibiting COX-2 because its selective role in inflammation, cancer cell initiation, and progression. Omega-6 fatty acids, which include arachidonic acid, are found in animal fats and linoleic acid, which is found in most vegetable oils. These eicosanoids are more inflammatory and can promote angiogenesis and cancer cell progression. Linoleic acid can be converted to arachidonic acid and produce the PGE2 series of prostaglandins, as well as the four series of leukotrienes that promote antiogenesis and cancer cell progression. Naturopathic strategies are to use omega-3 fatty acids that shunt the eicosanoid pathway away from PGE2 series of prostaglandins and into the PGE1,3 series of prostaglandins that are anti-inflammatory by nature.[28]

Neutrophils

The release of prostanoids and leukotrienes in an inflammatory event calls into play the normal cell migration of neutrophils and macrophages.[29] Neutrophils are dominantly called into play in early inflammation and die off early in the inflammatory process. They are replaced by macrophages, which are differentiated monocytes large enough to engulf foreign invaders as well as dead neutrophils and necrotic tissue.

When the tumor directs neutrophils into the cancer cells via chemotactic factors, the aberrant cell is then able to produce VEGF, IL-8, and other growth factors. These are directly involved in progressing tumor invasion and angiogenesis. Neutrophils are short lived in the pathology, leading to macrophage infiltration and ongoing inflammatory destruction of healthy tissue. These are phagocytic in function and effective as debris eating cells.

Macrophages and Monocytes

Macrophages also produce tumor necrosis factor (TNF), growth factors, and enzymes.[30] In cancer cell pathology, these secretions stimulate cancer cell growth, proliferation, angiogenesis, invasions, and metastasis. Some patients with cancer certain types of cancers, especially lung and colon, are more likely to have an associated monocytosis than people without cancer. In cancer patients, monocytosis may be associated with the presence of metastasis and therefore a shorter survival rate. Data has been shown to correlate patients with monocytosis and suppressed in vitro T-cell responses. On the other hand, lymphocytosis has been associated with lower recurrence rates and longer survival rates in cancer patients. The naturopathic strategy would be to promote lymphocytosis over monocytosis with therapeutics, such as a high soy diet and medicinal mushrooms, such as reishi that promote lymphocytes. Natural killer cells (NK) are specialized lymphocytes that may be enhanced by these lymphocyte promoting therapies.

The function of these immuno-responders is aberrant once induced into the cancer cell line. Monocytes and macrophages are directed into tumors by chemokines, which are substances secreted by the cancer cells to call in the monocyte/macrophage cells. The chemotactic factor, monocyte chemotactic protein – 1 (MCP-1), which calls in the monocytes from the host immune system, encourages macrophage infiltration into tumors instead of lymphocytes, thereby turning them into aberrant macrophages. MCP-1 also increases the production of MMP-9, a substance that promotes cancer invasiveness.[31] This aberrant macrophage is then preserved in the tumor by the tumor secreting its own macrophage colony stimulating factor, as well as by down regulation of the cell's biochemistry. Angiogenesis is then produced by growth factors that are secreted by the tumors, creating its own blood supply. Proteases are also secreted, and these proteases degrade the extracellular matrix of the healthy tissues, which, in, turn promotes tumor invasion (MMP-9 produced). Interleukins are then encouraged to be produced, such as IL 4-6, by tumor infiltrating lymphocytes over gamma-interferon. IL-6 is a potent growth factor that directly stimulates angiogenesis. Elevated serum levels of IL-6 are associated with metastases and increased mortality in many types of cancers, including lymphoma, myeloma, prostate, colorectal, and ovarian cancer. They may play a role in the promotion of cancer cachexia.[32]

Macrophagic activity in cancer tumor sites play a dual role at both induction and inhibition of angiogenesis and tumor progression. In healthy cell macrophagic activity, the macrophages phagocytose and create chemotactic factors for producing compounds that promote healing of the normally healthy tissue. These compounds, promoted by macrophages, are promoters of angiogenesis by compounds like tumor necrosis factor (TNF). TNF-α is produced by tumor associated macrophages and cancer cells and functions to produce MCP-1, IL-6, and promotes coagulation. TNF- α stimulates IL-6 production, which is a potent growth factor that directly stimulates angiogenesis. Clinical data has shown that elevated serum levels of TNF- α correlates with poor prognosis in some cancers,[32] such as NHL, CLL, hepatocellular carcinoma, myelogenous leukemia, prostate, and ovarian cancers. In ovarian cancer, the cancer cell lines were more invasive, with prostate cancer the loss of androgen responsiveness, and in breast cancer an increase of angiogenesis. TNF may be affected by the naturopathic strategies targeting it specifically with omega-3 fatty acids, soy isoflavones, and niacinamide.[19]

Other angiogenic factors include VEGF, bFGF, PDGF, and EGF in the presence of free radicals. The production of VEGF by macrophages is not only stimulated by the innate immune response, but also by the reperfusion of oxygen into the hypoxic cells. This oxygen reperfusion causes a high concentration of free radicals to exist, which in turn, stimulates VEGF production. Triggers of VEGF previously discussed include hypoxia, loss of tumor suppressor genes, and activation of oncogenes, such as *ras*, EGFR, and Bcl-2. VEGF serves to protect the growing neovasculature of the tumor from apoptosis while mediating the breakdown of the extracellular matrix to enhance further spread of the cancerous lesion. High levels of VEGF in the serum are associated with the more aggressive clinical progression of many types of cancer. An elevation of VEGF has been associated with an increase of a recurrence of cancer, noting that patients with lower VEGF levels have improved responses to chemo/radio therapies.

Naturopathic strategies that can alter the expression of VEGF are soy isoflavones and other bioflavonoids, ellagic acid, limonene, and vitamins.[19] All have been shown at different levels to alter VEGR expression. Transforming growth factor beta 1 (TGF-β1) elevated circulating levels have been found in patients with a variety of cancers and is associated with an increased progression, invasion and metastasis of the cancer.[33] Increased serum levels of TGF-β1 have been correlated with lower levels of circulating dendritic cells as well as an impairment in dendritic cell maturation. TGF-β1 is produced by IL-2 and is one of the most powerful immunosuppressive factors known.[33]

Fibrin

At the tumor site of inflammation, fibrin production and degradation continue non stop.[34] The fibrin does not evolve into mature connective tissue but instead surrounds the tumor and transforms into a chaotic mess of fibrin, immature blood vessels, and connective tissue conducive to angiogenesis and fibrinolysis. This ongoing production of a fibrin stroma may structurally support the growing tumor by encasing the lesion or clumps of cancerous cells. This has been seen in non solid tumor pathologies, such as lymphomas. Fibrin stroma can comprise up to 90% of a tumor's mass in some cancers. This fibrin stroma can also function to shield the tumor from the host's immuno-surveillance system. It has also been found that fibrin deposit on cancer cells promotes metastasis by increasing cellular adhesion, as well as stimulating angiogenesis. During chronic inflammation and tumor invasion, basic fibroblast growth factor (bFGF) is released into the extracellular matrix. This plays a direct role in tumor invasion and angiogenesis because liberated bFGF stimulates fibroblasts for angiogenesis and fibrin formation.[34]

Mast Cells

Histamine is generated by mast cells, which migrate toward tissue inflammation as a chemotactic factor response. Growth factor production calls in the mast cells toward the site, and once at the site the mast cells degranulate and release histamine. The histamine increases vascular permeability and angiogenesis. Strategies in cancer therapies are aimed at both stabilizing the mast cell so that degranulation does not occur, and inhibiting mast cell migration to start. Mast cells are called into an inflamed area by growth factors VEGF, bFGF, PDGF and EGF. Thus, strategies to inhibit these growth factor compounds will reduce mast cell migration to the site, therefore reducing angiogenesis. It is also worth noting that under hypoxic conditions lactic acid is produced, and lactic acid can stimulate the production of angiogenesis by macrophages.[35]

Proteases and Glycosidases

Enzymes are produced by the cancer cell that can help with the breakdown of the extracellular matrix, thus enabling angiogenesis and metastasis.[36] Proteases break apart protein structures and glycosidases break apart glycosaminoglycan chains. These are important in the cancer's progression and invasion into surrounding tissues. Hyaluronidases are glycosidases that break down hyaluronic acid; collagenases and proteases breakdown protein collagen. Some proteases at the site of inflammation can cause macrophage activity, which, in turn, produces more free radicals. For the cancer cell's strategy to proliferate, invade, and metastasize, the extracellular matrix must be penetrated into the surrounding capillaries. Once this penetration has happened, then angiogenesis can begin. Matrix met-alloproteinases (MMPs) are zinc-dependant enzymes that can degrade all components of the extracellular matrix. Blocking their action by tissue inhibitors of metalloproteinases (TIMPs) is a current strategy of chemotherapeutics, aiming at inhibiting tumor invasion and angiogenesis.[36]

Natural Killer Cells

Natural killer cells are immune cells that are specialized lymphocytes (non T, non B) that migrate to cancer cells and macrophages and destroy them. It has been shown that the more NK cells that are actively functioning in an immune system the less metastases are found. NK cells present as the first line of defense against metastatic spread. Prostaglandins, such as PGE2, inhibit NK activity, while cytokines, such as interferons and IL-2, can stimulate NK activity.[37]

Cytokines

Cytokines are soluble proteins secreted to control cellular proliferation as well as normal cell behavior. Some cytokines, such as tumor growth factor beta (TGF-β), inhibit cell proliferation. Cytokines are specific in the activation of the immune systems response. Interleukin 2 (IL-2) is the primary cytokine to instruct CD8 T cells (cytotoxic T8 cells) to proliferate. These stimulated CD8 cells also secrete other cytokines, such as interferon-gamma (IFN-gamma) and tumor necrosis factor (TNF-α and TNF-β). IFN-gamma is the primary cytokine that activates macrophages via the TH1 pathway. The activation of the macrophages then produces a variety of cytokines, such as TNF, IL-1, and IL-6. TH2 immune systems stimuli activate B cells by secreting specific cytokines, such as IL-4 and IL-5. Other cytokines produced by the TH2 cells include IL-3, IL-10, granulocyte macrophage colony stimulating factor (GM-CSF), and TGF-β. Cytokines also control the growth and activity of CD4 T cells (T4 helper cells).[38]

OTHER FACTORS
Autoimmune Factors

Suppressive autoimmune treatments may contribute to the development of cancer. Cancer is allowed to exist because of the ability of the cancer to escape the host immune defenses. If the host immune system cannot recognize the cancer as foreign if the critical immunostimulatory molecules of the cancer itself are not recognized. The inability of the host immune defenses to recognize cancer tumor is considered a state of anergy, which means there is a deletion of tumor specific lymphocytes that recognize the tumor.

Some of the more recent therapies, such as vaccines, are aimed at correcting this by stimulating the host immune response against the tumor cells.[39]

Infectious and Environmental Factors

Data from the 2000 census confirm the existence of geographic variability in cancer incidence, although this is not as marked as previously thought; for example, breast cancer rates in Marin County in California and in Washington State appear to be among the highest in the United States. Interestingly, the increased incidence is similar to that seen in higher socioeconomic groups with higher attained education, delayed childbearing, a lower rate of breastfeeding, and higher relative alcohol intake – and appears to primarily affect the white population. The contribution of environmental factors, exposure to toxins, and other dietary factors is not fully understood but clearly plays a role. Current research is focusing on the role of lifestyle factors and environmental exposures in childhood and adolescence to better understand the factors that increase risk of cancer in adulthood. "Interestingly, mortality from cancer also varies depending on the completed level of formal educational, with poorer survival seen in persons with less education (12 years) for unclear reasons."[6] It is accepted that radiation, benzenes, tetrahydrocarbons, and even household cleaning agents like chlorine at the right exposure levels are all environmental carcinogens.

Viral Factors

Certain cancers have a direct association to certain viral infectors, such as Epstein-Barr (EBV) virus infection and non Hodgkin lymphoma (NHL) and Burkitt's lymphoma. Human papillomavirus (HPV) has certain strains of the virus that directly produce cervical dysplastic changes that lead to cervical cancer, while other strains produce benign conditions. These oncogenic viruses have a direct link to the formation of the cancer above, but others have an associated risk for cancer with coinfection. Hepatitis B or C viruses have an associated risk of hepatocellular cancer while human herpes virus can be associated with Kaposi's sarcoma (KS).[40]

The finding of human herpesvirus-8 (HHV-8) DNA sequences in both AIDS associated KS and non AIDS associated KS, exemplifies the role the virus plays in the development of this cancer. The host immune system develops antibodies to HHV-8 and this is a direct link to the development of KS, and it is now postulated that the infection is necessary for the KS to develop.[41] Approximately 100% of women with cervical or anal cancer have evidence of HPV. HPV is a sexually transmitted virus and has 15 subtypes that have been identified with an increased risk of cervical cancer. HPV 16,18 are the most common and are associated with a 200x increased risk of cancer.[42] Although HPV is a common virus, many women do not develop cancer, with the exception of the previously mentioned strains. The viral-cancer connection is a slow progression with a persistent infection that lasts for over a decade or more. Other cofactors are associated with the cancer development like genetic or systemic cofactors, but the science is only partially understood. It is difficult to link exposures to the development of cancer since latency is usually long and the nature of the exposure is usually poorly documented.

Bacterial Factors

Bacterial infection has also been linked with an increased risk for certain cancers. Approximately 60% of gastric cancers are associated with *Helicobacter pylori (H. pylori)* infection. The infection of the bacteria is reported to increase the risk of cancer at the distal portion of the stomach six times as well as increase the risk for gastric lymphoma.[43] "Geographic variations in the incidence of gastric cancer appear to be influenced by geographic variations in the strain of *H. pylori*; strains that produce a specific protein are more likely to be associated with cancer than those that do not. Screening for and treatment of *H. pylori* may be a cost-effective way to prevent gastric cancer in high-risk populations."[6]

Hormone Replacement Therapy (HRT)

Using both estrogen and progesterone in combinations with each other or singularly has been associated with increase risk in certain cancers. The forms of these hormones most studied are the synthetic progesterone and conjugated horse equine estrogens (CEE). While there is much talk and publication stating the case for the use of biological (or biodynamic) natural hormone replacement (bHRT or NHRT) the research to validate these claims has not been gathered to compare effects to HRT or placebo.

Estrogen (CEE) is a common prescription for postmenopausal women, thought to decrease the onset and longevity of chronic disease associated with post menopausal women. The Women's Health Initiative (WHI) a large randomized clinical trial done in the United States with over 16,000 healthy volunteer women ages 50 to 79 years compared the effects of combined estrogen and progesterone to placebo. The trial was sponsored by the National Institutes of Health (NIH) and was abruptly halted in July 2002 when investigators reported that the overall risks of estrogen plus progestin (specifically Prempro) outweighed the benefits.[44]

At 6.8 years of follow-up, women treated with CEE had an increased risk of stroke, a decreased risk of hip fracture, and no difference in the rate of either coronary heart disease or breast cancer. The rate of incident disease events was equivalent in the placebo and CEE arms, indicating no overall benefit. However, longer term follow-up of women treated with CEE compared with placebo found a fascinating and striking 35% relative decrease in the incidence of invasive breast cancers in women without prior exposure to postmenopausal hormones, indicating that estrogen may have a protective effect against breast cancer. Women with a history of oophorectomy had a similar decrease in breast cancer risk. This marked contrast to the effects of combination hormone therapy is perhaps explained by the cancer promoting effects of progesterone. In women aged 65 years and older, CEE had an adverse effect on cognition, although there was no apparent increase in dementia.[44] An extension study is ongoing to continue to observe all women enrolled in the WHI study through 2010. In an observational study of over 40,000 women, those who used estrogen alone for 10 to 19 years were twice as likely to develop ovarian cancer as women who did not use menopausal hormones. For women who used estrogen for 20 or more years; longer follow-up from the WHI trial will be critical to understand this risk. To date, this study has not shown an increased risk of ovarian cancer in women taking CEE. "There are insufficient data on which to base a conclusion about whether combined estrogen and progesterone use affects the risk of developing ovarian cancer."[6]

Estrogen with progesterone, such as the pharmaceutical Prempro, was found to increase breast cancer incidence in post menopausal women. The WHI found that the cancer risk was an increase of 24% for breast cancer, although there were fewer cases of colon cancer in the treatment arm.[44,45] Heart disease and blood clots were also found to be at this increase risk while hip fractures were reported to be fewer in the treatment group. Recent data from the WHI indicates that the breast cancers that develop in women receiving combined hormonal therapy were significantly larger than those which developed in women in the placebo group, and were at a more advanced stage upon diagnosis than the placebo arm.[47] The WHI study also showed that almost twice the number of women receiving Prempro had abnormal mammograms at one year compared to the placebo group.[44,45] "The HABITS (hormonal replacement therapy after breast cancer) trial evaluated the safety of hormone replacement therapy (HRT) after a diagnosis of breast cancer. After a median follow-up of only 2.1 years, more than three times the number of women in the HRT group had developed a new breast cancer event compared to the women in the best treatment group. These dramatic differences led to early closing of the trial."[44-47]

References

1. Chabner BA Jr, Lynch TL, Longo DL. Harrison's Manual of Oncology. New York, NY: McGraw Hill Publ.;2007.

2. National Cancer Institute: National Institutes of Health (NIH). [Online.] Available http://www.nci.nih.gov

3. McKinnell RG, Parchment RE, Perantoni AO, Pierce GB. The Biological Basis of Cancer. New York, NY: Cambridge University Press;1988.

4. Moore JA. Science as a way of knowing: the foundations of modern biology. Cambridge, MA: Harvard University Press;1993.

5. Varmus H and Weinberg RA. Genes and the biology of cancer. New York, NY: Scientific American Library;1993.

6. McPhee SJ, Papadakis MA, Eds. Gonzales R, Zeiger R. Online Eds. CURRENT Medical Diagnosis & Treatment. 2004; 48th ed.:1535.

7. Vogelstein B, Kinzler KW. The genetic basis of cancer. New York, NY: McGraw Hill;1998.

8. Wulfkuhle JD et al. Proteomic applications for the early detection of cancer. Nat Rev Cancer. 2003 Apr;3(4):267-75.

9. Croce CM. Oncogenes and cancer. N Engl J Med. 2008 Jan;31;358(5):502-11.

10. Weinberg RA. Racing to the beginning of the road: The search for the origin of cancer. New York, NY: Harmony Books;1996.

11. Weinberg RA. September. How cancer arises. Scientific American, 1996 Sep;275(3):62.

12. Jemal A et al. Cancer statistics. CA Cancer J Clin. 2008 Apr;58(2):71-96.

13. www.asco.org.

14. www.seer.cancer.gov › Cancer StatisticsTrichopoulos D, Li FP, Hunter DJ. What causes cancer? Scientific American. 1996 Sep;275(3):80.

16. Rennie J, Rusting R. Making headway against cancer. Scientific American. 1996 Sep;275(3):56.

17. Boik J. Natural compounds in cancer therapy. Princeton, MN: Oregon Medical Press;2001.

18. Patterson JT. The dread disease: cancer and modern American culture. Cambridge, MA: Harvard University Press;1987.

19. Murray M, Birdsall T, Pizzorno J, Reilly P. How to Prevent and Treat Cancer with Natural Medicine. New York, NY; Riverhead Books;2002.

20. Riddihough G, Pennisi E. The evolution of epigenetics. Science. 2001 Aug 2001; 293(5532):1001-1208.

21. Bignold LP. The mutator phenotype theory can explain the complex morphology and behavior of cancers. Cell Mol Life Sci. 2002 Jun;59(6):950-58.

22. Toyokuni S, Okamoto K, Yodoi J, Hiai H. Persistent oxidative stress in cancer. FEBS Lett. 1995 Jan 16;358(1):1-3.

23. Coussens LM, Werb Z. Inflammation and cancer. Nature. 2002 Dec 19;420(6917):860-67.

24. Takahashi Y, Kitadai Y, Bucana CD, Cleary KR, Ellis, LM. Expression of vascular endothelial growth factor and its receptor, KDR, correlates with vascularity, metastasis, and proliferation of human colon cancer. Cancer Research.1995 Sep 15;55:3964.

25. Plate KH, Breier G, Weich HA, Risau W. Vascular endothelial growth factor as a potential tumour angiogensis factor in human gliomas in vivo. Nature. 1992 Oct 29;359:845-48.

26. Yang JC, Haworth L, Sherry RM, Hwu P, Schwartzentruber DJ, Topalian SL, Steinber SM, Chen HX, Rosenberg SA. A randomized trial of Bevacizumab, an anti-vascular endothelial growth factor antibody for metastatic renal cancer. New Engl J Med. 2003 July 31;349(5):427-34.

27. Lupulescu A. Prostaglandins, their inhibitors and cancer. Prostaglandins, Leukotrienes and Essential Fatty Acids. 1996 Feb;54(2):83-94.

28. Terano T, Salmon JA, Higgs G, Moncado S. Eicosapentaenoic acid as a modulator of inflammation: Effect on prostaglandin and leukotriene synthesis. Biochem Pharm. 1996 March 1;35(5):779-85.

29. Mantovani A. The yin-yang of tumor associated neutrophils. Cancer Cell. 2009 Sep;16(3):173-74.

30. Shih JY, Yuan A, Chen JW, Yang PC. Tumor associated macrophages: Its role in cancer invasion and metastasis. J Cancer Molecules. 2008;2(3):101-06.

31. Tsai CS, et al.Cilostazol attenuates MCP-1 and MMP-9 expression in vivo in LPS-administrated balloon injured rabbit aorta and in vitro LPS-treated monocytic THP-1 cells. J Cell Biochem. 2008 Jan 1;103(1):54-66.

32. Heikkila K, Harris R, et al. Association of circulating C-reactive protein and interluekin-6 with cancer risk: findings from two prospective cohorts and a meta-analysis. Cancer Causes and Control. 2008 July;20(1):15-26.

33. Grainger DJ, Heathcote K, Chiano M, Snieder H, Kemp PR, Metcalfe JC, Carter ND, Specter TD. Genetic control of the circulating concentration of transforming growth factor type ,1. Human Mol Genetics 1998;8(1):93-97.

34. Constantini V, Zacharski LR. The role of fibrin in tumor metastasis. Cancer and Metastasis Reviews. 1992;11(3-4):283-90.

35. Theoharides TC, Conti P. Mast cells the JEKYLL and HYDE of tumor growth. Trends in Immunology 2004;25(5):235-41.

36. Bernacki RJ, Niedbala MJ, Korytnyk W. Glycosidases in cancer and invasion. Cancer and Metastasis Reviews. 1985;4:81-102.

37. Anderson SK. Biology of Natural Killer cells: What is the relationship between natural killer cells and cancer? Will and increased number and/or function of natural killer cells result in lower cancer incidence. J Nutr. 2005 Dec;135:2910S.

38. Dranoff G. Cytokines in cancer pathogenesis and cancer therapy. Nature Reviews Cancer. Jan 2004;4:11-22.

39. Volkers N. Do autoimmune diseases raise the risk of cancer? J Nat Cancer Inst. 2011;91(23):1992-93.

40. Parkin DM. The global health burden of infection associated cancers in the year 2002. International J of Cancer. 2006;118(12):3030-44.

41. Pyakurel P, Pak R, Mwakigonija AR, Kaaya E, Biberfeld P. KSHV/HHV-8 and HIV infection in Kaposi's sarcoma development. Infectious Agents and Cancer. 2007;2:4.

42. www.cancer.gov/HPV

43. Correa P, et al. 2007. Carcinogenesis of Helicobacter pylori. Gastroenterology. 2007 Aug;133(2):659-72.

44. Anderson GL, et al. 2004. Effects of conjugated equine estrogen in postmenopausal women with hysterectomy: the Women's Health Initiative randomized controlled trial. JAMA. 2004 Apr 14;291(14):1701-12.

45. Hankinson SE, et al.2004. Towards an integrated model for breast cancer etiology: the lifelong interplay of genes, lifestyle, and hormones. Breast Cancer Res.2004;6(5):213-18.

46. Baron-Faust R. Breast cancer: What every woman should know. New York, NY: Hearst Books;1995.

47. McTiernan A, et al. 2005. Women's health initiative mammogram density study investigators. Estrogen-plus-progestin use and mammographic density in postmenopausal women: women's health initiative randomized trial. J Natl Cancer Inst. Sep 21;97(18):1366-76.

PART 2: NATUROPATHIC APPROACHES TO CANCER

Current research has not only revealed the molecular genetics of cancer, it has discovered the preventive and therapeutic role of specific lifestyle factors, including our diet and environment, stress management and physical exercise. What we eat and breath, what we worry about and what we do physically, can have an impact on the genesis and development of the aberrant cell that leads to cancer. Improving these lifestyle factors can also help prevent this development, and if the cancer has started, these factors can be therapeutic. Significantly, naturopathic medical modalities encompass these factors and provide the physician with a wide repertoire of treatment strategies.

Principles of Naturopathic Medicine

Naturopathic medicine is vitalistic, holistic, and eclectic, as shown in the six principles that inform this practice of medicine.

PRIMUM NON NOCERE

First, do no harm

This fundamental principle of naturopathic medicine is shared with allopathic physicians. In treating cancer, this principle is especially important because we are often using poisonous substances to arrest the progress of cancerous cells and to destroy them. The oncologist is always weighing the risk and benefits of treatments for their greater good. Naturopathic integrative treatments must not negatively influence the conventional therapeutics while attempting to enhance outcomes of the treatment and to reduce treatment side effects.

VIS MEDICATRIX NATURAE

Cooperate with the healing power of nature

Underlying the practice of naturopathic medicine is a profound belief in the healing power of nature that recognizes an inherent, or natural, ability in the body to heal itself. The *Vis* is a vital force that promotes recovery from illness and restores wellness, or homeo-balance. Naturopathic physicians act to identify and remove obstacles to recovery, and facilitate this healing ability by following established therapeutic protocols.

They help patients successfully complete their prescribed treatment schedule, by initiating protocols to safely prevent and treat side effects, and by minimizing negative outcomes of conventional treatments.

TOLLE TOTUM

Heal the whole person through individualized treatment

Naturopathic physicians treat each patient by taking into account physical, mental, emotional, genetic, environmental, social, and spiritual factors. Unlike some allopathic practices, their approach is not reductionist but rather holistic. They look for disturbances in the body-mind-spirit and "midwife" patients toward total health that extends beyond their specific cancer. Here the power of the spirit on the mind and emotions during active treatment offers the patient a sense of hope, and that hope is the medicine cancer patients need to endure the caustic treatment protocols designed to "kill" cancer. Outcomes research has shown that this sense of hope not only impacts the patients quality of life during active treatment but also after the therapeutic protocol is completed.

TOLLE CAUSEM

Identify and treat the cause

The exploration of the cause in naturopathic medicine goes beyond allopathic focus on suppressing symptoms, but in the case of cancer management, discovery of the cause may need to be put aside while we help patients with pressing symptoms. With cancer we need to look not only where the patient has been but, more importantly, where the patient is now. Most patients will be coming to our offices for help with their conventional cancer treatment protocols: patients seeking help from the side effects of a caustic treatment regimen designed to treat a very unnatural state of disease. We can lay the ground work *now* for investigating the cause and return to this inquiry during the active chemotherapy and radiation stages.

PREVINARE

Practice preventive medicine

Once patients have been successfully initiated into active chemotherapy and radiation treatments, naturopathic physicians refocus on the principle of disease prevention. Naturopathic medicine strives to create a healthy world in which humanity may thrive in symbiosis with the planet. This constitutes wellness, the establishment and maintenance of optimum health and balance. Wellness is a state of being healthy in body, mind, and spirit, characterized by positive emotion, thought, and action. Wellness is inherent in everyone, no matter what disease is being experienced; it is the innate ability to heal oneself, the *Vis medicatrix naturae*.

DOCERE
Teach the principles of healthy living
Naturopathic physicians educate patients about their health and encourage self-responsibility for health and well being. This is the core principle of patient-empowered medicine. This also acknowledges the therapeutic value inherent in the doctor-patient relationship and how that therapeutic milieu becomes part of the healing process for the patient.

Quality of life
Enabling the patient's inherent vitality, treating the whole person, not just the disease, enabling vitality, drawing on a variety of healing traditions, and midwifing hope – these are naturopathic strategies to help cancer patients reach homeobalance, or, at the least, enjoy a better quality of life. In this textbook, we will look at surgical, chemotherapy, and radiation therapies for different types of cancer and what naturopathic physicians can do to integrate their principles and practices of medicine with these conventional therapies to improve quality of life and provide a cure.

Naturopathic Practices
Naturopathic medical modalities have been shown in many scientific studies to be adjunctive to conventional cancer treatments, where nutritional and botanical medical modalities can, in some cases, work synergistically with chemotherapies and radiation therapies to enhance their effect and fight chemoresistance. Naturopathic medicine can help prevent or mitigate serious side effects from conventional treatments. Naturopathic medical modalities are also ideally suited to cancer prevention and chronic disease care. Seldom is one naturopathic modality used in isolation from another. Modalities often overlap and interact synergistically. Despite their eclecticism, all naturopathic modalities are ultimately focused on enabling the healing power of nature.

LIFESTYLE COUNSELING
Naturopathic lifestyle counseling for cancer prevention

Naturopathic medical modalities
- Lifestyle counseling
- Clinical nutrition
- Botanical medicine
- Homeopathic medicine
- Mind-body therapies
- Traditional medicines (Chinese, Ayurvedic, and Native)

involves advising patients how to avoid carcinogenic toxins in our environment and how to manage anxiety and stress. This counseling also addresses the emotional and mental health issues that arise in cancer case management, including coping with the prospect of death in palliative care. Lifestyle counseling often results in deploying one or more of the other modalities, most notably, clinical nutrition.

CLINICAL NUTRITION
Clinical nutrition involves dietary therapy and the administration of nutraceuticals. Diet plays a central role in the development of cancer and, in turn, its prevention and treatment. Naturopathic medicine recognizes the age-old maxim that food can be a poison and a medicine. "Let your food be your medicine and your medicine be your food," Hippocrates once wrote. In cancer care, diet not only addresses special nutritional needs but also provides immunotherapy, supporting the immune system in its fight against cancer. Clinical nutrition for cancer patients also involves taking nutritional supplements in therapeutic doses to support the immune system, enhance conventional chemotherapy, and address its side effects. Vitamins, minerals, amino acids, and other nutrients are used as nutraceuticals in conjunction with conventional pharmaceuticals.

BOTANICAL MEDICINE
Botanical medicine for cancer patients also involves using phytochemicals found in herbs and mushrooms to improve immune functions, to enhance conventional chemotherapy, and to manage side effects. These botanicals are used for their own medicinal properties and in conjunction with conventional pharmaceuticals.

HOMEOPATHIC MEDICINE
Homeopathic medicines for cancer are also used in an integrative manner in conjunction with conventional therapeutic strategies. Homeopathic remedies are used in acute dosing strategies to deal with pain, inflammation, GI distress, insomnia, and even the acceptance of the transition into death. The dosing

strategy is relatively low and needs to be repeated often due to interaction with the pharmaceutical treatments.

MIND-BODY THERAPIES

Mind-body therapies for cancer patients involve physical, emotional, and spiritual activities, such exercise programs, massage, reiki, yoga, meditation, deep breathing exercises, and prayer, that help alleviate anxiety and stress and offer palliative consolation.

Integrative Focus
Among these modalities of naturopathic medicine, lifestyle counseling, clinical nutrition, botanical medicines, and physical therapies have been most thoroughly studied in controlled clinical trials and most extensively practiced in cancer centers of excellence. They are the focus of this book as a result.

Naturopathic Treatment Protocols

Part of the art of integrating naturopathic and allopathic treatment of cancer is selecting and sequencing the various therapies that restore or improve health without risking harm to the patient. Recently, considerable research has been directed to studying naturopathic therapeutic protocols that can be applied to a wide range of conditions. For example, the *Foundations of Naturopathic Medicine* project has made these protocols one focus of their actvities. In his *Introduction to Principles & Practices of Naturopathic Medicine*, Dr Fraser Smith outlines an A,B,C pattern of naturopathic clinical reasoning:

A: Address fundamental health measures. Analyze the process of disease and process of healing to determine possible treatment strategies. Address the etiology, pathogenesis, and pathophysiology of the presenting condition, based on the results of the clinical assessment.

B: Build a basic plan of treatment measures in a logical sequence to promote self healing. Be sure that the necessary ingredients for good health are present or not impeded. In all but the most acute or simple cases, this involves a healthy diet, regular exercise, sleep hygeine, sunlight exposure, air quality, and sexual and work satisfaction. Some conditions or chronic diseases will dramatically improve or resolve entirely when patient and doctor address long-neglected basic ingredients of health and the proper conduct of life. Still, some patients need overall stimulation through homeopathy or other therapies that lead to increased vitality or activation of the *Vis medicatrix naturae.*

C: Consider specific treatment options for different individuals that enhance physiologic function and mitigate dysfunction. Case management involves an individualized treatment plan that allows the patient to move back toward health. This can range from giving some systems of the body a "tune up" to alleviating symptoms with nutritional supplements and botanical extracts that affect certain physiologic receptors in the body.

CANCER CASE MANAGEMENT
In cancer case management, this general naturopathic protocol applies. In Part 4 of this book dealing with specific cancers, this protocol is deployed with variations.

1. Enhance physiology using dietary therapy, nutraceuticals, and botanical medicines to activate the Vis mediatrix naturae as an anticancer agent. This protocol should arise logically from the pathophysiology of the cancer and the assessment of its kind and stage.

2. Support conventional cancer treatments with naturopathic approaches. The therapies chosen must be evidence based, proven to be effective and safe. The interaction of the therapies must be considered because many naturopathic treatments when taken in combinations are synergistic and when taken with conventional pharmaceuticals can interact adversely.

3. Mitigate side effects of conventional treatments with naturopathic therapies. These side effects include mucositis, cachexia, chronic pain, nausea and vomiting, constipation, hair loss, profound fatigue, neutropenia, anemia, sleep intrusion, and depression. Quality of life improves as a result, which, in turn, has been shown to improve outcomes.

4. Counsel long-term lifestyle changes to help prevent remission and short-term strategies for immediate palliation. This therapeutic protocol needs be individualized for the single patient. Each patient's tolerances and capabilities need to differentiated according to their vital force and for a willingness to adhere to and profit from a treatment program.

Lifestyle counseling is used by naturopathic physicians before, during, and after cancer therapy. Before treatment, the aim is preventive in reducing anxiety and stress, while promoting better nutrition. During treatment, counseling effort is focused on maintaining a sense of hope, avoiding possible depression. After treatment, the aim is to help patients achieve homeobalance by making long-term changes in their lives to address factors that caused their cancer and thus support remission. If the prognosis after treatment is for short-term survival, the naturopathic physician offers palliative counseling. Naturopathic physicians are well known for the time they allocate to lifestyle counseling, expecially stress management and clinical nutrition.

Physiological Stress

The concept of physiologic stress, aroused by multiple factors and giving multiple effects, was first articulated by Dr Hans Selye in a paper published in *Nature* on July 4, 1936, under the title "A Syndrome Produced by Diverse Nocuous Agents."[1] He discussed what he referred to as "stress induced illness" and coined the term "physiological alarm reaction" to identify the process the body uses to respond to situations of jeopardy. In subsequent publications, he found that this alarm reaction was the first of three stages of response to "nocuous" or stress-causing agents.[2]

1. Alarm Stage: The sympathetic nervous system is turned on by an increase in the adrenal medullary catecholamines, epinephrine and norepinephrine. This is the fight or flight response, resulting in emotions of anger, irritability, violence, anxiety, nervousness, and withdrawal. Physically, the person experiences an increase in heart rate and respiration.
2. Resistance Stage: This stage is the result of chronic stress and an increase in the production of glucocorticoids. Increased blood sugar levels, increased sense of well being, suppressed immune response, decreased immunity, and peptic ulcers are all significant clinical manifestations in this stage.
3. Exhaustion Stage: The adrenal glands are now depleted. Glucocorticoids no longer are adequately secreted. Postural or orthostatic hypotension occurs. If a continued increase in stress is

experienced during this phase, there is an increase in adrenalin secretion (by the norepinephrine signaling mechanism). Sweaty palms, anxiety, and related reactions are experienced along with poor digestion, palpitations, arrhythmias, and insomnia. When the adrenal cortex is exhausted, the medulla takes over and then an increase in blood sugar occurs. Simple sugar increases blood glucose, which provokes an increase in insulin. If blood sugar decreases in this phase, then an increase of glucocorticoid secretion occurs and the blood sugar is once again elevated with the corresponding increase in insulin levels. This maladaption is characteristic of the exhaustion phase.

A persistent elevation in cortisol also affects the immune system function by increasing neutrophils while decreasing lymphocytes, eosinophils, and monocytes. One of the most common causes of perpetuating

Non Specific Reactions that Characterize the Stress Response

- Rapid pulse and pounding heart
- General irritability, hyper-excitation, or depression
- Dryness of the throat or mouth
- Impulsive behavior
- Overpowering urge to cry or run away
- Inability to concentrate
- Weakness or dizziness
- Fatigue of unknown origin
- Floating anxiety
- Emotional tension
- Trembling and nervous ticks
- Being easily startled
- Nervous laughter
- Bruxism
- Hyperkinesis
- Sweating
- Salt craving
- Frequent need to urinate
- Diarrhea or indigestion
- Headaches
- Back pain
- Nightmares

allergic responses is adrenal exhaustion due to an elevated eosinophil and elevated IgE count. Due to the lower levels of adrenal functioning at the end of this exhaustion stage, a shift in the TH2 function occurs and the immune system becomes proinflammatory. This proinflammatory change is a co-factor in developing the aberrant cell.[3]

STRESS AS A SYNDROME

Selye's definition of stress was the nonspecific response of the body to any demand. Later, he recognized that the term "nocuous agents" was insufficient to describe the triggers of this syndrome and drew from a term in physics to describe these agents as stress. According to Selye, stress is not a disease.[4] It is a state of the system that creates a different physiological response to the world. In this sense, he refers to stress as a syndrome characterized by changes within the physiology of the organism resulting from altered environmental circumstances.[4-7]

Stressors

In an epigenetic context, stress has multiple effects on multiple genes, resulting in hormonal aberrations and a trend toward inflammation and immune irregularities that can cause disease, including cancer.[8] Hormones are activated or triggered by stressors in the hypothalamus-pituitary axis (HPA), which initializes a sympathetic nervous system response of arousal, adaption, and expression. The sympathetic response then affects other endocrine systems and parasympathetic nerves in the follicular cell fenestrations. Over time, these effects have an impact on genotypic and phenotypic expression.[9,10]

- ❖ Psychosocial (fear, loneliness, deprivation, isolation, rejection, anger, abuse)
- ❖ Chemical (xenobiotics, allergens, oxidative, clastogenic)
- ❖ Physical (trauma, malalignment, genomic)
- ❖ Environmental (radiation, time zones, noise, pollutants)
- ❖ Nutritional (dehydration, deficiency, toxicity, starvation)
- ❖ Inflammatory (dysbiosis, immune, vascular)

STRESS MODEL FOR THE ORIGIN OF DISEASE

Dr Selye's proposal was a revolutionary concept because it had previously been thought that each disease had its own specific cause. The discovery of stress-related diseases changed the face of medicine. The reactions to or signs of stress do not define a specific diagnosis; rather, they describe a functional state occurring across multiple organs that is related to an alteration in the expression of these psychoimmunoneuroendocrine responses. Over a prolonged period of exposure to these modulators, altered function results in a dysfunction of homeo-balance. This alteration to homeo-balance results in chronic disease via a shift in the TH2 immune system and inflammation as sequelae to that shift.

Selye was the first to propose that specific diseases, such as ulcers, immune collapse, nervous disorders, stroke, and heart disease, could be related to the general stress response. His model of disease describes a multifactorial approach that can result in a generalized response called the stress response. Over time, that stress response can produce a myriad of diseases, which differ in manifestation from person to person, depending on that person's unique set of susceptibility factors otherwise known as epigenetics. According to current models of this concept, the solution to overcoming age-related diseases is not in finding the single cause of each one but finding instead the multiple factors, antecedents, and triggers that result in changes that are then expressed phenotypically and genotypically in the body.[11]

CHRONIC STRESS

In prolonged stress, the hormonal response can become as damaging as the stressors themselves, depending on the individual and their epigenetics. In chronic stress, hormonal disease and imbalance lead to the individual becoming insulin resistant and slow to recovery after an injury or illness. What we now call metabolic syndrome, this illness becomes prolonged and can decrease the immune response. Libido and reproductive function diminish, and the muscles start to lose tone, with the body developing truncal obesity, the "apple" body shape, from the hormonal trigger of cortisol to store fat.[3,9]

Blood cholesterol, triglycerides, and blood pressure increase. Fatigue sets in, and sleep becomes restless and interrupted. The sleep continues to degrade and then insomnia accompanies the interrupted sleep issues. The person's mood slips toward depression or mood swings with anxiety and panic that then may lead to paranoia, all due to the alteration of neurotransmitters. Inflammatory response increases, and chronic inflammatory conditions arise. Immune defense against common infections decreases, while the spice of life is lost with the diminishing of T3 and the increase of cystokines like IL2, IL6, and TNF.

Usually the period from acute stress response to exhaustion varies depending on the individual. Always, there is a period of maladaption to stress in between excited and fatigued states. This maladaption often manifests with fatigue upon awakening, exhaustion in the afternoon, and a second wind in the evening, often accompanied with insomnia or sleep intrusion, usually between 2:00 and 3:00 a.m. This maladaption phase can be split into Phase 1 and Phase 2. Phase 1 maladaption is clinically expressed with fatigue either upon awakening or in the evening both accompanied by insomnia or sleep intrusion with normal DHEA levels. Maladaption Phase 2 is associated with more fatigue times and only one spike time in a day, typically at bedtime, with the associated sleep intrusion or insomnia and a slump in DHEA levels signifying a pregnenalone steal is in process.[8-11]

If the population of a society is experiencing a heightened state of stimuli, the average individual will translate this as stressful and the normal concentrations of the messenger molecules associated with the stress response are elevated to a point that is associated with the increase risk of age related chronic disease. In our culture today, many of us are over stimulated and under nourished. This lays the ground work for stress-related chronic disease, which we are now defining as normal.[12,13,14]

Psychoimmunoneuroendocrine Response

Robert Sapolisky recently defined the physiology of stress as the reaction of the body to imperfections in our world and the attempts of our bodies to get through them. He defines a stressor as any perturbation that disrupts homeostasis, and the stress response as a set of neural and endocrine adaptations that help reestablish homeostasis.[12-14]

Neuroendocrine changes aid in the adaptation to the struggle for survival of the species. This biochemical species preservation reaction produced glucose and adrenalin, which enabled the homo sapien to flee or kill its predators – fight or flight. There is a set of convergent physiological responses that occur during a stress response, no matter what the stress is. First, there is a secretion of sympathetic catecholamines, such as epinephrine and norepinepherine (adrenalin and nor adrenalin). In addition, glucocorticoids are secreted by the adrenal cortex. There is also a typical secretion of endorphin, vasopressin, and prolactin released by the pituitary gland, glucagons by the pancreas, and a few of the messenger molecules released under stress. These are all released so that the hormones turn on the "Fight or Flight" reflexive response, while the parasympathetic nervous system is shut down, as well as the sex hormone secretion and growth hormone secretion which eventually affects the thyroid gland. The catecholamines are released so that energy is mobilized in the form of the glucocorticoids from storage tissues…we are now getting

ready to run, jump, fly or fight! Next, the cardiovascular and pulmonary systems react and anabolism is suppressed as well as glycogen storage. Now, the sympathetic nervous system is turned on and digestion, growth, reproduction, and immunity are all suppressed, as well as T3 production.[12-14]

NERVOUS SYSTEM RESPONSE TO STRESS

The nervous system is an intricate system of positive and negative feedback loops that, when intact, keep and restore homeo-balance. In the context of holistic or integrative medicine, the spirit-mind-body connection plays a large role in how and even when the nervous system may be stimulated or depressed in function. The psyche is connected to the body via the cerebral spinal fluid and the nervous system.[15-19] The nervous system runs centrally through the spinal canal and peripherally through the nerve roots, from dermatomes and out to the peripheral nervous system. Many indigenous people believe the spirit lives in the spinal column or fluid.[20] The nervous system is made up of nerve cells called neurons, which consist of a cellular body and a long fiber tail called an axon. "Nerves" are in fact bundles of these fibers, with some axons being very long and running the length of the spinal cord from head to feet. The nerve cells (neuro-transmitters) transmit messages from one to the other via a synaptic cleft of neurotransmitters. This information process is always in flux as it undergoes regulation.

Central Nervous System and Peripheral Nervous System

There are two main parts to the nervous system: the central nervous system and the peripheral nervous system. The central nervous system includes the brain and the spinal cord. The peripheral nervous system includes the voluntary (somatic) and involuntary (autonomic) nervous systems. The voluntary system has 43 pairs of peripheral nerves that emerge from the central nervous system. The peripheral nerves are composed of two types: the sensory or afferent nerves, which conduct sensory information to the spinal cord and brain; and the motor or efferent nerves, which transmit instructions from the brain to the body. The brain and spinal cord receive information from the peripheral nerves then process and act of that information.

The autonomic nervous system govern reflexes such digestion, respiration, and blood circulation that must follow without thought automatically.[15,16] There are two parts to the autonomic nervous system: the sympathetic and the parasympathetic nervous systems. The sympathetic nervous system consists of nerves coming from the spinal cord in the trunk of the body. The parasympathetic nervous system consists of two groups of nerves, one emerging from the cranial region and one from the bottom of the spinal cord in the lumbar area of the body. This is the cranial-sacral connection.

The sympathetic nervous system response is a "fight or flight" reflexive response that prepares us for life-threatening danger, which is a hormonal response for species preservation. When we sense danger, the sympathetic nervous system facilitates the body's functions to prepare for battle or rapid movements by moving glucose into the blood stream to act as fuel. Glucose is mobilized into the bloodstream via the shunting of cortisol and the release of catecholamines, both of which aid in muscular activity while reducing any hindrance of muscle efficiency. Once this response is triggered, the digestive function is reduced and saliva ceases to flow, thus the production of dry mouth and urge to micturate. The skin becomes pale as blood is withdrawn and shunted to the muscles. Sweat glands step up their secretion to cool the body down, while the heart rate and respiration rates increase. Pupils dilate to improve vision. The system is ready to go on high alert (fight or flight).

The parasympathetic system acts to regain balance once the crisis is over and starts by slowing down the breathing and heart rate in order to begin to relax the muscles. Blood is shunted back to all areas of the body, and the catecholamines are diminished and no longer active in the body. The GI begins to relax.

This is the normal nervous response to stressful situations which is designed to function for a matter of

PTSD Neurophysiology

In post traumatic stress disorder (PTSD) neurophysiology, the HPA axis activation is the same as chronic disease: hypothalamus increases secretion of CRF; an attenuated ACTH release from the pituitary creates an excessive release of cortisol; and the exaggerated cortisol effects the anterior pituitary and the hypothalamus in the feedback loop mechanism – the same as the inflammatory cytokines of chronic disease activate the same feedback loop. Excessive stress causes this negative feedback loop activation, and the arousal phase has a global effect on the physiology of the thyroid and gonads via the HPA and sex binding hormone globulin. These are the neuro-immuno-endocrine effects that chronic stress creates as cortisol excretion increases but not the release of ACTH release, causing desensitization to the ACTH receptor. Acute stress is different because the ACTH receptor in the feedback mechanism functions and is not desensitized.[14-16]

seconds and then dissipate, but in our modern stressful lives, the sympathetic system goes into overdrive, perpetuating itself with its own neurotransmitters. The sensory system of the central nervous system (CNS) receives information from sight, sound, touch and even non-ionizing radiation, and translates these stimuli into neurological and chemical signals. These signals can communicate either bliss or alarm to distant tissues.[14-19]

BIOCHEMICAL RESPONSE TO STRESS

Corticorotrophin-releasing hormone (CRH) secretion occurs within seconds of exposure to a stressor and triggers pituitary release of ACTH within about 15 seconds. CRH is just one messenger molecule that causes ACTH to release. In descending order, the other triggers are vasopressin, oxytocin, and the catecholamines. Chemical messages are transmitted through the corticorotrophin-releasing hormone (CRH) of the hypothalamic gland to the hypothalamic-pituitary-adrenal (HPA) axis and the hypothalamic-pituitary-thyroid axis. Several key hormones function in the state of the stress system reaction, including CRH, norepinephrine, serotonin, acetylcholine, gamma-butyric acid (GABA), arginine, vasopressin and the glucocorticoids, cortisol and DHEA.

The hypothalamic-pituitary-adrenal (HPA) axis is responsible for the stress response and plays an important role in an individual's long-term response to stress and the genotypic expression of that long-term effect. Once ACTH is released, it rapidly triggers adrenocortical synthesis and the release of glucocorticoids. With the onset of stress, the glucocorticoid concentration rises within a few minutes from the secondary release of the catecholamines. Glucocorticoids react with cytosolic receptors that act to bind the hormone, to translocate to the nucleus, and to regulate gene expression. Glucocorticoids can increase or decrease the transcription of particular genes associated with the stress, thus effecting epigenetics with aberrant genotypic expression, lending itself toward the creation of the aberrant cell that becomes cancer.[11-17]

Gut Control

With acute stress response, glucocorticoids block energy storage and help mobilize energy from storage sites, increase cardiovascular tone, and inhibit anabolic processes, such as growth, repair, reproduction, and immunity. In a chronic stress response, the chemical messaging system has a graded response depending on the type and magnitude of the stimuli. It has a fine tuned control system for letting out the response according to the magnitude of the stimuli.

The response is not linear but exponential, so once the stress response arrives at a certain point, the next level of increased stimuli can result in significant increases in the output of messenger alarm molecules. HPA and inflammatory mediators increase immune responses and rheumatoid expressions (hypervigilant system response equals autoimmune disease). Stress induced injury to HPA ties into PTSD, CFS, FMS and multiple chemical sensitivities due to elevated levels of IgE, nitric oxide, and peroxynitrite from highly driven cortisol and increased proinflammatory cytokine mediators in mitochondrial-rich tissues of the body: brain, heart and bowel. The GALT immune system in the gut, if influenced by food reactions, translates cortisol to the immune system of the brain (microglia), causing increased inflammation in an otherwise pristine environment: a stressed gut equates to poor brain function.[18-24]

IMMUNE SYSTEM RESPONSE TO STRESS

Chronic stress causes activation of the neuroendocrine system, which influences the immune system. Once the immune system is activated, it influences the neuroendocrine system. The central nervous system produces neurotransmitters, such as serotonin and catecholamines, for which there are receptors on the surface of specialized immune cells. The immune system produces cytokines as well as antibodies that influence the activity of receptor sites on the blood/brain barrier. The gastrointestinal mucosa, which has a large cluster of immune tissue (GALT), has receptors for the brain-derived neurotransmitters, and the brain has receptors for the gastrointestinal messenger molecules – the gut/brain connection.

It has been recently demonstrated that chemical, allergic, and psychological stresses cause alteration in the GI mucosa, which results in the uptake or release of agents that influence nervous system function such as inflammatory cytokines. These inflammatory cytokines, such as IL-1, IL-2, and TNF suppress hypothalamic activity. Thus, the chronic long-term exposure to increased catecholamine and glucocorticoid secretion by the HPA from exposure to stressors results in an effect on the function of the immune system. The effect is to increase the production of inflammatory cytokines from the immune system, while simultaneously reducing immunological vigilance against infectious organisms and formation of the aberrant cell.[21-24]

GLUCOMINERALCORTICOID PATHWAY

The reproductive and adrenal cortical steroids are produced from cholesterol. Low plasma cholesterol could have an impact on the production of adrenal and gonadal steroids due to the lack of the molecular backbone of cholesterol available from the diet. The conversion of cholesterol to pregnenolone is a rate-limiting step in adrenal hormone production and the major site of ACTH action on the adrenal glands. The production of adrenal androgens from pregnenolone and progesterone occurs in the reticularis and fasciculate layers of the adrenal cortex.

DHEA (and its sulfate), as well as androstenedione, are major androgens produced in the adrenal gland cortex. They are converted to testosterone by peripheral conversion. In males, this occurs in the testes, and in women, it occurs principally in adrenal glands, the breast, and adipose tissues (via aromatization). In females, ovarian androgen production is low; the adrenal glands substantially contribute to total androgen production by peripheral conversion of androstenedione to testosterone. In menopausal women, the adrenal production of androgen precursors results in 100% of the available molecules that can be converted to testosterone by peripheral tissues. In menstruating females, hyperinsulinemia/insulin resistance increases the ovarian production of androgens and can result in acne, facial hair, menstrual irregularities, and, in severe cases, polycystic ovarian syndrome with reproductive failure. Progesterone conversion from pregnenolone is also altered and usually deficient.[3,9,24]

Generally, the adrenal glucocorticoids inhibit the synthesis of DNA and messenger RNA, creating an inhibitory influence on genomics. In the adrenal medulla, the catecholamines are synthesized from N-acetyl tyrosine. Tyramine, which is found in foods like chocolate, coffee, some cheeses, red wine and bananas, can stimulate the release of norepinephrine. Norepinephrine is converted to epinephrine in the adrenal medulla and in a few specialized neurons in the central nervous system by methylation requiring S-adenosylmethionine, which is produced in the folate cycle. If there is an inborn error or folic acid metabolism, then the process of methylation is compromised. High levels of glucocorticoids induce methylation, which indicates chronic stress conditions characterized by an increased level of cortisol, and can increase the activity of epinephrine, creating insulin resistance over time.[3,9,10,24]

In detoxification of epinephrine, there must be adequate amounts of S-adenosylmithionine derived from 5-methyltetrahydrofolate with the help of vitamin B-6. The catecholamines bind to many different receptor sites in tissues and influence their functions. Alpha 1 and alpha 2 adrenergic receptors and the beta receptors regulate vasoconstriction, cardiac force of contraction, lipolysis, thermogenesis, insulin release, glycogenolysis, and gastrointestinal motility. The beta 1 receptor mediates inotropic and chronotropic effects of catecholamines on cardiac muscle, whereas beta 2 receptor mediates smooth muscle relaxation of the vasculature. Catecholamines also increase rennin release, which is involved in the conversion of angiotensin I and angiotensin II, at the kidney.[3,9,24]

Chronic stress also has an impact on the synthesis and activity of the mineralocorticoids and aldosterone. Its production is controlled primarily by the rennin/angiotensin system, although it is slightly activated by sodium and potassium levels, ACTH, and catecholamines. The principal effects of aldosterone are on the maintenance of normal sodium and potassium concentrations and extracellular fluid volume. Elevations in aldosterone result in retention of sodium and fluid and loss of potassium.[3,9,13-25,29]

Cortisol Reactions

Cortisol itself in high levels acts as a mineralocorticoids with adverse effects:
- Aging
- Chronic stress
- Hypothyroidism
- HPA and HPT effected by stress
- HPA stress induced adaptation and cell mediated immune system goes down but the inflammatory process increases and more chronic disease and inflammatory reactions affect reproduction, metabolism and growth/repair.
- Increased arthralgias and myalgias due to chronic stress and pro-inflammation changes

CRH Response

The CRH response to a given stimulus is specific to the individual but in general CRH output may result in the following changes:
- Hyperinsulinemia, hypercortisolemia, hyperchatecholaminemia=metabolic syndrome
- Increased visceral fat deposition=truncal obesity
- Reduced testosterone, reduced estrogen, reduced progesterone=decreased libido and reproductive vitality
- Increased oxidative stress, increased inflammatory mediators=genetic mutations and possible cancers
- Increased activation of detox pathways like methylation, sulfation, and glucoronicadation=NASH syndrome, liver dysfunction

CHOLESTEROL AND STRESS

Lipemia develops with acute stress reactions and resolves over a day but chronic stress has a long-term effect, raising the blood cholesterol. Over time, metabolic dysfunctions cause this effect on the triglycerides in particular, showing the effects of the inflamed and dysfunctional immune system. CoQ10 levels in mitochondrial respiratory chain goes down with increased anaerobic metabolism happening, causing increased lactate and pyruvate, which is produced as a waste product of the anaerobic metabolism, and causing increased muscle cramping, fatigue, and fibromyalgia-like symptoms.[3,9,10,11]

THYROID AND STRESS

Thyroid disease has an increased incidence of autoimmune thyroiditis associated with increased autoimmune antibodies, subclinical hypothyroidism, depression, and chronic fatigue syndrome all associated with the effects of the stress hormones on the thyroid feedback and production mechanism. Chronic stress response of the thyroid function starts out in one of two usual methods: either through the hypervigilant immune dysfunction causing autoimmune disease of the thyroid; or subclinical hypothyroidism by down-regulation of T3 production. Thyroid releasing hormone (TRH) from the hypothalamus is affected by CRH, which also stimulates GH, and then will have a secondary effect on the pituitary hormone thyroid stimulating hormone (TSH). TSH goes directly to the thyroid to stimulate the production of T4 by instructing the gland to iodinize and thyroid peroxidase to form the hormone. Most of the T4 hormone (approximately 85%) is bound with only a very small percent left unbound and free to be converted peripherally to T3, the most active form of the thyroid hormone. Every cell in the body and brain has some form of receptor site for T3. Selenium is known to work in the conversion of T4 to T3 in the liver, with a small amount converted in the kidneys and brain. Subclinical states show within normal limits of these indices, but the clinical picture shows fatigue, immune suppression, weight gain, hair loss, hyperlipidemia, hypertension, dysglycemia, NASH syndrome, and more.[3,9-11]

TSH can be used as a measurement, but T3 is a much better assay. Subclinical hypothyroid patients put on only T4 find that the hormone replacement is not effective because there must be a balance of T4 and T3 (and remember in a chronically stressed out system T3 is down-regulated and underproduced in response to the chronic stress hormones produced). T3 has a very specific effect on neuropsychological function and helps to prevent premature death from

THE EFFECTS OF STRESS AND NUTRITIONAL SUPPORT ON THE HPA/HPT AXES

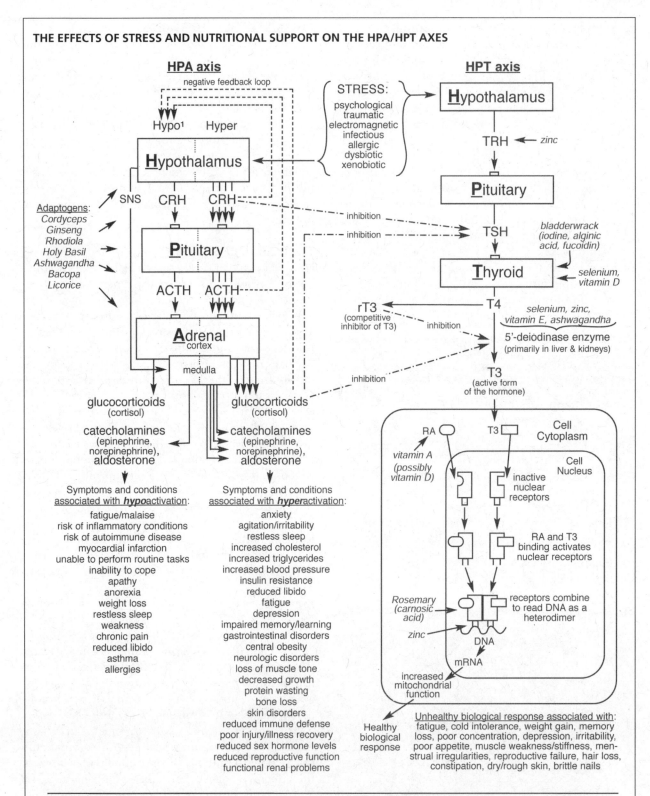

1. **Contributors to *hypo*activation of HPA**: a) reduced biosynthesis of CRH, ACTH, and cortisol due to organ hypofunction or depleted hormone precursors, b) CRH hypersecretion causing down-regulation of pituitary CRH receptors and reduced secretion of ACTH, c) increased negative feedback sensitivity, d) morphological changes (e.g., adrenal atrophy).

Acronym Key: ACTH: adrenocorticotropin hormone; CRH: corticotropin-releasing hormone; DNA: deoxyribonucleic acid; mRNA: messenger ribonucleic acid; RA: retinoic acid; rT3: reverse triiodothyronine; SNS: sympathetic nervous system; T3: triiodothyronine; T4: thyroxine; TRH: thyrotropin-releasing hormone; TSH: thyroid-stimulating hormone.

heart attacks, hypertension, and cardiovascular disease. T3 increases peripheral circulation due to vasodilation and lowers vascular pressure and affects the heart at a cellular level and must absolutely be delivered to these receptor sites. T3 works at the level of the mitochondria and is more biologically active than growth hormone. In healthy aging, there is low autoimmune Abs to thyroid with blood levels showing higher amounts of iodine, tyrosine, and other thyroid hormone precursors. T3 can be supported by botanical and glandular therapies.[3,9,10,11,14,17]

Cholesterol and Thyroid

T3 influences mitochondrial uptake of cholesterol through its binding to mitochondrial receptor sites. Therefore, low thyroid function increases Apo-A-1 gene and increases LDL due to low T3 (good T3 levels increase the HDL/LDL levels), thus affecting total cholesterol level, with the LDL receptor gene influenced by T3 showing an inverse relationship between CVD and thyroid hormone levels of T3.[13,14]

Clinical Applications

Chronic disease affected by lifestyle, psyche, stress, and physiological markers has an effect on the phenotypic expression of the genome. Aging, chronic disease, and cancer all show a natural increased stress response with a decreased ability to repair. There is also a noted lower expression of metabolic and biosynthetic genes that then leads to increased catabolic activity, showing the tell-tale signs of unhealthy aging, chronic disease, and terminal illness. All three of these issues also show increased inflammatory processes in the brain, with hyperinsulinemia altering the expression of genes, proteins, and kinases. In chronic stress induced dysfunction, this process happens faster and more virulently.

In clinical presentations, we see the loss of fine sensory motor skills, like vibratory sensation, loss of low and high frequency hearing, loss of memory recall and quick reflexive response, loss of balance and equilibrium, loss of dexterity, loss of endurance and muscle strength, and loss of lean body mass, all equating to the measurement of biological age and aging.

Measures for Fighting Cancer

Most cancer patients receive the news that they have cancer with a stress response as an initial part of the reaction. Some handle this news with great difficulty, while others have a more accepting nature. A stress response returns with each step of the process from diagnosis through treatment, and then upon follow-up visits. The stress response in palliative situations is no less physiologically or emotionally challenging. The physician can help control these stress responses with proactive lifestyle counseling (including good sleep hygiene), dietary hormone- balancing measures, and spiritual practices.

A new model of cancer survivorship needs to be created in response to the current improvement of cancer treatments, integrative strategies and early diagnosis all leading to improved cure rates and long-term survival. Each time a cancer patient returns to their oncologist for a follow-up screening exam, their psyche worries if they will be free of cancer or not. Long-term follow up strategies and survivor programs can change the current model.

PHYSIOLOGICAL MANAGEMENT

1. **Eat protein by 8 a.m. each morning and every 4-5 hours while awake: if you wake early in the morning make sure to eat protein within one hour upon awakening.**

Cortisol levels start to rise whenever you do not eat for 5 hours in response to a drop in glucose. During our daily overnight fast, cortisol levels begin to rise to the level needed for us to "bounce out of bed" around 3 a.m. to hit peak around 7 a.m. If you eat later than 8 p.m., then the peak cortisol elevation needed for easy wakening may be delayed, and you are likely to feel tired in the morning and not experience adequate energy to function properly until later in the day. Likewise, if you do not eat by 7 or 8 a.m., then the morning cortisol level continues to rise and may overshoot the normal range. Add a cup of hot stimulant to the adrenals like caffeine on an empty stomach and the cortisol shoots through the roof in response.

When the cortisol level overshoots its goal any time during the day, it is often difficult to bring the cortisol level back down in time to achieve the lower range needed in the evening for sleep to go below REM and into slow gamma wave restorative sleep. Thus, the fatigue problem perpetuates itself by causing an insomnia or sleep intrusion.

Some individuals who tend to skip breakfast do so unwittingly in order to use short-term starvation as a stimulus to secrete cortisol and thus bring subnormal morning cortisol levels up to normal. This approach has the disadvantage of stimulating epinephrine, and if you add a cup of coffee and a cigarette, the average American breakfast becomes a cortisol-inducing nightmare. Sleep will be interrupted if we have inadequate glycogen stores to provide the brain with energy throughout the night while we are sleeping. Every time we eat protein we replete glycogen stores, or if we eat on a low glycemic scale every 4-5 hours during the daytime. When a meal is skipped, glycogen stores in the liver are depleted a little, and if we eat more carbohydrates than proteins within a 4-5 hour span. If meals are skipped habitually or we eat excess starches and sugars, the inflammatory response is turned on and sleep is automatically disrupted. There is a high metabolic need for proteins. A protein snack of a predigested protein, like yoghurt, will balance the blood sugar, feed the brain, and promote restful sleep by balancing blood glucose overnight.

2. Go to Bed and Sleep by 10 p.m.

Sleep is one of the most important factors in the strategies for fighting cancer. By going to bed by 10 p.m., you utilize the naturally high point of the excretion of the hormone melatonin from the pineal gland. Sleep is the easiest way to turn on this hormone. You are likely to feel more refreshed with 5 hours of sleep between 10 p.m. and 3 a.m. than with 5 (or more) hours sleep that do not begin until 3 a.m. because of this natural melatonin level. Of note is that some immune system protective functions do not even engage until one has had 7 or more hours of continuous sleep. Chronic sleep deprivation takes a toll on immune surveillance, thus the recommendation for at least 8 hours of sleep.

3. Control Pain Promptly

Pain is the single most impressive factor in terms of sharply elevating cortisol levels and suppressing the immune system while causing inflammation. Patients who suffer with acute and chronic pain soon display the signs and symptoms of cortisol excess: physical and mental fatigue, weight gain around the middle, muscle weakness (in excess of the weakness expected from lack of exercise alone), abdominal bloating, easy bruising, sleep disturbance, digestive abnormalities, and increase in mucous membrane infections (sinusitis, bladder infection, bronchitis, etc.), and ultimately immune suppression. These symptoms are detrimental to cancer survival and cannot be reversed until the pain is controlled. Sometimes with cancer pain only pharmaceutical intervention will be sufficient.

4. Correct the Circadian Rhythm

Once it has been determined that the circadian rhythm is abnormal, multiple therapeutic approaches are available. The treatment regimen is aimed at correcting the depressions or elevations in cortisol at each particular time of day. Phosphorylated serine helps to elevate lower secretory IgA to normal, while re-sensitizing the ACTH receptor in the hypothalamus. Phosphorylated serine helps to lower cortisol by

these two mechanisms and is safe while effective. Use the protocol to prime the aberrant sleep cycle 1-2 hours before bedtime, at bedtime and as needed when sleep is interrupted during the night. After retraining the sleep cycle, less and less of the phosphorylated serine would be needed but always keep at least one dose at bedtime to keep receptor site sensitivity. Sometimes melatonin supplementation is needed to reset the sleep cycle.[26-36]

CONNECTIVITY

Stress affects the health of the whole person – body, mind, and spirit. To manage stress, we need to address these connections. We need this same interconnectivity if we are to thrive; if we are not connected spiritually and with each other in a "tribal community," we do not feel supported, valued, or healthy. When working with the diseased patient, these aspects of connection become very important. Outcome studies have shown that the more connected cancer patients are to their loved ones, caregivers, and community, the longer they survive their cancers.[35]

SPIRITUALITY

Countless studies have shown the act of faith strengthens the immune system and turns off fight or flight mechanisms. Spiritual practices and a belief system enhance the immunomodulators to fight cancer cells, even changing the neuroendocrine hormones released in this response. The endorphins released from the feeling of being loved or of being in love have the same physiological effects on the immune system as an anti-inflammatory. The act of faith gives the patient a belief in something greater than the self and that in turn gives Hope. Hope, laughter, love, and a sense of the divine have been shown to increase not only the quality of life but also longevity.[19,35]

References

1. Selye H. A syndrome produced by diverse nocuous agents. Nature. 1936 July 4;138:32.

2. Selye H. The general adaptation syndrome and the diseases of adaptation. J Clin Endocrinol. 1946 Feb;6(2):117-234.

3. Jones DS. Textbook of Functional Medicine. Gig Harbor, WA: Institute for Functional Medicine; 2005.

4. Selye H. Stress and disease. Science. 1955 Oct 7;122:625-31.

5. Selye H. From Dream to Discovery: On Being a Scientist. New York, NY: McGraw-Hill; 1964.

6. Selye H. Hormones and Resistance. Berlin; New York: Springer-Verlag, 1971.

7. Seyle H. Stress without Distress. Philadelphia, PA: J. B. Lippincott Co.;1974.

8. Daruna JH. Introduction to Psychoneuroimmunology. San Diego, CA: Elsevier Academic Press; 2004.

9. Habib KE, Gold PW, Chrousos GP. Neuroendocrinology of stress. Endocrinol Metab Clin North Am. 2001 Sep;30(3):695-728.

10. Lamounier-Zepter V, Ehrhart-Bornstein M, Bornstein SR. Metabolic syndrome and the endocrine stress system. Horm Metab Res. 2006;38:437-41.

11. Wilson J. Adrenal Fatigue: The 21st Century Stress Syndrome. Petaluma, CA: Smart Publications; 2005.

12. Sapolsky R. Stress in The Wild. Scientific American. 1990 Jan;262(1):106-13.

13. Sapolsky R, Lewis CK, McEwen BS. The neuroendocrinology of stress and aging: the glucocorticoid cascade hypothesis. Science of Aging Knowledge Environment. 2000 Sep 25;38:21.

14. Sapolsky R, Romero M, Munck AU. How do glucocorticoids influence stress responses? integrating permissive, suppressive, stimulatory, and preparative actions. Endocrine Reviews. 2000;21(1):55-89.

15. Sapolsky R, Rodrigues SM. Disruption of fear memory through dual-hormone gene therapy. Biol Psychiatry. 2009;65(5):441-44.

16. Sapolsky R, Mitra R. Effects of enrichment predominate over those of chronic stress on fear-related behavior in male rats. Stress. 2009;12(4):305-12.

17. Sapolsky, R, Cheng MY, Sun G, Jin M, Zhao H, Steinberg GK. Blocking glucocorticoid and enhancing estrogenic genomic signaling protects against cerebral ischemia. J Cereb Blood Flow Metab. 2009;29(1):130-36.

18. Benson, H, Greenwood, AB, Klemchuk, AB. The relaxation response: psychopysiologic aspects and clinical applications. Intl J Psychiatry Med. 1975;6(1/220); 87-97.

19. Moritz S, Quan H, Rickhi B, Liu M, Angen M, Vintila R, Sawa R, Soriano J, Toews J. A home-study-based spirituality education program decreases emotional distress and increases quality of life: a randomized controlled trial. Altern Ther Health Med. 2006 Nov/Dec;12(6) 26-35.

20. Sharma AK. Panchakarma therapy in Ayurvedic medicine. Mishra LC (ed.) Scientific Basis for Ayurvedic Therapies. New York, NY: CRC Press; 2004:43-61.

21. Stam R, Ekkelenkamp K, FrankhuijzenAC, bruijnzeel AW, Akkermans LMA, Wiegant VM. Long-lasting changes in central nervous system responsivity to colonic distention after stress in rats. Gastroenterology. 2002;123(4):1216-25.

22. Holzer P. Neural injury, repair, and adaptation in the GI tract II. The elusive action of capsaicin on the vagus nerve. Am J Physiol Gastrointest Liver Physiol. 1998 July; 275(I): G8-G13.

23. Tougas G. The autonomic nervous system in functional bowel disorders. Gut. 2000;(Suppl IV)47: iv78-iv80.

24. Porges SW. Orienting in a defensive world: Mammalian modifications of our evolutionary heritage: a polyvagal theory. Psychophysiology 1995;32:301-18.

25. Brown RP, Gerbarg PL. Sudarshan kriya yogic breathing in the treatment of stress, anxiety, and depression: part I - neurophysiologic model. J Altern complement Med. 2005 Aug;11(4):711-17.

26. Bada LJ, Cook WH, Hoag JB. The role of autonomic nervous system in rapid breathing practices. Indian J Physiol Parmacol. 1996;40:4318-324.

27. Rege NN, Thatte UM, Dahanukar SA. Adaptogenic properties of six rasayana herbs used in Ayurvedic medicine. Phytother Res. 1999;13:275-91.

28. Mishra LC, Singh BB, Dagenais S. Scientific basis for the therapeutic use of Withania somnifera (Ashwagandha): a review. Altern Med Rev. 2000 Aug;5(4):334-46.

29. Archana R, Namasivayam A. Antistressor effect of Withania sominfera. J Ethnopharmacol. 1999 Jan;64(1): 91-93.

30. Bhattacharya SK, Bhattacharya A, Chakrabarti A. Adaptogenic activity of Siotone, a polyherbal formulation of Ayurvedic rasayanas. Ind J Exp Biology. 2000 Feb;38: 119-128.

31. Goyal RK, Singh J, Lal H. Asparagus racemosa– an update. Indian J Med Sci. 2003 Sep;57(9):408-14.

32. Srikumar R, Parthasarathy NJ, Manikandan S, Narayanan GS, Sheeladevi R. Effect of Triphala on oxidative stress and on cell-mediated immune response against noise stress in rats. Mol Cell Biochem. 2006 Feb;283(1-2):67-74.

33. Singh N, Singh SM, Prakash, Singh G. Restoration of thymic homeostasis in a tumor-bearing host by in vivo administration of medicinal herb Tinospora cordifolia. Immunopharmacol Immunotoxicol. 2005;27(4):585-99.

34. Bhattacharya SK, Bhattacharya A, Chakrabarti A. Adaptogenic activity of Siotone, a polyherbal formulation of Ayurvedic rasayanas. Ind J Exp Biology. 2000 Feb;38:119-128.

35. Carlson LE, Speca M, Patel KD, Goodey E. Mindfulness-based stress reduction in relation to quality of life, mood, symptoms of stress and levels of cortisol, dehydroepiandrosterone sulfate (DHEAS) and melatonin in breast and prostrate cancer outpatients. Psychoneuroendocrinology. 2004;29(4):448-74.

36. West J, Otte C, Geher K, Johnson J, Mohr DC. Effects of Hatha yoga and African dance on perceived stress, affect, and salivary cortisol. Ann Behav Med. 2004 Oct;28(2):114-18.

The discipline of clinical nutrition comprises the study of food nutrition, or diet, and the study of nutrient supplements used medicinally. In the case of cancer, clinical nutrition as a naturopathic medical modality includes dietary and nutritional therapy as adjuncts to conventional cancer treatments, though in some cases, clinical nutrition can be a first-line therapeutic, and for the cancer-fighting patient, it may even be a biological response modifier. It is a cost-effective, non-toxic, scientifically proven adjuvant therapy for the cancer patient. Patients have the advantage in the fight against cancer if they have a strong nutritional status.

The goals for this first-line therapy are to prevent and treat malnutrition, to enhance tumor kill while reducing chemotherapy and radiation toxicities, to stimulate immune responses, and to selectively starve tumors.

Dietary Therapy

Dietary therapy can be preventive or therapeutic in the case of cancer. Procarcinogens in our food supply need to be avoided to prevent cancer, and therapeutic diets can strengthen immunity to carcinogens and genetic factors.

PREVENTIVE DIETS

The safety of our food supply has become compromised by the use of carcinogenic herbicides, pesticide, and chemical fertilizers. Our food has also become excessively processed, often losing the nutritional value of whole, natural food sources. Replacing carcinogenic food with organic food and eating whole, fresh foods can help prevent cancer development.

Non-Carcinogenic Food Sources

Evidence shows that the environment of the cell is a dominant cofactor in the transformation of a proto-oncogene into an oncogene. Pesticides, herbicides, growth hormones, antibiotics, PCBs, and many other byproducts of factory farming and industrialization are known procarcinogens in many different mutation processes.

Organic Food

Organic food is grown and processed without these procarcinogens, as defined by the United States Department of Agriculture (USDA). Look for the USDA certified organic label when buying food.[1]

The evidence continues to grow supporting organically grown meats, dairy, fruits, vegetables, and grains that are less procarcinogenic more nutritious. Simply by removing the pesticide, herbicide, and inorganic fertilizers, the foods become safer for the consumer and the environment. They also become and tastier.

Organic Certification[1]

The USDA (United States Department of Agriculture) regulates organic labeling and defines organic as:

- Any milk, meat, poultry, and eggs made from animals given no antibiotics or growth hormones and fed organic feed. These animals also must live in an environment with conditions that are able to move freely in and out of shelter. The organic label also includes the processing of these animal products by a processor that is certified and machinery that is not cross contaminated with non organic animal products.
- For any plant product no chemical fertilizers or sewage sludge can be used to fertilize crops. No pesticides, genetic engineering, or irradiation to kill germs is allowed, nor can crops be harvested prematurely. Plant diseases and pests can only be treated with non-chemical methods, such as natural insect predators, traps, or natural repellants.
- No chemical herbicides are to be used on any organic plant products. Mulching, weeding, or mechanical cultivation can used to control weeds with growing strategies of companion planting instead of herbicides.

Whole Foods

Replacing highly processed foods with whole foods also lowers the procarcinogenic load and the glycemic index of the diet. Highly processed foods have additives and preservatives that again are known procarcinogens. Eating locally reduces the need for more processed foods that require added preservatives to survive the long route from farm to table.

Locally, the sustainability of the local farmer is helped, and globally, the strain on fossil fuel resources, the production of toxic emissions, and other costs of mass production farming and transportation are reduced. The benefits are transformational: producing healthy food, healthy people, and a healthy planet.

MACRONUTRIENT THERAPEUTIC DIETS

The goal of a therapeutic diet is to keep patients as healthy as possible while undergoing conventional treatments and experiencing possible side effects. Therapeutic diets involve increasing macronutrient content, including fiber.

With cancer patients, macronutrients (proteins, carbohydrates, and fats) are needed in larger amounts than recommended in standard food guides, such as the USDA *MyPyramid* guide and Health Canada's *Eating Well for Good Health* guide. The average 150 lb. female cancer patient will require a 2,000 kcal diet rather than the food guide recommended 1800 kcal to maintain a healthy weight during active treatment. Most patients in active treatment require 2,500 kcal delivered in a nutrient dense, high-protein diet.[2]

GI Side Effects

Many of the side effects of conventional drug and radiation therapies target the gastrointestinal system. This is partly due to the nature of the gut's cells. The mucosa of the GI system is rapidly dividing, sloughing off and replacing cells approximately every three to four days. Chemotherapy and radio therapies are also targeting rapidly dividing cells that are cancer. Mucositis is a common side effect of chemotherapy and radio therapy on the GI, producing nausea, vomiting, stomatitis, taste changes, anorexia, and cancer cachexia. Nutraceutical interventions, glutamine, for example, can not only treat but prevent these treatment side effects of the GI.

High-Protein Diet

The importance of proteins in the diet of the cancer patient and cancer survivor cannot be overemphasized. Proteins are the building blocks of our bodies, used to repair tissues and build the immune system, enzymes, muscles, and hormones. The basic building block for proteins is the amino acid, also known as a peptide. There are approximately 20 major amino acids and eight are considered essential, which means they cannot be made by the human body and must be ingested. By eating complete proteins, these essential amino acids are acquired through the diet.

When proteins are digested, they are broken down by stomach acid into subunits of amino acids and are absorbed into the blood stream. The amino acids then reassemble into chains called polypeptides. These chains of polypeptides link to one another in various configurations. These various configurations form thousands of different proteins, all coming from only 20 amino acids.

All of the macronutrients are important in the diet, but only proteins can supply the essential amino acids. They also supply basic elements, such as nitrogen, which is essential to all living beings. Among the essential amino acids, glutamine is key for the cancer patient in active treatment.

Glutamine

Glutamine is the most abundant of the essential amino acids and has more metabolic activity than the rest. Glutamine has been found to be important in preventing mucositis and cachexia and as the chief source of fuel for the rapidly dividing cells lining the gastrointestinal tract. It also is an important nutrient for proper immune system white blood cell function.[2] Glutamine should be considered an essential amino acid in the cancer patient undergoing active cancer treatments. It has been shown that this amino acid can prevent and treat chemo/radiation induced mucositis, stomatitis, and cachexia.[3]

Protein Deficiency

Daily protein intake requirements increase with the metabolic increase associated with cancer and cancer treatments. Cancer cells, like all cells of the body, require protein in order to exist, but cancer cells do not succumb to protein deprivation in the diet. If there is a deficiency of protein in a cancer patient's diet, the muscle will be broken down in response to the metabolic need of the system enhanced by the rapidly dividing cancer cell's increased metabolism. Cachexia is the medical term for this activity. It is a common sequelae of conventional chemotherapies and radiation. The weight loss that often accompanies cancer can be from several different cofactors, but often it is accompanied by muscle wasting, or cachexia.

Generally, the daily protein requirement for a patient actively in conventional treatment is between 75 and 100 grams per day in divided doses. If there are any kidney issues or if the patient has a decreased kidney function, the dose should be lowered appropriately. The "right" amount of protein required should be determined by the individual patient's needs matching the current nutritional status with

PROTEIN FUNCTIONS[5]

1. Immune system proteins. Immunoglobulins and antibodies (AB) are proteins made by the immune system, specifically by white blood cells called B cells, in response to a foreign substance or antigen (AG). ABs bind to AGs and create immune complexes (AB/AG) that can be recognized by the immune system and destroyed. Immunoglobulins and antibodies detect bacteria, viruses, protozoan, or other exogenous invaders. They can also mistake these invaders as self in autoimmune reactions.

2. Enzymes. Enzymes are simple proteins that direct chemical reactions and changes within the cell for proper function. Each of the thousands of biochemical changes happening within a cell at any given moment requires a very specific enzyme for proper action. Daily processes, such as digestion, energy (ATP) production, oxygenation, muscle contraction, and memory, all require an individual, specific enzyme to complete its task.

3. Hormones. Hormones are important in the self- regulation of each bodily system. Hormones are responsible for balancing the whole body via neuro-immuno endocrine reactions that biofeedback to the brain. These functions are considered essential. The regulation of an imbalanced system will cause either an excess or deficiency of the hormones used in that system's checks and balance. Daily functions of body temperature regulation, digestion, glucose regulation, sexual function, and weight loss or gain are a direct effect of hormones in flux.

4. Transport proteins. Transport proteins are literally what their name implies; they transport other substances throughout the body. For example, albumin, a transport protein found in the blood stream, is the most abundant protein in the blood. Albumin acts as a transport protein and carries zinc, calcium, fatty acids, and vitamin B-6 throughout the system.

5. Structural proteins. Structural proteins make up muscles, ligaments, cartilage, hair, and nails. Additional proteins are used structurally within the cell membranes, providing architecture as well as communication channels between the inside and outside environments of the cell. If there is a deficiency of proteins in the diet, the body will breakdown muscle tissues to provide the needed proteins to meet its requirements.

the type, location, stage of the cancer and the conventional treatment therapies utilized. Undergoing conventional cancer therapy may require as much as 50% more protein than usual.[4]

People with cancer have a different calculation used for the daily requirement needed: Intake between .45 to .9 grams per pound of body weight per day. This means that a cancer patient weighing 150 lbs would require 67-135 grams of protein per day, while a healthy person weighing the same amount would only require 54 g.[2]

Protein Absorption

How able the patient is in absorbing proteins must also be considered. There are at least three factors to take into consideration: the quality of proteins in the diet, the quantity of proteins in the diet, and the ability of the gastrointestinal tract to break them down.

The densest and most absorbable source of proteins is in the form of meats. The ability of the gastrointestinal system to break down these proteins begins with the acidity of the stomach. If insufficient amount of hydrochloric acid (stomach acid) and digestive enzymes are produced, then hindrance of protein breakdown and absorption ensues. Second line interventional strategies include digestive aids to help the

gastrointestinal system enhance its function. Animal meats, if eaten alone, will create a more acidic blood pH. This acidity/alkalinity is a determinant factor in fighting the cancer cells *in vivo*. This acidic effect can be neutralized by eating vegetables with proteins. Vegetables, especially the leafy greens, are alkalizing to your blood pH. By combining proteins and vegetables, the blood pH becomes balanced in its acid/base.[6] Animal meats overall do have more arachadonic acid and fatty acids that can be proinflammatory overall, especially if the source is a factory farmed animal product. Wild red meats are leaner than poultry and some fish: deer, elk, bison, and even grass feed bovine can be beneficial lean red meats that should be eaten in a diet that is omnivorous and includes plant proteins, such as legumes, seeds and nuts.

Dietary Sources of Protein
- Lean proteins, such as are available in:
- Organic wild meats
- Seafood
- Legumes
- Egg
- Organic dairy products
- Nuts
- Seeds

Glycemic Index and Glycemic Load of Common Foods[8]

Glycemic Index High > 70 (poor) Low < 55 (good)	Common Food Item	Glycemic Load High > 20 (poor) Low < 10 (good)
75	Whole white wheat bread	7
35	Fresh bing cherries	8
86	Rice milk	29
37	Skim milk	4
24	Kidney beans	3
61	Honey	6
78	White potato	26
63	Sweet potato	11
36	Fresh apple	6
67	Millet	22
68	Brown rice	21

(Adapted from www.mendosa.com)

The Right Carbohydrate Diet

The description of a cancer cell as an "obligate glucose metabolizer" is not far from the truth. Several cancer cell lines have growth strategies that particularly use glucose as fuel for rapid cellular division. Therefore, not only consideration of the source of the simple carbohydrate but also how fast it metabolizes into glucose once inside of the body should be evaluated.

Carbohydrates are essential to the daily function of the body. They provide fuel for both the body and the brain. There are two basic types of carbohydrates, simple and complex. Complex carbohydrates include whole grains, fruits, and vegetables. Simple carbohydrates are also known as simple sugars and are found in processed foods, such as fruit juices, white processed flour products, and junk foods. Encouraging a diet high in complex carbohydrates and low in simple carbohydrates can be considered a first line strategy in preventing and actively fighting of cancer.

Glycemic Index and Glycemic Load

Glycemic index is a ranking system of carbohydrates based on how quickly they increase the body's blood glucose. A low glycemic index is a carbohydrate that breaks down slowly once ingested, and releases glucose at a slow rate into the blood stream. A high glycemic index is a carbohydrate that breaks down quickly once ingested, and releases glucose into the blood stream at a fast rate causing spikes and dips in the blood sugar response. Eating lower on the glycemic index helps to regulate the blood glucose level over time.

The glycemic index (GI) is a numerical system of measuring how much of a rise in circulating blood sugar a carbohydrate triggers – the higher the number, the greater the blood sugar response. So a low GI food will cause a small rise, while a high GI food will trigger a dramatic spike. A GI of 70 or more is high, a GI of 56 to 69 inclusive is medium, and a GI of 55 or less is low.[7]

The glycemic load (GL) is a relatively new way to assess the impact of carbohydrate consumption that takes the glycemic index into account, but gives a more comprehensive picture. A GI value tells you only how rapidly a particular carbohydrate turns into sugar. It doesn't tell you how much of that carbohydrate is in a serving of a particular food. You need to know both things to understand a food's effect on blood sugar. That is where glycemic load comes in. The carbohydrate in watermelon, for example, has a high GI. But there isn't a lot of it, so watermelon's glycemic load is relatively low. A GL of 20 or more is high, a GL of 11 to 19 inclusive is medium, and a GL of 10 or less is low. Foods that have a low GL almost always have a low GI. Foods with an intermediate or high GL range from very low to very high GI.[7-8]

Dietary recommendations of eating low on the glycemic index while maintaining a relatively low glycemic load (GL) can be met by eating a variety of whole grains, fruits, vegetables, and organic proteins. Low GI/GL choices help the body to feel full or satiated longer while prolonging physical endurance and refueling carbohydrate stores after exercise.

Tips for choosing low GI/GL foods are basic: choose whole grains, breads made from whole grains, sprouted grains and seeds, and cereals. Whole grains include the bran of oats, millet, barley, quinoa, buckwheat, triticale, spelt, kamut, and amaranth. Alternating these grains that are glutenous with non-glutenous grains also decreases the generation of an inflammatory response from the components of the whole cereals.

Encourage eating a variety of whole organic fruits and vegetables while reducing high GI/GL foods, such as white potatoes, in the diet. By adding vegetables and fruits with seeds and nuts a perfect snack of proteins, carbohydrates, and fats can be accomplished easily.

Using whole grains and alternating grains several times a week not only adds a complex carbohydrate that is generally low in glycemic index but also high in fiber content. Ways to use a variety of grains include creating pilafs by sautéing vegetables in a little olive oil (omega-9) and adding cooked grains and spice for flavoring or serving whole grains as a side dish with vegetables and fruit toppings. Combining legumes, meats, poultry, or fish with a whole grain to create an entrée or marinated grains added to tossed green salads are easy combinations that add complex carbohydrates to the diet. Using ground whole grains instead of processed flours in baked casseroles, stuffing, and soups is also an easy substitution that adds more nutritional content to the meal.[9]

Dietary Sources of Whole Grains
- Brown rice: non-glutenous grain that is much more nutritious than white rice stripped of its bran. The brown rice is high in germ, bran, B vitamins, minerals, and fiber.
- Amaranth: gluten-free whole grain that is high in protein and minerals. It can be also used as a wheat flour or cereal substitute.

- Barley: whole grain that can be used in soups and broths to give a high mineral content.
- Millet: low glutenous grain that is high in protein and minerals. It makes great hot cereal and can be added to granola or added to soups and homemade breads.
- Quinoa: gluten-free grain that has the highest protein content. It is also a good source of B vitamins and fiber. It is a great flour substitute and can also be used in place of rice or cracked wheat in tabouli.
- Spelt: ancient wheat with lower gluten but high in both fiber and proteins. Spelt breads are easily found as substitutes for white flour breads.
- Wheat: hard wheat is higher in protein but also in gluten, while sft wheat is usually refined white fours.
- Oats: whole (groats) or steel cut oats (oatmeal) are high in B vitamins, minerals, and fiber.

High-Fiber Diet

Fiber is extremely important in the diet and helps to prevent diseases as well as reduce risk for certain cancers. Some diseases, such as diabetes, heart disease, obesity, and cancer, have shown reduction in incidence of morbidity as well as mortality by increasing fiber content in the diet.

Fiber is generally divided into two categories, soluble and insoluble. Insoluble fiber is found in the bran of whole grains as well as in the form of cellulose from fruits and vegetables. The insoluble fiber content of a food affects the glycemic index by lowering the rate of glucose release into the blood stream.

Soluble fiber is commonly found in the whole grain itself or in fruit pectin. Oatmeal, psyllium seed, guar gum, and gum Arabic are all forms of soluble fiber. Fiber when consumed regularly decreases risk of certain cancers, such as colon cancer, as well as decreasing the risk of constipation and diarrhea in cancer treatment.[10] The average American consumes 10 to 15 grams of fiber daily, while the recommendation for a healthy diet is 25 to 35 grams daily.[11] This healthy dietary amount should include sources of fiber from both categories of soluble and insoluble fiber sources.

Dietary Sources of Fiber
- Legumes (the bean family): an excellent source of fiber and proteins. Soluble forms of legumes lower cholesterol as well as stabilize blood glucose.
- Whole fresh fruit: valuable soluble fiber know as pectin. Pectin is usually found in the skin and

pulp of the fruit. Figs, prunes, and raspberries have the highest fiber content.

- Whole green leafy vegetables: great sources of soluble and insoluble fiber as well as other micronutrients needed to fight cancer.
- Root vegetables: excellent sources of fiber and low glycemic index choices like sweet potatoes, turnips and yams can replace high glycemic potatoes.
- Cooked or stewed fruit: may be used instead of dried fruits, which have more associated preservatives and yeast growth.
- Whole grains: excellent sources of fiber as well as complex carbohydrates. By retaining its outer shell layer, the bran and germ are preserved, which are especially rich in the B vitamins.

The Right Fat Diet

Fats are an essential part to any diet, but there are some fats that are not. Saturated fats and trans fatty acids should be limited or avoided as much as possible in a cancer-fighting diet.

A fatty acid is an organic acid molecule consisting of a chain of carbon molecules and a carboxylic acid (COOH) group. Fatty acids are found in fats, oils, and as components of a number of essential lipids, such as phospholipids and triglycerides. Fatty acids can be burned by the body for energy.[12] Total daily dietary fat intake should be about 30% of calories ingested, with a daily fat intake for a 2,000 kcal diet being about 65 grams.[11]

Trans Fats

Trans fatty acids are created synthetically by heating unsaturated fats (like vegetable oils) in the presence of hydrogen. This is done to make the liquids solidify (as in margarine, for example), which in turn makes the oils more stable, enabling a longer shelf life with the trans fat. Foods made with these trans fats can remain as prepackaged processed foods on the shelves of consumers for extremely long periods before spoiling.

The issue with the trans fatty acid is not only the amount of saturation but the denaturing of the molecule that results from this saturation. The molecule of the fatty acid becomes more linear which then is less able to be metabolized by the body. These trans fats then can be incorporated into the cellular structure, like the cell membrane, and impede biological functions. This is the direct link between trans fatty acids and inflammatory reactions and cancer.

Trans fatty acids have been in the headlines with some cities, such as New York City, banning them from restaurant use in 2006.[13] As of January 1, 2006 food manufacturers were required to list both saturated and trans fat amounts on food labels. In reality, there will be a small remnant amount of trans fats found in any product that has been hydrogenated.[13]

Saturated Fats

Processed, prepared foods are higher not only in trans fats but also in saturated fats. Saturation refers to the number of hydrogen atoms linked to the carbon atom making a backbone of a fatty acid. The more hydrogen atoms attached to the bonds, the more saturated the fat. Monounsaturated fats have one double bond between carbons that makes one less hydrogen bond (hence the mono). Polyunsaturated fats have many double bond links between carbons, resulting in as few hydrogen atoms as possible.

Most vegetable oils are a combination of mono and polyunsaturated fats. Olive oil and canola (rapeseed) oil are monounsaturated fats, which makes them more stable with high heat applications. Thus, they are better cooking oils than the polyunsaturated vegetable oils, which can become damaged with high heat. The higher amount of polyunsaturated fats, the more damage by heat there can be, and the more formation of dangerous biocompounds that are considered procarcinogenic. Omega-3 and flax seed oils should never be heated because of this denaturing.[14]

Saturated fats are found in animal products, such as beef, chicken with skin, dairy products, shortening, fatty meats, and snack foods. Highly processed pre-prepared foods, such as prepackaged snack foods, are high in plant saturated fats, such as coconut, palm and palm kernel oils, as well as animal lards and shortening. These "bad" fats push the prostaglandin 2 series (PGE2), which is proinflammatory and associated with an increase risk of some cancers. These bad fats are also associated with increasing insulin resistance over time with long-term ingestion, causing dysglycemia, which is directly linked to cancer cell growth. Studies continue to show that diets high in saturated animal fats are directly linked to increased cancer risk.

Unsaturated Fats

Unsaturated fats are healthy fats that are needed for the body's proper function. Unsaturated fats include olive, corn, flax, hemp and canola (rapeseed) oils, nuts (almonds and walnuts), avocados, and soy oil products.

Encourage a diet high in unsaturated fats with adequate protein intake accompanied with plant carbohydrate and fiber for a balanced, glucose stabilizing diet. Small frequent meals five to six times per day, each including carbohydrate, fat and protein is the optimal strategy for the cancer fighting patient.[15]

Essential Fatty Acids

Essential fatty acids are the omega-3 and omega-6 series of fats. These are considered essential because they are needed for the body's daily function and cannot be made endogenously. Every living cell in the plant and animal kingdoms, down to phytoplankton and cyanobacteria, have the essential omega-3 oil in their structure.

Although humans and other mammals can synthesize saturated and some monounsaturated fatty acids from carbon groups in carbohydrate and protein, they lack the enzymes necessary to insert a cis double bond at the n-6 or the n-3 position of a fatty acid. Consequently, omega-6 and omega-3 fatty acids are essential nutrients. The parent fatty acid of the omega-6 series is linoleic acid (LA; 18:2n-6) and the parent fatty acid of the omega-3 series is alphalinolenic acid (ALA; 18:3n-3).[12]

Omega-3 and omega-6 fatty acids are considered polyunsaturated fatty acids (PUFAs) and can be found in fish, shellfish, flax and hemp seeds as well as sea vegetables.

These EFAs are linked directly to the two parent fatty acids, which also cannot be manufactured by the body: ALA and LA. From these two parent fatty acids the body can manufacture the other EFAs of the omega-3 and omega-6 series. Humans can synthesize long-chain (20 carbons or more) omega-6 fatty acids, such as dihomo-gamma-linolenic acid (DGLA; 20:3n-6) and arachidonic acid (AA; 20:4n-6) from LA and long-chain omega-3 fatty acids, such as eicosapentaenoic acid (EPA; 20:5n-3) and docosahexaenoic acid (DHA; 22:6n-3) from ALA.[12]

Essential fatty acids are needed for many metabolic, immunological, and hormonal functions in the body. These EFAs are present in every organ, tissue, and cell membrane for proper system function. Even though the body can synthesize all the other series 3 and 6 omega acids from the parent fatty acids, there is an associated metabolic cost. Also, the therapeutic doses required in cancer and chronic disease would be hard for this patient population to ingest from food sources, with most of plant and ocean sources containing highest levels of ALA with

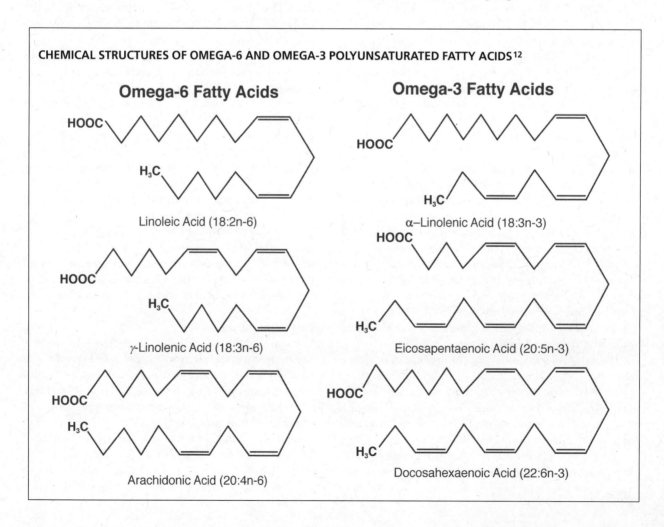

CHEMICAL STRUCTURES OF OMEGA-6 AND OMEGA-3 POLYUNSATURATED FATTY ACIDS[12]

Omega-6 Fatty Acids

Linoleic Acid (18:2n-6)

γ-Linolenic Acid (18:3n-6)

Arachidonic Acid (20:4n-6)

Omega-3 Fatty Acids

α–Linolenic Acid (18:3n-3)

Eicosapentaenoic Acid (20:5n-3)

Docosahexaenoic Acid (22:6n-3)

much reduced amounts of EPA/DHA. Therefore, it is considered an essential supplement in the fight against cancer to directly consume EPA and DHA daily.[16]

Omega-6 to Omega-3 Ratio

It has been estimated that the ratio of omega-6 to omega-3 fatty acids in the diet of early humans was 1:1, but the ratio in the typical Western diet is now almost 10:1 due to increased use of vegetable oils rich in LA and declining fish consumption. A large body of scientific research suggests that increasing the relative abundance of dietary omega-3 fatty acids may have a number of health benefits.[12]

Elevated intake of omega-6 series of EFAs can be considered a proinflammatory diet. Essential fatty acids are transformed into prostaglandins, which are regulatory compounds that regulate inflammation, pain, and edema and play a role in the regulation of blood pressure, blood clotting, heart, kidney, and digestive function. These prostaglandins are formed via the eicosanoid pathway.

Eicosinoids are chemical messengers derived from the PUFAs that play a critical role in immune function and inflammatory responses. During an inflammatory response DGLA, AAM, and EPA in cell membranes can be metabolized by the enzymes cyclooxygenase and lipoxygenase to form prostaglandins and leukotriene series. Western diets high in AA found in cell membranes result in the formation of more eicosanoids derived from the AA, which is more inflammatory by promoting prostaglandin series 2 formation. Diets higher in EPA, rather than AA, promote the formation of prostaglandin series 1 and 3, which are considered to be anti-inflammatory, less vasoconstrictive, and have less of a coagulation factor.[16]

Prostaglandins

Prostaglandins are participatory in response to allergens, production of steroids, and other hormones and help control nerve conduction and signal transduction. Prostaglandins derived from the omega-6 series of fatty acids also tend to stimulate cancer cell growth and promotion, while the omega-3 series inhibits cancer.[17]

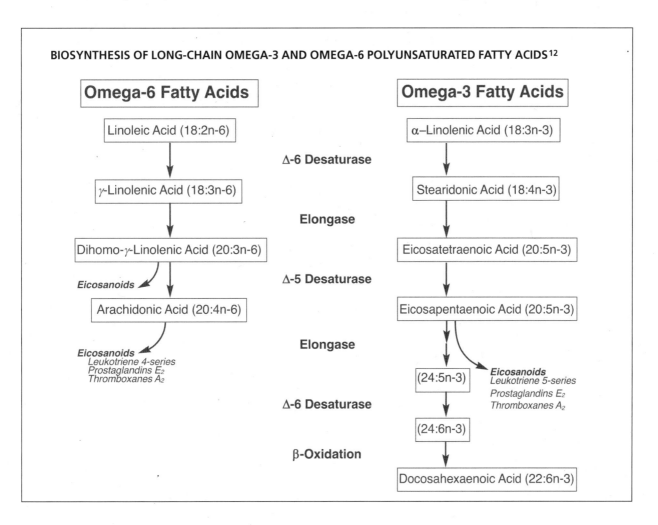

BIOSYNTHESIS OF LONG-CHAIN OMEGA-3 AND OMEGA-6 POLYUNSATURATED FATTY ACIDS[12]

Cell membranes are made up of mostly fatty acids arranged in a bi-phospholipid layer. The type of fat consumed can directly determine the type of fat found in the cell membrane. Hence the trans fat mutation that can be linked to protooncogene turn on, due to the alteration of the function of the cell membrane which leads to cell injury or death. Without this healthy cell membrane cells lose their ability to hold electrolytes, water and vital nutrients as well as their ability to communicate with one another. Also lost is the ability of the cell to be controlled by regulatory hormones, which in turn leads to the hyperplasia associated with cancer.[17]

Omega-3 and omega-6 EFAs are considered essential because the body needs a balance of both series in order to properly function. In the correct ratio of these omega oils it has been shown not only to aid in cancer prevention and cancer support but also psychoneuro-immuno-endocrine functions. Omega-3 series has been shown to improve the cardiovascular system, reduce hypertension, act as an anti-inflammatory, and improve rheumatoid arthritis and autoimmune disease, and even reduce depression. The improved immuno modulation and anti-inflammatory functions with omega-3 series can be thought of as anticarcinogenic in strategy or preventive.[16-17]

Sources of Omega-3 Series Fatty Acids
- Wild game: Deer, buffalo, elk, moose, and other small game are high in omega-3 fatty acids as well as lean and low in saturated fats. This is due to their natural lifestyle and diet.
- Marine sources: Salmon, halibut, tuna, cod, snapper are all cold water fish that are high in omega-3 oils naturally. It would be more preferable to eat smaller cold water fish, such as herring, sardines, mackerel, and flounder, due to the amount of tainted contaminates found in the fish secondarily from human waste and pollution of the oceans. Servings should be limited to two or three weekly because of toxicity issues with contaminates found in the marine foods.
- Plant sources: Walnuts, hemp seed, flax seed, leafy green vegetables, and rapeseed oil are excellent sources of omega-3 oil. The plant sources of omega-3 also yield a higher level of omega-6 oils, with hemp giving the highest plant source of omega-3 to 6 in ratio.
- Enhanced foods: Omega-3 enriched eggs, which are obtained by feeding the hens a diet rich in the essential fatty acid.
- Supplements: It is preferable to get the therapeutic doses of omega-3s needed to prevent and treat cancer integratively with supplements due to the high residues of PCBs, mercury, and other toxins found in our marine foods. This exposure is from human pollution that has compromised the marine ecology. Supplements should be assayed for these contaminants and be free of any form of toxins.

ANTICANCER FOODS

There are many preventive and anticancer agents found in whole foods. These constituents do not work alone, but work in synergy with each other within the perfect combination found in the whole food itself. We can isolate certain therapeutic constituents from plant sources and use them in a treatment regimen.

Synergism

Whole foods include anticancer modulators, such as beta-carotene, lycopene, retinols, lutein, and chlorophyll. More than 500 mixed carotenoids 600 bioflavonoids are found within the plant food itself. It has been shown that a small glass of orange juice taken daily, with only 37 mg of vitamin C, is twice as likely to lower the chances for stomach cancer than taking 1000 mg of vitamin C daily. There is something about the whole, freshly squeezed orange juice that is synergistically stronger than the individual parts.[18]

Part of this synergism is not only due the nutritional value of the food, but also due to its growth and vitality. Organic foods are more nutritious not only because they are nutrient dense, but because they do not have any pesticide or herbicide residue while being given healthy fertilizer to grow. This raises the vitality, or vibrational synergism of the plant, which affects the macrocosmic circle of life. The consumer's vitality thereby is affected by the vitality of the food consumed. Nature has spent tens of thousands of years perfecting the synergism and nutrition of the plants. These foods are only just beginning to be identied. The body's own defense mechanism is an immuno-surveillance team of over 20 trillion cells looking for antigens, including cancer cells. A diet with the proper amount of proteins, carbohydrates, essential fatty acids, and fiber provides the building blocks to keep the immune system at peak surveillance and its response accurate.

These super foods have a positive nutritional synergism that when taken in combinations augment the healing effect. Nutrient to nutrient combinations enhance the activity of each other, while nutrient to pharmaceutical combinations decrease medication side effects and in some cases even reverse chemo/radio cellular resistance.[19]

DIETARY SOURCES OF SUPER FOODS

Garlic: Stimulates the natural protection against cancer tumor cells. It is toxic to invading pathogens being not only antimicrobial but also anti-cancer in its activity toward cancer cells, while remaining harmless to healthy cells. Constituents of allinin, allicin, s-allyl cysteine, selenium bioflavonoids like quercitin may be components of how garlic can actually revert a cancer cell back to a healthy cell in vitro. Garlic also induces biotransformation of the cancer cell, thought to be an effect of selenium.[2,4-5,16-17]

Yogurt: Scientists have found that the active cultures of bacteria in yogurt actually enhance and fortify the immune system. Lactobacillus spp., the active culture in yogurt, was found to triple the body's own production of interferon, which is used by the immune system against cancer cells. Yogurt also has been shown to raise the endogenous levels of natural killer cells, enhancing cancer kill. Yogurt has been proven to slow down tumor growth and progression in the GI tract, while improving the immune system's ability to destroy cancer cells.[2,4-5,16-17]

Carotenoids: Plants with abundant colors are associated with high carotenoid levels and are full of bioflavonoids and carotenoids, which have been shown to function as anti-inflammatories, antioxidants, and detoxifying agents. They potentiate the immune system and there is some evidence that they are toxic to cancer cells. They inhibit tumor promotion by inhibiting covalent DNA binding, and induce biotransformation towards a healthy cell. Beets, carrots, tomatoes, spinach, squash, and other vegetables with vibrant, rich, deep colors are pigments that are phytochemicals. More than 800 carotenoids and 20,000 bioflavonoids act as immune stimulants, antioxidants that offer protection to healthy cells and cytotoxicity to cancer cells.[2-5,10,17]

Cruciferous vegetables: Broccoli, cabbage, brussel sprouts, cauliflower, all have an active ingredients called indoles that have been shown to be preventive against cancer. They act as detoxifying agents and help the body to increase its own production of important protective enzymes.[2,4-5,10,17]

Legumes: These seed foods have a unique ability to envelop tumor cells and prevent their growth. Soy, garbanzo, kidney, pinto, and other beans are rich in protease inhibitors like inositol hexaphosphate that are specific anti-cancer fighters. Geinstein has been shown to have an anti-angiogenic affectively stunting the creation of blood vessels from tumors. Legumes also are high in lignans, which aid in the body's own detoxification via promotion of methylation as well as aiding in dietary fiber content.[2,4-5,10,17]

Purple fruits: All of the fruits that have a red-blue (purple) color are high in antioxidants, ellagic acids and proanthocyanidins (pycnogenols), all classified as a larger group of plant pigments known as flavonoids. These phytochemicals function not only as antioxidants but also as multifunctional modulators of the detoxification system in the body. These phytonutrients can act on modulating specific phase I cytochrome P450s and phase II conjugases independently or simultaneously, to balance the detoxification function. These bioflavonoids can have chemoprotective effects, protecting against neoplastic, mutagenic, and other toxic effects when exposed to various carcinogens.[5,10,19,20]

In Dr Abram Hoffer's book *Healing Cancer*, coauthored with Linus Pauling, this concept of nutritional synergism is explained in detail.[20] The patient outcomes show not only improved survival statistics as determined by time (months to years past prognosis stats), but also an improved overall quality of life by those survivors.

How to Build a Meal

These guidelines can be used in counseling cancer patients on how to implement and maintain an anti-cancer macronutrient diet.

Most patients in active chemo/radio therapies can achieve their needed nutritional status by consuming 3 meals a day at approximately 75 grams of protein each, and 2-3 snacks, which would include the additionally needed 25 grams of protein. If this mark cannot be met by eating these meals, protein shakes can be used to help. These 'shakes' should be high in digestible proteins, complete with all essential amino acids and the protein source chosen to meet the specific indications of each patient's nutritional status, cancer diagnosis, and conventional treatment strategies. In addition, they should take in consideration the glycemic burden and be palatable![15-20]

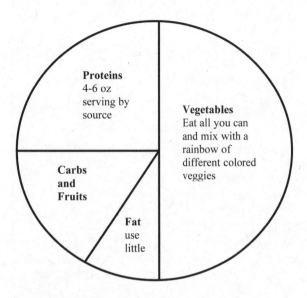

How many servings?
The daily diet should consist of the following amounts:
- Vegetables should be at least 5 and up to 10 servings a day (blended green drinks and juicing can help meet this quota)
- Proteins at least 3 servings a day
- Seeds, nuts, etc. should be around 4 servings a day
- Whole grains range from 3 to 6 servings a day
- Legumes can be protein supplements and should range from 2 to 3 servings a day
- Fruits range from 2 to 3 servings a day
- Dairy (always organic) should be limited to only 1 to 2 servings a day

What is a serving? Basic guidelines for the above recommendations:
- Vegetables are 1 cup of uncooked green leafy veggies, ½ cup of uncooked, non leafy veggies, ½ cup of cooked veggies or ½ cup of fresh veggie juice
- Proteins 4-6 oz depending on the source of the animal proteins, red meats are typically more dose dense per ounce in proteins, with wild meats being more dose dense while also lower in fats than poultry sources
- Seeds or nuts are ¼ cup per serving
- Whole grains range in serving size dependant on the grain itself, but typically a serving is equal to 1 slice of whole wheat or rye loaf bread, ½ cup of cooked whole grain cereal, ½ cup of whole grain pasta, 1 ear of corn
- Legumes typically are ½ cup per serving unless they are the only protein source for the meal, then serving size should be readjusted to fit the protein needs
- Fruits can be one medium sized fruit, ½ cup cut up fruit, 1 cup of purple berries, ¼ cup of dried fruit or 4 oz of fruit juice
- Dairy should always be organic and 1 cup of milk, yoghurt or cottage cheese is a serving size, or 1 ounce of hard cheese
- Oils should equate to about 1 tablespoon per serving

Hydration
Water essential to stay alive and needed to enable all cancer therapies. Proper hydration can aid in the detoxification of the byproducts of chemotherapies while aiding in the removal of other toxins and dead cells.

Approximately 65% of the human body is made up of water. Water is needed to transport oxygen and nutrients to the cells while eliminating cellular waste. Water is needed for proper digestion and absorption of food in order to maintain the muscles, organs, tissue and skin. Water is essential in the regulation of body temperature.[2,4,11,21]

Dehydration is a big concern with people who are going through chemo/radio therapies. Proper hydration becomes critical to this population, especially for patients experiencing any side effects of conventional treatment like diarrhea and vomiting. The long-term effect of dehydration leads to electrolyte imbalances, including sodium, potassium, and calcium, which are all important in keeping homeobalance within the system.

Signs of dehydration – dark-colored urine, dry skin and lips, and dizziness – should be monitored. Skin turgor can be monitored for preliminary signs of dehydration.[22]

The recommendation for cancer patients undergoing conventional treatments is a minimum of 6-8 glasses of filtered water daily. In addition, herbal teas should be 3-4 cups daily. This gives a total of 9-12 glasses of liquid taken in daily.[2,4,11,21]

Filtered water is recommended for the cancer patient undergoing conventional treatments in order to remove and reduce harmful contaminants found in our water supplies. Contaminants found in our water supplies include but are not limited to: Lead, chlorine, molds and algae, mercury, chlordane, pesticides, herbicides, chemocides, benzene, asbestos, carbon tetrachloride, tricholerthene, total trihalomethenes, various micro-organisms that create turbidity.

Immunotherapy
The source of caloric intake for the cancer patient will also influence the patient's inherent immune system. There is a complex array of substances in whole organic foods that act as biological response modifiers (BRMs). BRMs are substances that stimulate the

body's response to infection and disease. The body naturally produces small amounts of these substances. Scientists can produce some of them in the laboratory in large amounts for use in treating cancer, rheumatoid arthritis, and other diseases. Once study concludes, "We have seen a surge in the use of immunotherapy for the treatment of cancer. Biological response modifiers can act passively by enhancing the immunologic response to tumor cells or actively by altering the differentiation or growth of tumor cells. Active immunotherapy with cytokines, such as interferons (IFNs) and interleukins (IL-2), is a form of nonspecific active immune stimulation. The use of IL-2 has recently been approved by the United States Food and Drug Administration (FDA) for the treatment of renal cell carcinoma and metastatic colorectal cancer."[19]

BRM Strategies

Cancer affects critical biological responses that usually maintain homeo-balance. The integrative approach to cancer care is built on the foundation of a healthy diet, positive lifestyle, including spiritual and emotional health, and healthy daily hygienics (sleep, elimination, hygiene, exercise, meditation). The holistic principle that the whole is greater than the sum of its parts applies directly in the integrative approach to cancer treatment. The nature of cancer is to outgrow its boundaries and go beyond its original borders, so, too, must integrative approaches.

Integrative interventions

Integrative treatment aims to intervene in the development and growth of cancer cells, as well as in the promotion of tumor progression. This involves affecting immune function, gluccocorticoid pathways, hormonal status, inflammation, insulin resistance, allergies or atopy, digestion, and elimination: endopsychoimmuno therapies. To promote BRM activity and cancer immunity, consider these strategies:

Immunotherapies

Various medicinal herbs, nutraceuticals, and other supplements can be used to aid detoxification and support the immune system in preventing and treating cancer. If patients show signs of lowered immunity, consider these therapies to:

- Stimulate immunity: medicinal mushrooms, medicinal herbs, glandulars, homeopathics, nutraceuticals
- Alter genetic expression of cancer: vitamins D-3, C, E, B-12, folic acid, herbals

- Promote cell membrane fluid dynamics: calcium, magnesium, essential fatty acids (EFAs), omega-3 EFAs (EPA, DHA), CoQ10 enzyme, phosphatidylated amino acids (serine, inositol, choline, ethanolalamine), lecithin, evening primrose oil (EPO)
- Assist cellular Inter-Communication: vitamin A, retinoids, betacarotene, lycopene, herbs, glandulars, homeopathics, glycoproteins
- Balance Steroid Hormonal Influences: Indole-3-carbinol, Diim, lignans, kudzu, Omega 3 oils, bioflavonoids, EPO, herbals for detoxification, calcium-D-glucarate, glutathione
- Encourage Prostaglandin Synthesis: EPO, EFAs/EPA, vitamins A,C,E,D, herbal antiflammatories and Cox1&2 inhibitors, perilla seed, bioflavonoids, glycemic index
- Enhance Detoxification: herbals for specific pathway enhancement (garlic, milk thistle, grape seed, calcium-D-glucarate, glutathione, selenium, CoQ10, allinin/allicin, EDTA/DMSA)
- Provide Antioxidants: Endogenous vs. Exogenous: Endogenous vitamin A, C, D, E, alpha-lipoic acid, CoQ10, melatonin, selenium, glutathione. Exogenous EGCG (green tea), curcumin (tumeric), EPA, EPO, beta-carotene, lycopene, beta-sitosterols, ginkgo, quercitin, proanthocyanidins, resveratrol
- Activate anti-proliferative mechanisms: vitamins A, Bs, C, D, E, K, medicinal mushrooms, EPA/DHA, ginkgo, quercitin, curcumin, modified citrus pectin
- Alter Tumor Invisibility/Protection: modified citrus pectin, EGCG, herbals, medicinal mushrooms
- Bolster Energetic Dynamics: oxidative stress responders, adaptogens, chromium, GTF, CoQ10, thiamin, niacin, riboflavin, B-6, B-12, alpha lipoic acid, breathing techniques (Qi Kung, Prana Yama), spirituality/prayer

MICRONUTRIENT THERAPY

Macronutrients are not the only source of cancer-fighting agents in our food. Micronutrients, such as vitamins, minerals, amino acids, and enzymes, can also play a therapeutic role when given at high doses. Some of these micronutrients can be derived from food sources, but larger doses may need to be taken as a supplement. Cancer patients usually require a therapeutic dose of micronutrients, more than the disease prevention amounts recommended in food guides.

Phytochemicals

Phytochemicals include pycnogenol, resveratrol, limonene, beta-carotene, ubiquinone, indole-3-carbinol, ethnanolalamine, and ellagic acids. Phytochemicals are found in whole foods (fruits, grains, vegetables, herbs, and spices) influence cell-to-cell signaling.[23] This influence is crucial in maintaining healthy cellular function. When this cell-to-cell communication is lost, an aberrant cell can be formed. This progenitor cell then can lead to an offspring of progeny that becomes cancer.

However, once the aberrant cell has developed, these phytochemicals can disrupt cancer cell signaling, potentially stopping cell growth and causing apoptosis.[23] We must look for ways to increase these phytochemicals in the diet of cancer-fighting patients and supplement the diet if deficient. Many of the dietary strategies already discussed increase phytochemicals in the diet. To enhance the diet specifically to meet the patient's needs is the next line of nutritional intervention. By opening up the palate and creating a wide variety of choices from whole foods, herbs and spices with a variety of combinations enhances the phytochemical content in the diet. Eating more vegetables with a wide variety of colors at every serving and juicing upgrades the phytochemicals in the diet. Researchers at M.D. Anderson Cancer Center in Texas found that extensive research during the last half of the century has found multiple molecular targets where phytochemicals can be used not only for the prevention of cancer but also for treatment.[24]

ANTIOXIDANTS

Antioxidants are phytochemicals that work specifically to scavenge free radicals within the body. The natural processes of our physiological and biochemical functions create free radicals. Free radicals are dangerous, especially to mitochondria DNA and lipid-rich membranes that are predominant in the nervous system and the brain. Free radicals cause oxidative stress and have common targets for free radical damage: lipid cell membranes, cell receptor site complexes, enzymes, DNA, mitochondria, structural proteins, and the normal functions of viruses and bacteria. Free radicals can impact inflammation, xenotoxins, and stress.[25-28]

Primary and Secondary Antioxidants

Primary antioxidants include vitamins C and E, alpha lipoic acid, N-acetylcysteine, and any other compound whose primary therapeutic effect is to increase intracellular antioxidant stores.[29]

Secondary antioxidants include flavonoids and other plant constituents that have anticancer effects

Key properties of antioxidants
- The antioxidant system of the body relies on a complex interplay of many different dietary antioxidants.
- Taking any single antioxidant nutrient is not enough. Total protection requires a strategic, comprehensive supplement program.
- Although dietary supplements are important, they cannot replace the importance of consuming a diet rich in antioxidants.[25-28]

through mediated kinase inhibition or other nonantioxidant actions. Most phytochemicals have an antioxidant activity, which in turn protects our cells from oxidative stress, reducing the certain types of cancer. Phytochemicals, such as carotenoids, flavonoids, and polyphenols, all show this potent effect.[25-28]

Endogenous Antioxidants

These are antioxidants that are normally produced within the body's systems.[30]

Co-enzymeQ10 (ubiquinone): This enzyme is found in the mitochondrial membrane within a cell. CoQ10s activity in this membrane passes along electrons through an oxidation/reduction series, which at the end produces ATP and O_2 by splitting H_2O. These are the components of a cell required for cellular energy, repair, and rejuvenation.[31-33]

Alpha Lipoic Acid: This amino acid not only acts as an antioxidant but also enhances the effects of other antioxidants, for example, vitamins C and E.[34]

Folic Acid: This B vitamin has been shown to be involved in DNA repair after oxidative stress has damaged the DNA.[35]

Selenium: This mineral not only acts as an antioxidant but also promotes the body's own production of antioxidants.[36,37]

Melatonin: This endogenous hormone is secreted by the pineal gland and helps maintain the circadian sleep/wake cycle. When taken in higher than physiological doses, it acts as an antioxidant.[39-45]

L-Carnitine: This amino acid is synthesized in the liver, skeletal, and heart muscle and is essential for energy production and fat metabolism. It works to suppress oxidative damage in the brain, heart, skeletal muscle, and liver.[46]

Food sources of phytochemicals

Phytochemicals	Food Source	Anticancer Benefit
Vitamins		
Vitamin A Carotenoids (Beta-carotene)	Carrots, peppers, mangoes, apricots, tomato, red peppers	Antioxidant, immune stimulant, cancer prevention, induce cell differentiation, inhibit tumor growth[47-49]
Vitamin C	Peppers, broccoli, strawberries, etc.	Antioxidant, immune stimulant and modulator, anticancer strategy, stabilize p53[50-52]
Vitamin D	Dark green leafy veggies, cold water fish, dairy	Antioxidant, antiproliferation, immune modulator[53,54]
Vitamin E	Whole grains, nuts, and seeds	Antioxidant, inhibits tumor growth and progression, induce apoptosis[55-57]
Folic acid, lectins	Legumes, nuts, seeds, asparagus and spinach	Immune stimulant and modulator, antioxidant[58]
Minerals		
Calcium	Dairy, almonds, watercress, sea vegetables, bone broth, sesame seeds	Some cancers indicated for cancer prevention increase tumor kill[59]
Magnesium	Bran, whole grains, nuts, figs and tofu	Essential electrolyte for chemo/radio prevention[60]
Potassium	Oranges, potatoes, bananas, lima beans, avacados	Essential electrolyte for chemo/radio prevention pre and post treatment[61]
Selenium	Brazil nuts, whole grains, orange juice, pumpkin seeds	Antioxidant, apoptotic, chemopreventative[36,37]
Zinc	Oysters, pumpkin seeds, pecans, ginger root	Antioxidant, apoptotic, chemopreventative[38,62]
Botanicals		
Flavonoids	Multi-colored fruits and veggies	Anti-inflammatory, antioxidant, apoptotic, immune enhancing[63-64]
Dialyl sulfide, S-allyl cysteine, allicin and allinin	Garlic and onions	Immune stimulant, antioxidant, enhance detoxification[65-69]
Lycopene	Tomato, red peppers	Antioxidant, immune stimulant, chemopreventive, slows tumor progression[70-72]
Indoles (Indole-3-carbinol), Isthiocynanate	Cruciferous vegetables: broccoli, cabbage, cauliflower	Binds tumor promoting hormones for excretion, inhibits cancer growth[73]
Beta-Glucan	Medicinal mushrooms	Immune stimulator[73-76]

Phytochemicals	Food Source	Anticancer Benefit
Ace and Beta Mannan	*Aloe vera* juice	Immunostimulatory, increases wound healing and recovery[77-78]
Polyphenols, Ellagic acid, resveratrol	Blueberries, blackberries, strawberries, grapes, pomegranate, purple fruits	Antioxidant, immune stimulant, aids in liver detox, apoptosis[79]
Proanthocyanidines (proanthocyanidolic oligomers), resveratrol	Grape seed, red wine, pine bark	Immune stimulant, apoptosis, antioxidant, slows tumor progression[80]
Polyphenols (ECGC) and catechins	Green Tea	Antioxidant, apoptosis, slows tumor growth, inhibits cancer[81-86] EGFR receptors modulator
Proteolytic enzymes	Pineapple, kiwi, papaya	Stimulate immune system and help to break up complexes, inhibit tumor growth and progression[87]
Cinnamic acid	Cinnamon	COX-2 inhibitor, inhibits cancer growth[88]
Gingerol, gingerenone	Ginger	Reduces chemo/radio associated nausea, improves digestion, immune stimulant and anti-inflammatory[89] COX-2 inhibitor
Capsaicin	Hot red peppers	Inhibits metastasis, immune stimulant, inhibits clot formation[90]
D-Limonene, citrus pectin, bioflavonoids	Citrus fruit (orange, lemon, lime)	Inhibits metastasis, immune stimulant, antioxidant[91]
Curcumin	Tumeric	Antioxidant, anti-inflammatory, inhibits metastasis, chemopreventative[92-98]
Genistein, daidzein, isoflavonoids, phytosterols, protease inhibitors, lectins	Soybean	Chemopreventive for some cancers, inhibits cancer growth and promotion, enhances detoxification, hormone blockade for some cancers[99-104]
Chlorophyllin, glutathione	Collards, spinach, kale and greens	Antioxidant, immune stimulatory, enhances liver detoxification[105]
Eugenol	Cloves	Antioxidant, immune stimulant, antimicrobial[106-107]
Silymarin, silybum	Milk thistle	Inhibit cancer cell growth, antioxidant, enhances liver detoxification, COX-2 inhibitor[108-110]
Ursolic acid	Apples, pears, prunes	Antioxidant, immune stimulant, apoptotic[111]
Diosgenin	Wild yam, fenugreek	Antioxidant, apoptotic[112]
Lignins, alpha linolenic acid	Flax seed (meal)	Anti-inflammatory, immune stimulant, binds excess estrogens and aids in detoxification; anti-estrogen[113]

Exogenous Antioxidants

These are antioxidants that are not normally produced within the body's systems. According to Dr Abram Hoffer, "Human beings, cows, horses, mice, rats, guinea pigs, and all other mammals (also fish and reptiles) all require vitamin A, vitamin B-1, and vitamin C. These species have lost the ability to make these vitamins themselves, even though their ancestors likely could by eating plants, which manufacture all of these substances, and hence derive from their food enough vitamins to satisfy their needs to the extent sufficient to keep them alive long enough to have progeny, without the need for them to use energy and materials to make additional amounts of these substances. Only a few species of animal have lost this ability." Vitamins A, B, and C are considered exogenous antioxidants because as a human species we cannot manufacture or extract enough optimally from the foods we eat.[20]

EGCG (epigallocatechin gallate): This flavonoid is found in *Camelia sinensis* (green tea) and acts not only as an antioxidant but also promotes apoptosis in cancer cells.[81-86]

Curcumin (tumeric): This medicinal and culinary herb, found in the plant *Curcuma longa* and other species, reduces lipid peroxidation caused from free radicals.[92-98]

***Coriolus versicolor* (turkey tails):** This medicinal mushrooms polysaccharides fractions that act as antioxidants towards specific cancer growth.[114]

Calcium-D-Glucarate: This calcium salt, found in many fruits and vegetables, inhibits beta-glucoronidase, and elevated beta-glucoronidase activity is associated with an increased risk for hormone dependent cancers.[115]

Indole-3-carbinol: This is the main metabolite of diindoylmethane and stimulates the production of detoxifying enzymes. It works as a strong antioxidant, protecting DNA and enhancing repair of cell structures.[73]

DIM (diindolylmethane): is a natural compound formed during the breakdown of glucobrassicin present in the Brassica genus of plants (cabbage, broccoli, brussel sprouts, cauliflower and kale). Indole-3 carbinol is a immediate precursor of DIM.[116]

Vitamin A: This vitamin functions metabolically to affect vision, gene transcription, immune function, embryonic development, reproduction, bone metabolism, skin health, and antioxidant activity.[47-49]

Vitamin C: This vitamin protects against oxidative damage, but it is a water soluble vitamin, which in high doses can cause bowel irritation. It may be used intravenously to reach the high doses needed to treat certain disease processes.[50-52]

Vitamin E: This vitamin has been shown to inhibit the COX-2 pathway of inflammation, and also affects precursory pathways prior to the expression of COX-2. It is a fat soluble vitamin, so oral administration is adequate, although it can effect platelet aggregation in high doses.[55-57]

References

1. www.usda.gov/wps/portal/usda/usdahome?navid=ORGANIC

2. Alshuler L, Gazella KA. Definitive Guide to Cancer. 2nd Ed. Berkley, CA: Celestial Arts, Ten Speed Press; 2007:522.

3. Noe, JE. L-glutamine use in the treatment and prevention of mucositis and cachexia: a naturopathic perspective. Integr Cancer Ther. 2009;8:409-15.

4. Murray M, Birdsall T, Pizzorno J. How to Prevent and Treat Cancer with Natural Medicine. New York, NY: Riverhead Books, Penguin/Putnam; 2002:409.

5. http://www.brighthub.com/science/medical/articles/6050.aspx

6. www.edgarcayce.org/are/holistic_health/data/reaba11.html Foster-Powell K, Holt S, Brand-Miller, J. International table of glycemic index and glycemic load values: American Journal of Clinical Nutrition. 2002;76(1):5-56.

8. www.mendosa.com

9. Donaldson M. Nutrition and cancer: a review of the evidence for an anti-cancer diet. Nutrition Journal. 2004;3:19.

10. Thompson HJ, et al. Effect of increased vegetable and fruit consumption on markers of oxidative cellular damage. Carcinogenesis 199;20(12):2261-66.

11. Dietary Guidelines for Americans. 2008. http://www.healthierus.gov/dietaryguidelines

12. Oregon State University Linus Pauling Institute online: http://lpi.oregonstate.edu/infocenter/othernuts/omega3fa/index.html

13. Jones C, Hellmich N. 2006. NYC bans trans fats in restaurants. USAToday.com. Available at http://www.usatoday.com/news/health/2006-12-04-trans-fat-ban

14. Colomer R, Menendez JA. Mediterranean diet, olive oil and cancer. Clinical and Transitional Oncology 2006;8(1):15-21.

15. National Cancer Institute. 2008. Nutrition in Cancer care. http://www.cancer.gov/cancertopics/pdq/supportivecare/nutrition

16. MacLean H, et al. Effects of omega-3 fatty acids on cancer risk: a systematic review. Journal of the American Medical Association 2006;295(16):403-15.

17. Jones DS (ed). Textbook of Functional Medicine. Gig Harbor, WA: Institute of Functional Medicine;2006.

18. Eaton SB, et al. Paleolithic Prescription. New York, NY:Harper & Row;1988.

19. Purabi R, Gupta G, Kohli K. Biological response modifiers in cancer. From Medscape General Medicine:MedGenMed Hematology-Oncology - Clinical Review. Posted 11/14/2006

20. Hoffer A, Pauling L. Healing Cancer: Complementary Vitamin & Drug Treatments. Toronto, ON:CCNM Press;2004.

21. U.S. Department of Agriculture. Anatomy of My Pyramid. http://www.mypyramid.gov/professionals/pdf_anatomy.html

22. MedicineNet.Com

23. Cole WC, Prasad KN. Contrasting effects of vitamins as modulators of apoptosis in cancer cells and normal cells: a review. Nutr. Ca. 1997:29(2);97-103.

24. Bharat B, et al. Potential of Spice-Derived Phytochemicals for Cancer Prevention. pdf publication. Affiliation Cytokine Research Laboratory, Department of Experimental Therapeutics, The University of Texas M. D. Anderson Cancer Center, Houston, TX;2008.

25. Bagchi K and Puri S. Free Radicals and antioxidants in health and disease. Eastern Mediterranean Health Journal. 1998;4(2):350-60.

26. Belkacémi Y, Touboul E, Méric JB, Rat P, Warnet JM. Radiation-induced cataract: physiopathologic, radiobiologic and clinical aspects. Cancer Radiother. 2001 Aug;5(4):397-412.

27. Weiss JF, Landauer MR.Radioprotection by antioxidants.Ann N Y Acad Sci. 2000;899:44-60.

28. Lamson DW, Brignall MS. Antioxidants and cancer therapy II: quick reference guide. Altern Med Rev. 2000 Apr;5(2):152-63.

29. Donnerstag B, Ohlenschläger G, et al. L- glutathione and S-acetylglutathione as selective apoptosis-inducing agents in cancer therapy. Institute for Medical Virology, Johann Wolfgang Goethe University Hospital, Frankfurt, Germany; Elsevier. Cancer Letters 1996;110:63-70.

30. Kamat JP, Devasagayam TPA, Priyadarsini KI, Mohan H. Reactive oxygen species mediated membrane damage induced by fullerene derivatives and its possible biological implications. Toxicology. 2000;155:55-61.

31. Okada K, Yamada S, Kawashima Y, et al. Cell injury by antineoplastic agents and influence of coenzyme Q10 on cellular potassium activity and potential difference across the membrane in rat liver cells. Cancer Res. 1980 May;40(5):1663-67.

32. Folkers K, Brown R, Judy WV, Morita M. Survival of cancer patients on therapy with coenzyme Q10. Biochem Biophys Res Commun. 1993 Apr 15;192(1):241-45.

33. Folkers K, Osterborg A, Nylander M, Morita M, Mellstedt H. Activities of vitamin Q10 in animal models and a serious deficiency in patients with cancer. Biochem Biophys Res Commun. 1997 May 19;234(2):296-99.

34. Packer L, Witt EH, Tritschler HJ. Alpha-lipoic acid as a biological antioxidant. Free Radic Biol Med. 1995 Aug;19(2):227-50.

35. Kruman I, Kumaravel TS, Lohani A, Pedersen WA, Cutler RG, Kruman Y, Haughey N, Lee J, Evan M, Mattson M. Folic acid deficiency and homocystenine impair DNA repair in hippocampal neurons and sensitize them to amyloid toxicity in experimental models of Alzheimer's disease. The Journal of Neroscience 2002 Mar 1, 22(5):1752-62.

36. Rao L, Pusehner B, Prolla TA. Gene expression profiling of low selenium status in the mouse intestine: transcriptional activation of genes linked to DNA damage, cell cycle control and oxidative stress. J Nutr . 2001;131:3175-81.

37. Büntzel J. [Experiences with sodium selenite in treatment of acute and late adverse effects of radiochemotherapy of head-neck carcinomas. Cytoprotection working group in AK supportive measures in oncology within the scope of MASCC and DKG] [Article in German] Med Klin (Munich). 1999 Oct 15;94 Suppl 3:49-53.

38. Nagler RM, et al. Redox metal chelation ameliorates radiation-induced bone marrow toxicity in a mouse model. Radiation Research. August 2001;156(2):205-09.

39. Lissoni P, Barni S, Meregalli S, Fossati V, Cazzaniga M, Esposti D, Tancini G. Modulation of cancer endocrine therapy by melatonin: a phase II study of tamoxifen plus melatonin in metastatic breast cancer patients progressing under tamoxifen alone. Br J Cancer. 1995 Apr;71(4):854-56.

40. Lissoni, P, Barni, Cazzaniga M, ARdizzoia A, Rovelli F, Brivio F, Tancini G. Efficacy of the concomitant administration of the pineal hormone melatonin in cancer immunotherapy with low doses of IL-2 in patients with advanced solid tumors who had progressed on IL-2 alone. Oncology. 1994 Jul-Aug;51(4):344-47.

41. Lissoni P, Cazzanga M, Tancini G, et al. Reversal of clinical resistance to LHRH analogue in metastatic prostate cancer by the pineal hormone melatonin: efficacy of LHRH analogue plus melatonin in patients progressing on LHRH analogue alone. Eur Urol 1997;31:17881.

42. Steinhilber D, Brungs M, et al. No title. J. Biol. Chem. 1995;270:7037-40.

43. Neri B, De Leonardis V, Gemelli MT, et al. Melatonin as biological response modifier in cancer patients. Anticancer Res 1998;18:132932.

44. Lissoni P, Brivio O, Brivio F, et al. Adjuvant therapy with the pineal hormone melatonin in patients with lymph node

relapse due to malignant melanoma. J Pineal Res. 1996;21:23942.

45. Lissoni P. Is there a role for melatonin in supportive care? Support Care Cancer. 2002 Mar;10(2):110-16.

46. Neri B, Neri GC, Bandinelli M. Differences between carnitine derivatives and coenzyme Q10 in preventing in vitro doxorubicin-related cardiac damages. Oncology. 1988;45(3):242-46.

47. Prasad KN, Edwards-Prasad J, Kumar S, Meyers A. Vitamins regulate gene expression and induce differentiation and growth inhibition in cancer cells their relevance in cancer prevention. Arch Otolaryngol Head Neck Surg. 1993;119(10):1133-40.

48. Gundimeda U, Hara S, Anderson WB, Gopalakrishnakone R. Retinoids inhibit the oxidation modification of protein kinase C induced by oxidant tumor promoters. Arch Biochem Biophys 1993;300:576-630.

49. Ehrenpreis ED, Jani A, Levitsky J, Ahn J, Hong J. A prospective, randomized, double-blind, placebo-controlled trial of retinol palmitate (vitamin A) for symptomatic chronic radiation proctopathy. Dis Colon Rectum. 2005 Jan;48(1):1-8.

50. Elsendoorn TJ, et al. Chemotherapy-induced chromosomal damage in peripheral blood lymphocytes of cancer patients supplemented with antioxidants or placebo. Mutation Research/Genetic Toxicology and Environmental Mutagenesis. 2001 Nov;498(15):145-58.

51. Gundimeda U, Hara S, Anderson WB, Gopalakrishnakone R. Retinoids inhibit the oxidation modification of protein kinase C induced by oxidant tumor promoters. Arch Biochem Biophys 1993;300:576-630.

52. G. Muralikrishnan, V. Amalan Stanley, K. Sadasivan Pillai. Dual role of vitamin C on lipid profile and combined application of cyclophosphamide, methotrexate and 5-fluorouracil treatment in fibrosarcoma-bearing rats. Cancer Letters. 2001 Aug;169(2):115-20.

53. Dalhoff K, Dancey J, et al. A phase II study of the vitamin D analogue Seocalcitol in patients with inoperable hepatocellular carcinoma. Br J Cancer. 2003 Jul 21;89(2):252-57.

54. Holt PR, Arber N, Halmos B, et al. Colonic epithelial cell proliferation decreases with increasing levels of serum 25-hydroxy vitamin D. Cancer Epidemiol Biomarkers Prev. 2002 Jan;11(1):113-19.

55. Neuzil N, et al. Induction of cancer cell apoptosis by-tocopheryl succinate: molecular pathways and structural requirements. The FASEB Journal. 2001;15:403-15.

56. Rose AT, McFadden DW. Alpha-tocopherol succinate inhibits growth of gastric cancer cells in vitro. J Surg Res. 2001 Jan;95(1):19-22.

57. Mutlu-Türko_lu U, Erbil Y, Oztezcan S, Olgaç V, Toker G, Uysal M. The effect of selenium and/or vitamin E treatments on radiation-induced intestinal injury in rats. Life Sci. 2000 Apr 7;66(20):1905-13.

58. Branda RF, Nigels E, Lafayette AR, Hacker M.Nutritional folate status influences the efficacy and toxicity of chemotherapy in rats. Blood. 1998 Oct 1;92(7):2471-76.

59. Wu K, Willett WC, Fuchs CS, Colditz GA, Giovannucci EL. Calcium intake and risk of colon cancer in women and men. Journal of the National Cancer Institute 2002; 94(6):437-46.

60. www.cancer.org/Cancer/ColonandRectum-Cancer/.../colorectal-cancer

61. www.cancer.org/Treatment/TreatmentsandSideEffects/.../potassium

62. Cai L, Cherian MG, Iskander S, et al. Metallothionein induction in human CNS in vitro: neuroprotection from ionizing radiation. Int J Radiat Biol. 2000 Jul;76(7):1009-17.

63. Hofmann J, Fiebig HH, Winterhalter BR, Berger DP, Grunicke H. Enhancement of the antiproliferative activity of cis-diamminedichloroplatinum (II) by quercetin. Int J Cancer. 1990;45(3):536-39.

64. Pan X, Wang, H, and Lee RJ. Boron delivery to a murine lung carcinoma using folate receptor-targeted liposomes. Anticancer Res. 2002;22:1629-33.

65. Dorant E, van den Brandt PA, Goldbohm RA. Allium vegetable consumption, garlic supplement intake, and female breast carcinoma incidence. Breast Cancer Res Treat. 1995;33:163-70.

66. Van er Logt EMJ, Roelofs HMJ, Nagengast FM, Peters WHM. bgg117Induction of rat hepatic and intestinal UDP-glucuronosyltransferases by naturally occurring dietary anticarcinogens. Carcinogenesis 2003;24(10):1651-56.

67. De S, Chakraborty RN, Ghosh S, Sengupta A, Das S. Comparative evaluation of cancer chemopreventive efficacy of alpha-tocopherol and quercetin in a murine model. J Exp Clin Cancer Res. 2004 Jun;23(2):251-58.

68. Knowles LM, Milner JA. Diallyl disulfide induces ERK phosphorylation and alters gene expression profiles in human colon tumor cells. J Nutr. 2003;133(9):2901-06.

69. Broekmans WMR, Klopping-Ketelaars IAA, Schuuman CRWC, Verhagen H, van den Berg H, Kok FJ, van Poppel G. Fruits and vegetables increase plasma carotenoids and vitamins and decrease homocysteine in humans. J Nutr. 2000;130:1578-83.

70. Saada HN, Azab KS. Role of lycopene in recovery of radiation injury to mammalian cellular organelles. Pharmazie. 2001 Mar;56(3):239-41.

71. Cole, W.C., Prasad, K.N. Contrasting effects of vitamins as modulators of apoptosis in cancer cells and normal cells: a review. Nutr. Cancer. 1997;29: 97 103.

72. Yan, et al. No Title. Mol. Cell. Biol. 1993;13:4513-22.

73. Auborn KJ, Saijun F, Rosen EM, Goodwin L, Chandraskaren A, Williams D, Chen DZ, Carter TH. Indole-3-Carbinol is a negative regulator of estrogen. J. Nutr. 133:2470S-2475S; July 2003 Supplement: Nutritional genomics and proteomics in cancer prevention.

74. Taguchi T, Furue H, Kimura T, Kondo T, Hattori T, Ito I, et al. End-point results of Phase III study of Lentinan. Gan To Kagaku Ryoho. 1985;12:366-80.

75. Jiang J, Slivova V, Valachovicova T, Harvey K, Sliva D. Ganoderma lucidum inhibits proliferation and induces apoptosis in human prostate cancer cells PC-3 International Journal of Oncology.2004;24:1093-99.

76. Liu WK, Ng TB, Sze SF, Tsui KW. Activation of peritoneal macrophages by polysaccharopeptide from the mushroom Coriolus versicolor. Immunopharmacology. 1993;26:139-46.

77. Gribel NV, Pashinski VG. Antimetastatic properties of aloe juice.Vopr Onkol. 1986;32(12):38-40.

78. Su CK, Mehta V, Ravikumar L, Shah R, Pinto H, Halpern J, Koong A, Goffinet D, Le QT. Phase II double-blind randomized study comparing oral aloe vera versus placebo to prevent radiation-related mucositis in patients with head-and-neck neoplasms.Int J Radiat Oncol Biol Phys. 2004 Sep 1;60(1):171-77.

79. Jang, M. and Pezzuto, J.M. Resveratrol blocks eicosanoid production and chemically-induced cellular transformation: implications for cancer chemoprevention. Pharm. Biol. 1998;36:28-34.

80. Nadakumar V, Singh T, Katiyar SK. Multi-targeted prevention and therapy of cancer by proanthocyanidins. Cancer Lett. 2008 October 8; 269(2): 378-87. Published online 2008 May 23.

81. Kuroda Y, Hara Y. Antimutagenic and anticarcinogenic activity of tea polyphenols. Mutat. Res. 1999;436:69-97.

82. Weisburger JH, Hara Y, Dolan L, Luo F-Q, Pittman B, Zang E. Tea polyphenols as inhibitors of mutagenicity of major classes of carcinogens. Mutation Res. 1996;371:57-63.

83. Ebata J, Fukagai N, Furukawa H. Mechanisms of antimutagenesis by catechins towards N-nitrosodimethylamine. Environ Mutagen Res. 1998;20:45-50.

84. Klaunig JE, Xu Y, Han C, et al. the effect of tea consumption on oxidative stress in smokers and nonsmokers. Proc Soc Exp Biol Med. 1999;220:249-54.

85. Seely D, Mills EJ, Wu P, Verma S, Guyatt GH. The effects of green tea consumption on incidence of breast cancer and recurrence of breast cancer: a systematic review and meta-analysis. Integra Cancer Ther. 2005;4:144-55.

86. Lin JK, Liang YC, Lin-Shiau SY. Cancer Chemoprevention by tea polyphenols through mitotic signal transduction blockade. Biochem. Pharmacol. 1999;58:911-15.

87. Dale PS, Tamhankar CP, George D, Daftary GV. Co-medication with hydrolytic enzymes in radiation therapy of uterine cervix: evidence of the reduction of acute side effects. Cancer Chemother Pharmacol. 2001 Jul;47 Suppl:S29-34.

88. Kwon HK, Hwang JS, So JS, Lee CG, Sahoo A, Ryu JH, Jeon WK, Ko BS, Im CR, Lee SH, Park ZY, Im SH. Cinnamon extract induces tumor cell death through inhibition of NFkappaB and AP1.BMC. Cancer. 2010 Jul 24;10:392.

89. Frondoza CG, Sohrabi A, Polotsky A, Phan PV, Hungerford DS, Lindmark L. An in vitro screening assay for inhibitors of proinflammatory mediators in herbal extracts using human synoviocyte cultures. In Vitro Cell Dev Biol Anim. 2004;40:95-101.

90. Min JK, Han KY, Kim EC, et al. Capasaicin Inhibits in Vitro and in Vivo Angiogenesis. Cancer Res 2004;64:644-651. Published online January 26, 2004.

91. Lu XG, Zhan LB, Feng BA, Qu MY, Yu LH, Xie JH. Inhibition of growth and metastasis of human gastric cancer implanted in nude mice by d-limonene.World J Gastroenterol. 2004 Jul 15;10(14):2140-44.

92. Dinkova-Kostova A, Paul Talalay P.. Relation of structure of curcumin analogs to their potencies as inducers of Phase 2 detoxification enzymes. Carcinogenesis. 1999; 20(5): 911-14.

93. Radhakrishna Pillai G, Srivastava AS, Hassanein TI, Chauhan DP, Carrier E. Induction of apoptosis in human lung cancer cells by curcumin. Cancer Lett. 2004;208:163-170.

94. Chendil, D., Ranga, RS, Meigooni D, Sathishkumar S, Ahmed MM. 2004. Curcumin confers radiosensitizing effect in prostate cancer cell line PC-3. Oncogene Feb.26;23(8):1599-607

95. Adams BK, Cai J, Armstrong J, et al. EF24, a novel synthetic curcumin analog, induces apoptosis in cancer cells via a redox-dependent mechanism. Anticancer Drugs. 2005 Mar;16(3):263-75.

96. Karunagaran D, Rashmi R, Kumar TR. 2005. Curr Cancer Drug Targets. Mar; 5(2):117-29.

97. Manson MM, Farmer PB, Gescher A, Steward WP. Innovative agents in cancer prevention. Recent Results Cancer Res. 2005;166:257-75.

98. Corpet DE, Pierre F. Point: From animal models to prevention of colon cancer. Systematic review of chemoprevention in min mice and choice of the model system. Cancer Epidemiol Biomarkers Prev. 2003 May;12(5):391-400.

99. Bemis DL, Capodice JL, Desai M, Buttyan R, Katz AE. A concentrated aglycone isoflavone preparation (GCP) that demonstrates potent anti-prostate cancer activity in vitro and in vivo. Clin Cancer Res. 2004 Aug 1;10(15):5282-92.

100. Kumar NB. The Specific Role of Isoflavones in Reducing Prostate Cancer Risk. H. Lee Moffitt Cancer Center and Res. Inst., Tampa, Fl;2004.

101. Maggiolini M, Bonofiglio D, Marsico S, Panno ML, Cenni B, Picard D, Ando S. Estrogen receptor alpha mediates the proliferative but not the cytotoxic dose dependant effects of two majo phytoestrogens on human breast cancer cells. Mol Pharmacol. 2001 Sep;60(3):595-602.

102. Jones JL, Daley BJ, Enderson BL, Zhou JR, Karlstad MD. 2002. Genistein inhibits tamoxifen effects on cell proliferation and cell cycle arrest in T47D breast cancer cells. Am Surg. Jun;68(6):575-7; discussion 577-78.

103. Sarkar FH, Li Y. Soy isoflavones and cancer prevention. Cancer Invest. 2003;21(5):744-57.

104. Upadhyay S, Neburi M, Chinni SR, et al. Differential sensitivity of normal and malignant breast epithelial cells to genistein is partly mediated by p21(WAF1). Clin Cancer Res 2001;7:1782-89.

105. Singh A, Singh S, Bamezai R. Molecular epidemiology and cancer prevention: modulatory influence of chlorophyllin on the mouse skin papillomagenesis and xenobiotic detoxification system. Carcinogenesis.1996;17 (7): 1459-63.

106. Banerjee S, Panda CK, Das S. Clove (Syzygium aromaticum L.), a potential chemopreventive agent for lung cancer. Carcinogenesis. 2006;27(8): 1645-54.

107. Bat-Chen W, Golan T, Peri I, Ludmer Z, Schwartz B. Allicin purified from fresh garlic cloves induces apoptosis in colon cancer cells via Nrf2. Nutr Cancer. 2010;62(7):947-57.

108. Scambia G, De Vincenzo R, Ranelletti FO, Panici PB, Ferrandina G, D'Agostino G, Fattorossi A, Bombardelli E, Mancuso S. Antiproliferative effect of silybin on gynaecological malignancies: synergism with cisplatin and doxorubicin Eur J Cancer. 1996 May;32A(5):877-82 (Cell Culture Study).

109. Bokemeyer C, Fels LM, Dunn T, Voigt W, Gaedeke J, Schmoll HJ, Stolte H, Lentzen H. Silibinin protects against cisplatin-induced nephrotoxicity without compromising cisplatin or ifosfamide anti-tumour activity.Br J Cancer. 1996 Dec;74(12):2036-41.

110. Tyagi A Silibinin causes cell cycle arrest and apoptosis in human bladder transitional cell carcinoma cells by regulating CDKI-CDK-cyclin cascade, and caspase 3 and PARP cleavages. Carcinogenesis. 2004 Sep;25(9):1711-20. Epub 2004.

111. Shan JZ, Xuan YY, Zheng S, Dong Q, Zhang SZ. Ursolic acid inhibits proliferation and induces apoptosis of HT-29 colon cancer cells by inhibiting the EGFR/MAPK pathway. J Zhejiang Univ Sci B. 2009 Sep;10(9):668-74.

112. Huo R, Zhou QL, Want BX, Tashiro SI, Onodera S, Ikejima T. Diosgenin induces apoptosis in HeLa cells via activation of capase pathway. Acta Pharmacol Sin. 2004 Aug;25(8):1077-82.

113. Aehle E, Müller U, Eklund PC, Willför SM, Sippl W, Dräger B. Lignans as food constituents with estrogen and antiestrogen activity. Phytochemistry. 2011 Dec;72(18):2396-405. Epub 2011 Sep.

114. Lamproglou I, Boisserie G, Mazeron JJ, Bok B, Baillet F, Drieu K. [Effect of Ginkgo biloba extract (EGb 761) on rats in an experimental model of acute encephalopathy after total body irradiation]. Cancer Radiother. 2000 May-Jun;4(3):202-06.

115. Schmittgen TD, Koolemans-Beynen A, Webb TE, etal. Effects of 5-fluorouracil, leucovorin, and glucarate in rat colon-tumor explants. Cancer Chemother Pharmacol. 1992;30:25-30.

116. Eun Ji Kim, et al. Oral administration of 3,3'-diindolylmethane inhibits lung metastasis of 4T1 murine mammary carcinoma cells in BALB/c mice. Journal of Nutrition. 2009 Dec:139(12):2373-79.

Like nutraceuticals, some medicinal herbs can be deployed as first-line therapy and others work to enhance conventional therapies.

Medicinal Herbs
BOTANICAL ANTIOXIDANTS

Curcuma longa

Traditionally, tumeric has been used as an anti-inflammatory agent and for wound healing and longevity. The root contains curcumin, which has been investigated for its chemopreventive activities.

One identified mechanism is the ability of curcumin to induce Phase 2 detoxification enzymes, especially glutathione transferases and quinone reductase, while inhibiting procarcinogen activating Phase I enzymes, such as cP4501A1 (in-vivo).[1] Studies have also shown that it sensitizes prostate cells to radiation,[2] induces apoptosis of prostate cancer cells,[3] and overcomes chemoresistance.[4] Curcumin has been shown to be chemopreventive and can help prevent recurrence.[5,6]

Camellia sinensis

Green tea contains a polyphenol called epigallocatechin-3-gallate (EGCG), as well as catechins, epicatechin (EC), epicatechin-3-gallate (ECG), and epigallocatechin (EGC). Oral consumption of green tea polyphenols inhibited prostate cancer development in mice transfected with prostate cancer cells. EGCG induced apoptosis in prostate cancer cells occurred via regulation of p53 and NF-kappaB.[7]

Cimicifuga racemosa (Black cohosh)

This herb suppresses cell proliferation. Cimicifuga extracts induce cell cycle arrest at G1.Cyclin D1 promotes transition from G1 to S and is overexpressed in 50% to 60% of primary human breast carcinomas. Cimicifuga, actein in particular, decreases cyclin D1. This growth inhibition was demonstrated with alcoholic extract of cimicifuga for both ER+ and ER- cells. The effect in humans and required dose is unknown,[8] and it is still unclear if Cimicifuga is safe for use in women with active breast cancer or a history of breast cancer. However, there is no convincing data demonstrating harm or risk. Cimicifuga is not a phytoestrogenic plant, but may have other tumor promoting activities. The safest course of action may be to use it for a relatively short term use (1-12 months) in a women without active disease.[9]

Silybum marianum (Milk thistle)

This herb has anticancer potential to suppress cell proliferation. It also inhibits human prostate carcinoma DU145 cells, due to impairment of cell signaling pathways. Milk thistle consists of a family of flavonoids: silybin, isosilybin, silychristin, silydianin, and taxifoline. Numerous studies have indicated that silymarin is a chemopreventive agent *in vivo* against a variety of carcinogens and tumor promoters, including UV light, DMBA, PMA, and others.[9]

Silymarin

Silymarin has also been shown to sensitize tumors to chemotherapeutic agents through the down regulation of the MDR protein and other mechanisms. It binds to both estrogen and androgen receptors, and down regulates PSA. Silymarin exhibits its own anti-tumor activity against human tumors (prostate and ovary) in animal studies.[10]

Silymarin can suppress the proliferation of a variety of tumor cells: prostate, breast, ovary, colon, lung, and bladder. This suppression is accomplished through cell cycle arrest at the G1/S-phase and induction of cylin-dependent kinase inhibitors, such as p15, p21, and p27. Suppression also occurs by down regulation of anti-apoptotic gene products (Bcl-2, Bcl-xl), inhibition of cell survival kinases (AKT, PKC, MAPK), and inhibition of inflammatory transcription factors (NF-kappaB).[11] Silymarin can also down-regulate gene products involved in the proliferation of tumor cells (cyclin D1, EGFR, COX-2, TGFβ, IGF-IR), invasion (MMP-9), angiogenesis (VEGF), and metastasis (adhesion molecules). The anti-inflammatory effects are mediated through suppression of NF-kappaB regulated gene products, including COX-2 and LOX, inducible iNOS, TNF, and IL-1.[12]

Various clinical trials have indicated that silymarin is bioavailable and pharmacologically safe, with studies in progress to demostrate the clinical efficacy

GREEN TEA STUDIES

In one study, oral intake of green tea polyphenols in mice transfected with prostate cancer resulted in:

- Reduced levels of Insulin-like Growth Factor[14]
- Inhibition of markers of angiogenesis/metastasis, including Vascular Endothelial Growth Factor, Urokinase Plasminogen Activator, and matrix metalloproteinases 2 and 9[15]
- Oral treatment with green tea reduced elevated PSA levels in human study[16]
- EGCG inhibits COX-2

Green tea has been shown to be chemopreventive for oral and colon cancers. Oral consumption of green tea reduces PGE2 in a dose-dependent manner in colonic cells. PGE2 is elevated in colon cancer cells and stimulates growth signaling pathways, and is additionally associated with invasiveness properties.[17]

In a 6 mo. RCT (n=59) of subjects with oral leukoplakia, 3 g tea (capsules) and mixed tea in glycerin was applied topically to lesions TID. Partial regression of lesions occurred in 37.9% of tea-treated group and artial regression of lesions in 10% of placebo group.[18]

Green tea has inhibitory actions on almost all steps of carcinogenesis. Clinical trials bear this out. A published meta-analysis of all cohort and case-control studies assessing breast cancer incidence and breast cancer recurrence resulted in 7 observational reports that met inclusion criteria. The pooled relative risk for the highest levels of green tea consumption on the risk of developing breast cancer was 0.79 (95% CI, 0.62-1.01; p=0.064). The highest levels of green tea consumption (typically >5 cups daily) showed a pooled relative risk of 0.56 (95% CI, 0.38-0.83; p = 0.0041) for stage I and II disease.[19]

EGCG has been demonstrated in a number of in-vitro models to increase DNA repair. This effect is the result of EGCG's influence on the excision-repair system.[15] Rats exposed to heterocyclic amines demonstrated significantly reduced mutagenicity and increased DNA repair in hepatocytes when fed green tea extract.[20]

Catechins, ECG, and EGCG have demonstrated antimutagenic effects against bacterial mutagens (in-vivo). EGCG counters the carcinogenic effects of chemical carcinogens (such as benzenes).[20]

Green tea polyphenols capture and detoxify radicals of various promoters of carcinogenesis and radicals produced from exposure to radiation and light. C, EC, ECG, EGCG suppress formation of free radicals, specifically reducing hydroxyl radicals (in vivo).[21] This antioxidant effect has also been demonstrated in humans. Urinary and WBC markers of oxidative stress were analyzed for smokers and non-smokers and compared to a control group. Green tea consumption (3 gm as tea t.i.d.) for 7 days resulted in significant decreases in oxidative DNA damage and lipid peroxidation and free radical generation in smokers (also in non-smokers).[21]

against various cancers.[22] Silibinin and silymarin each inhbit DNA synthesis by arresting cells in G1. This has been demonstrated in skin, prostate, and breast cancer models.[23] Silybin inhibits the growth of ovarian cells in a dose-dependent manner. The growth of these cells was arrested in the G1 phase of cell division.[13]

Silybinin

The flavanoid silibinin inhibits receptor and non-receptor tyrosine kinase signaling pathways that inhibit TNF-α mRNA expression.[25] These actions result in decreased cell growth and DNA synthesis in human prostate, breast and, cervical carcinoma cells.

Genestein and daidzein (Soy bean)

Genistein is a major component of soy with antiproliferative action. Genistein produces cell cycle arrest in human prostate cancer cell line. It decreases growth of prostate cancer tissue in a dose-dependant manner. Genistein has been found to modulate

multiple cellular pathways that are mediated by the androgen receptor, which is important in prostate carcinogenesis.[22] It potentiates inhibition of tumor growth by radiation. Genistein combined with radiation caused a significantly greater inhibition of tumor growth (87%) compared with radiation (73%) or genistein (30%) alone.[23]

Genistein binds to ERα on MCF-7 (ER+ breast cancer cells) and stimulates transcription and proliferation of MCF-7 cells. At concentrations up to 1 μM, genistein is a full ERα agonist.[24] Long-term exposure may promote breast cancer development and stimulate progression of ER+ tumors.[25] Genistein blood levels in humans on a high-soy diet are reported at 1μM - 6μM.[26] At concentrations above 10μM, other mechanisms cause cytotoxic effects. The maximum concentration that can be reached physiologically is reported to be 18.5μM.[26] At high concentrations (largely unachievable through diet) of 50 μM – 100 μM, Up-regulate heat shock protein mRNA (involved in apoptotic signaling) and down-regulate mRNA expression of ERa. Decreases tyrosine kinase expression and downstream regulators.[27] Causes cell-cycle arrest in G0-G1 and G2-M by up-regulating p21. A protein called p21 acts as the molecular switch that triggers telomere-initiated senescence.[24]

Daidzein is converted by intestinal bacteria into equol. At experimental levels that correlate with prostatic concentrations of equol from men living in Asia and consuming their traditional diets that include significant soy, equol arrests prostate cancer cell lines in the G0/G1 phase.[27] Of interest is that Asian men convert diadzein to equol more effectively than do North American men. This is likely the result of different diets and consequent differences in gut ecology.[23]

Soy studies

Early stage prostate cancer patients were supplemented with 60 mg of soy isoflavones to look at changes in hormonal and proliferative risk factors implicated in prostate cancer promotion. In this study, 76 patients with Gleason scores of 6 or below, between the ages of 50 and 80, were randomized for supplementation or placebo for 12 weeks. PSA changes and steroid hormone levels were analyzed at baseline and post intervention. Of the 76, 59 competed the 12-week intervention with serum free testosterone reduced or showing no change in 61% of the isoflavone group compared to 33% in placebo group. Serum PSA levels were decreased or unchanged in 69% of the isoflavone group compared to 55% in placebo group . And 19% of the isoflavone group reduced total PSA by 2 points or more during the 12-week period. Data suggest supplementation with soy isoflavones in early stage prostate cancer alters surrogate markers of proliferation, such as serum PSA and free testosterone.[28]

Isoflavones are poorly absorbed in glycosylated forms. Soy with Basidiomycetes provides an enriched, biologically active aglycone isoflavone in prostate and bladder cancer in vitro and in vivo. Growth of cells in vitro inhibited by 72 hours of treatment with induction of apoptosis were detected in cells with p53+. In mice whose diets consisted of 2% of this fermented isoflavone, tumor growth suppression occurred. Best results in vivo and in vitro was with wild type p53, which activated both cell cycle suppression and apoptotic signaling. This can be an effective chemopreventive and/or therapeutic for prostate and bladder cancers.[23]

Ginkgo biloba

Ginkgo biloba extract (GBE) contains 24% phytoestrogens (PEs), including kaempferol, quercetin, and isorhamnetin).GBE and its PEs bind to both ERβ and ERα, with a higher affinity for ER. In one study, GBE and the PEs induced cell proliferation in ER-positive MCF-7 cells.[29]

Glycyrhiza glabra (Licorice)

Glycyrrhiza contains phytoestrogenic flavonoids. However, licorice extracts have demonstrated antiestrogen effects when given with estradiol, notably in E-dependent endometrial carcinoma cells in an animal model. The postulated mechanism is the suppression of estrogen-induced c-fos/jun mRNA expression and the expression of corresponding proto-oncogene proteins in the uterine tissue. It is conceivable that this effect overshadows the phytoestrogenic effect of licorice extracts.[30]

Indole-3-carbinol

This compound, found in Brassica vegetables, is theoretically synergistic with aromatase inhibitors (herbal and conventional): Arimidex, Femara, Aromasin). Indole-3-carbinol (I3C) converts estrone to 2-OH metabolites that are antiproliferative and apoptotic, and inhibits transcription of genes driven by ERα binding. I3C induces apoptotic genes.[31]

Scutellaria baicalensis (Chinese skullcap)

One of the seven herbs in PC-SPES, which is moderately successful in lowering PSA values,[32] *Scutellaria baicalensis* has the strongest antineoplastic activity, attributable to its flavonoids.[33]

Ganoderma lucidum

This botanical medicine suppresses invasive cell migration, inhibits cell proliferation, and induces apoptosis. These effects are due, in part, to downregulation of NF-kappa and upregulation of p21.[34]

Beta-Sitosterol

This type of phytosterol is antiproliferative and proapoptotic on prostate tissue. In one study, beta-sitosterol or cholesterol was applied to prostate cancer cells. Beta-sitosterol decreased growth by 24% and induced apoptosis fourfold as compared to cholesterol.[35] It is found in soy foods and nuts, such as pumpkin seeds, almonds, walnuts, hazelnuts, wheat germ, and avocado.[37]

Studies have shown that beta-sitosterol is antiproliferative with pro-apoptotic effects on prostate tissue. Mice implanted with prostate cancer cells were fed either a high phystosterol or a high cholesterol diet. Mice fed phytosterol diet had tumors 40% to 43% smaller than those fed the cholesterol diet. The number of mice with lymph node and lung metastasis was almost one-half that of the cholesterol-fed group.[36]

Anticancer Medicinal Herbs

Medicinal Herb Latin Name Common Name	Anticancer Action	Interactions Cautions	Therapeutic Dose
Nepeta spp. Catnep, catnip	Carminative	None	1-3 tsp in 1 cup water steep and use for antinausea 15-30 minutes before meal as needed
Curcuma longa Tumeric	Cox 1&2 inhibitor, lox inhibitor, chemosensitizer, apoptotic	Some with certain chemotherapies prohibited	Constituent based to activated curcuminoids 100-300mg per dose
Camelia spp. Tea, Green Tea	Gallic acids, EGCG, etc. Chemopreventative, chemo/radio sensitizing, apoptotic, anti-angiogenic	Maybe with Curcumin ??? some chemotherapies	Green tea must have polyphenols (not decaf) 5-10 cups per day or equivalent
Vaccinium spp. Blueberries, bilberries, etc.	Proanthocyanadin, (OPC), antioxidant, apoptotic, chemopreventative	None	Resveratrol (100% trans) 100-300 mg; CoQ10 100-1200mg in a lysozymed form (water soluble)
Scuttelaria bicalensis, spp skullcap	Cox 1&2 inhibitor, Lox inhibitor, chemopreventative, chemosensitizer, apoptotic	None	Recommended dose variable and patient dependant

Another study found that it inhibited 5-alpha reductase, with a 33% to 44% decrease in hepatic and prostatic 5-alpha reductase activity.[37] Beta-sitosterol also stimulates immune system. It was shown that it caused stimulation of human peripheral blood lymphocyte proliferation *in vitro*.[38] Ingestion by human volunteers resulted in enhancement of T-cell proliferation.[39]

Medicinal Mushrooms (Mycomedicinals)

Several fungi have been used as anticancer medicines in Native North American and traditional Chinese medical practices. Considerable research has been conducted on the efficacy and safety of mycomedicinals. More than a dozen species have proven to be therapeutic in cancer care.

Medically accepted mushroom species[40]
Ganoderma lucidum (Reishi or Ling Zhi)
Lentinus (Lentinula) edodes (Shiitake)
Phellinus linteus (Mesima)
Porio cocos
Auricularia auricula
Hericium erinaceus (Lion's mane)
Grifola frondosa (Maitake)
Inonotus obliquus (Chaga)

Grifola frondosa (Maitake)
Flammulina velutipes
Pleurotus ostreatus (Oyster mushroom)
Trametes (Coriolus) versicolor (Turkey tails)
Tremella fuciformis
Schizophyllum commune
Cordyceps sinensis (non mushroom caterpillar fungus).

Polysaccharides

Recent improvements in chemical technology have enabled the isolation and purification of the relevant compounds of specific interest called polysaccharides, which exhibit demonstrable anticancer activities. Most appear to act as immune system enhancers, though some can have direct cytotoxic effects on cancer cells. Only a small number have progressed successfully to objective clinical assessment in human trials.[40] The anti-tumor polysaccharides isolated from mushrooms (fruit-body, submerged, cultured mycelial biomass or liquid culture broth) are either water-soluble -D-glucans, -D-glucans with heterosaccharide chains ofxylose, mannose, galactose or uronic acid or -D-glucan-protein complexes - proteoglycans.[40-45] Mushroom-derived glucan and polysaccharo-peptides can act as immunomodulators. The ability of these compounds to enhance or suppress immune responses

Anticancer medicinal mushrooms

Cancer	Medicinal Mushroom
Breast	Grifola frondosa, Lentinula elodes, Trametes versicolor
Cervical/Uterine	Agaricus blazei, Inonotus obliquus, Phellinus linteus, Schizophyllum commune, Trametes versicolor
Colorectal	Agaricus blazei, Grifola frondosa, Phellinus linteus
Gastric/Stomach	Hericium erinaceus, Phellinus linteus, Schizophyllum commune, Trametes versicolor
Leukemia	Cordyceps sinensis, Ganoderma lucidum, Grifola frondosa, Polysporus umbellatus, Trametes versicolor
Liver	Ganoderma lucidum, Grifola frondosa, Lentinula edodes, Phellinus linteus, Polysporus umbellatus, Trametes versicolor
Lung	Cordyceps sinensis, Ganoderma lucidum, Grifola frondosa, Polysporus umbellate, Trametes versicolor
Lymphoma	Cordyceps sinensis, Flammulina veluptipes
Melanoma	Lentinula edodes, Phellinus linteus
Prostate	Flammulina veluptipes, Ganoderma lucidum, Grifola frondosa, Lentinula edodes, Trametes versicolor
Sarcoma	Agaricus blazei, Ganoderma lucidum, Pleurotus ostreatus

(Adapted from fungiperfecti.com)

depends on a number of factors, including dosage, route of administration, timing and frequency of administration, mechanism of action, and the site of activity. Some are orally bioavailable.[40-45]

Literature Review

The main medically important polysaccharide compounds that have undergone clinical trials include lentinan from *Lentinus edodes*, schizophyllan from *Schizophyllum commune*, PSK and PSP from *Trametes versicolor*, and Grifron-D from *Grifola frondosa*.[40]

Several mushroom compounds have shown to potentiate the non-specific and specific immune responses and activate many kinds of immune cells that are important for the maintenance of homeobalance in the immune system: host cells (such as cytotoxic macrophages, monocytes, neutrophils, natural killer cells, dendritic cells) and chemical messengers (cytokines such as interleukins, interferon, colony stimulating factors) trigger complement and acute phase responses.[40-50] They can also be considered as multi-cytokine inducers able to induce gene expression of various immunomodulatory cytokines and cytokine receptors. Lymphocytes governing antibody production and cell mediated cytotoxicity (T-cells) are also stimulated.[40-50]

Lentinan and schizophyllan are T-cell oriented immunopotentiators and require a functional T-cell component for biological activity by way of increasing helper T-cell production, increased macrophage production leading to a stimulation of acute phase proteins and colony stimulating factors which in turn affect proliferation of macrophages, neutrophils and lymphocytes, and activation of the complement system.[40-50]

PSK and PSP (polysaccharides) are potent immunostimulators with specific activity for T-cells and for antigen-presenting cells, such as monocytes and macrophages. Their biological activity is characterized by their ability to increase white blood cell counts, interferon-y, and interleukin-2 production and delayed type hypersensitivity reactions.[40-45] This ability to effectively increase white blood cell counts helps in the integrative strategy with lymphoma/ leukemia as these white cell lines are often affected in the combination chemotherapeutics creating a neutropenia that may interfere with the sequence and amount of chemo to be administered.[40-50]

There have been extensive *in vivo* studies demonstrating the anticancer activity of the glucan polysaccharides and polysaccharide-peptides in animal probands. These studies strongly indicate an immunomodulating mode of action from these polysaccharides. However, in *in vitro* studies on various cancer cell lines, there is even stronger evidence for direct cytotoxic effects on the cancer cells for some, but not all, of the polysaccharides.[41-50]

Many of the mushroom polysaccharides have proceeded through Phase I, II and III clinical trials mainly in Japan and China but now in the United States.[46] Lentinan (*L.edodes*) has demonstrated strong antitumor activity in a wide range of cancers and with human clinical trials it has proven successful in prolonging the survival rates, especially those patients with gastric and colorectal cancer.[40,42,48] Lentinan has been approved as a drug in Japan and is considered an important adjuvant treatment for several cancers.[40] Schizophyllan (*S. commune*) has proved useful for recurrent and inoperable gastric cancer, as well as increasing survival times of patients with head and neck cancers.[51,52] Neither of these compounds show any significant sideeffects.[46,47] There are several on-going clinical trials with Grifron-D, GD (*G. frondosa*) on breast, prostate, lung, liver and gastric cancers underway in Japan and in the United States showing promising results.[53,54] In *in vitro* studies GD appears to inactivate glyoxalase I, an enzyme believed to metabolize chemotherapeutic compounds used against cancer cells thus potentially enhancing their bioavailability and possible chemoresistance.[52] Two compounds, PSK and PSP (derived from mycelial cultures of *T. versicolor*), have evident anticancer properties when given with conventional chemotherapeutic agents, yielding no increase in sideeffects.[52]

PSK has successfully been used in Phase I, II and III clinical trials with cancers of the stomach, esophagus, nasopharynx, colon, rectum, lung, and breast cancer.[42,43,47,48] PSK gave protection against the immunosuppression that normally is associated with surgery and long-term chemotherapy effecting not only the WBC line but keeping the innate as well as acquired immune function intact.[40-42] PSK continues to be used extensively in Japan as an adjunct to standard chemotherapies and radiation.[52] PSP has been extensively studied by Chinese scientists and oncologists, with little evidence of side-effects. Clinical trials have shown efficacy in gastric, esophageal, and nonsmall cell (NSCLC) lung cancers,[40-50] and PSP has been recognized as a drug by the Chinese Ministry of Public Health.[52]

A significant observation from these studies is the apparent ability of all of the above mushroom-derived polysaccharides when administered with radiotherapy and/or chemotherapy to significantly reduce the side-effects so often encountered by patients from these cytoxic strategies.[50,52] A dose response *in vitro* study showed almost complete cell death (95%) within 24 hours of exposure to Maitake D-fraction ($\geq$480 mcg/ml). Combinations of Maitake D-fraction in a concentration as low as 30-60 mcg/ml with 200 microM of vitamin C were just as effective as GD alone at 480 mcg/ml: all have cytoxic cell death >90%.[51] It was found that the bioactive β-glucans from the Maitake mushroom have the cytoxic effect, presumably through oxidative stress that leads to apoptosis and ultimately cancer cell death.[51] β-glucan was also demonstrated to sensitize cytotoxic cells to carmustine (BCNU) in PC-3 cells. This activity created an associated (80%) inactivation of the glutathione dependent detoxifying enzyme, glyoxalase I (Gly-I). Thus, the BCNU/beta-glucan combination may be specific to target the Gly-1 enzyme and improve current treatment efficacy.[52]

References

1. Dinkova-Kostova A, Talalay P. Relation of structure of curcumin analogs to their potencies as inducers of Phase 2 detoxification enzymes. Carcinogenesis. 1999;20(5):911-14.

2. Chendil D, Ranga RS, et al. Curcumin confers radiosensitizing effect in prostate cancer cell line PC-3. Oncogene. 2004 Feb.26;23(8):1599-607.

3. Adams BK, Cai J, Armstrong J, et al. EF24, a novel synthetic curcumin analog, induces apoptosis in cancer cells via a redox-dependent mechanism. Anticancer Drugs. 2005 Mar;16(3):263-75.

4. Karunagaran D, Rashmi R, Kumar TR. Curr Cancer Drug Targets. 2005 Mar; 5(2):117-29.

5. Barnard RJ, Aronson WJ. Preclinical models relevant to diet, exercise, and cancer risk. Recent Results Cancer Res. 2005;166:47-61.

6. Corpet DE, Pierre F. Point. From animal models to prevention of colon cancer. Systematic review of chemoprevention in min mice and choice of the model system. Cancer Epidemiol Biomarkers Prev. 2003 May;12(5):391-400.

7. Sah JF, Balasubramanian S, Eckert RL, Rorke EA. 2004. Epigallocatechin-3-gallate inhibits epidermal growth factor receptor signaling pathway: evidence for direct inhibition of ERK1/2 and AKT kinases. J Biol Chem 279:12755-62.

8. Einbond LS, Shimizu M, Xiao D, et al. Growth inhibitory activity of extracts and purified components of black cohosh on human breast cancer cells. Breast Cancer Res Treat. 2004;83(3):221-31.

9. Agarwal R, Agarwal C, Ichikawa H, et al. Anticancer potential of silymarin: from bench to bed side. Anticancer Res. 2006;26:4457-98.

10. Bhatia N, Zhao J, Wolf DM, Agarwal R. Inhibition of human carcinoma cell growth and DNA synthesis by silibinin, an active constituent of milk thistle: comparison with silymarin. Cancer Lett. 1999 Dec 1;147(1-2):77-84.

11. Scambia G, De Vincenzo R, Ranelletti FO, Panici PB, Ferrandina G, D'Agostino G, Fattorossi A, Bombardelli E, Mancuso S. Antiproliferative effect of silybin on gynaecological malignancies: synergism with cisplatin and doxorubicin Eur J Cancer. 1996 May;32A(5):877-82 (Cell Culture Study).

12. Zhao JJ and Agarwal RR. Tissue distribution of silibinin, the major active constituent of silymarin, in mice and its association with enhancement of phase II enzymes: implications in cancer chemoprevention. Carcinogenesis. 1999;20(11);2101-08.

13. Zi XL, Zhang J, Agarwal R and Pollak M. Silibinin up-regulates insulin like growth factor binding protein 3 expression and inhibits proliferation of androgen independent prostate cancer cells. Cancer Res. 60:5617-20.

14. Weisburger JH, Rivenson A, Aliaga C, Reinhardt J, Kelloff GJ, Boone CW, Steele VE, Balentine DA, Pittman B, Zang E. Effect of tea extracts, polyphenols, and epigallocatechin gallate on azoxymethane-induced colon cancer. Proc Soc Exp Biol Med. 1998 Jan;217(1):104-08.

15. Lee YK, ND Bone, AK Stege, TD Shanafelt, DF Jelinek and NE Kay. VEGF receptor phosphorylation status and apoptosis is modulated by a green tea component, epigallocatechin-3-gallate (EGCG), in B-cell chronic lymphocytic leukemia. Blood. 2004 August 1; 104(3):788-94.

16. Ebata J, Fukagai N, Furukawa H. Mechanisms of antimutagenesis by catechins towards N-nitrosodimethylamine. Environ Mutagen Res.1998;20:45-50.

17. Jianping L, Jianmin X, Yutong F. Green tea (Camellia sinensis) and cancer prevention: a systematic review of randomized trials and epidemiological studies. Chinese Medicine. 2008;3:12.

18. Weisburger JH. Tea and health: the underlying mechanisms. Proc Soc Exp Biol Med. 1999;220:271-75.

19. Seely D, Mills EJ, Wu P, Verma S, Guyatt GH. The effects of green tea consumption on incidence of breast cancer and recurrence of breast cancer: a systematic review and meta-analysis. Integra Cancer Ther. 2005;4:144-55.

20. Kuroda Y, Hara Y. Antimutagenic and anticarcinogenic activity of tea polyphenols. Mut Res. 1999;436:69-97.

21. Klaunig JE, Xu Y, Han C, et al. The effect of tea consumption on oxidative stress in smokers and nonsmokers. Proc Soc Exp Biol Med. 1999;220:249-54.

22. Sarkar FH, Li Y. Soy isoflavones and cancer prevention. Cancer Invest. 2003;21(5):744-57.

23. Bemis, DL, Capodice, JL, Buttyan, R., Katz, AE. Botanicals in the Treatment of Prostate Cancer: Pre-clinical research. New York, NY: Columbia University Medical Center, 2004.

24. Upadhyay S, Neburi M, Chinni SR, et al. Differential sensitivity of normal and malignant breast epithelial cells to genistein is partly mediated by p21(WAF1). Clin Cancer Res 2001;7:1782-89.

25. Maggiolini M, Bonofiglio D, et al. Estrogen receptor alpha mediates the proliferative but not the cytotoxic dose dependant effects of two majo phytoestrogens on human breast cancer cells. Mol Pharmacol. 2001 Sep;60(3):595-602.

26. Jones JL, Daley BJ, Enderson BL, Zhou JR, Karlstad MD. 2002. Genistein inhibits tamoxifen effects on cell proliferation and cell cycle arrest in T47D breast cancer cells. Am Surg. Jun;68(6):575-77; discussion 577-78.

27. Sarkar FH, Li Y. Soy isoflavones and cancer prevention. Cancer Invest. 2003;21(5):744-57.

28. Kumar NB. The Specific Role of Isoflavones in Reducing Prostate Cancer Risk. H. Lee Moffitt Cancer Center and Res. Inst., Tampa, Fl;2004.

29. Oh SM, Chung KH. 2004. Estrogenic activities of Ginkgo biloba extracts. Life Sci. Jan 30;74(11):1325-35.

30. Mori H, Niwa K, Zheng Q, Yamada Y, Sakata K, Yoshimi N. Cell proliferation in cancer prevention; effects of preventive

agents on estrogen-related endometrial carcinogenesis model and on an in vitro model in human colorectal cells. Mutat Res. 2001 Sep 1;480-81:201-07.

31. Auborn KJ, Fan S, Rosen EM, Goodwin L, Chandraskaren A, Williams DE, Chen D, Carter TH. Indole-3-carbinol is a negative regulator of estrogen J Nutr. 2003 Jul;133(7 Suppl):2470S-2475S.

32. Hsieh TC, Lu X, Chea J, Wu JM. Prevention and management of prostate cancer using PC-SPES: a scientific perspective. J Nutr. 2002 Nov;132 (11 Suppl):3513S-3517S.

33. Zhang DY, Wu J, Ye F, et al. Inhibition of cancer cell proliferation and prostaglandin E2 synthesis by Scutellaria baicalensis. Cancer Res. 2003: 4037-43.

34. Jiahua J, et ak. Ganoderma lucidum inhibits proliferation and induces apoptosis in human prostate cancer cells PC-3. Int. Journal of Oncology.2004; 24: 1093-99.

35. von Holtz RL, Fink CS, Awad AB. beta-Sitosterol activates the sphingomyelin cycle and induces apoptosis in LNCaP human prostate cancer cells. Department of Physical Therapy, Exercise, and Nutrition Sciences, State University of New York at Buffalo 14214-3000, USA. Nutr Cancer. 1998;32(1):8-12.

36. Awad A B, Fink CS, Williams H, Kim U. In vitro and in vivo (SCID mice) effects of phytosterols on the growth and dissemination of human prostate cancer PC-3 cells. European Journal of Cancer Prevention. 2001 Dec;10(6):507-13 (Research Papers).

37. Awad A B, Downie A, Fink CS, Kim U. Dietary phytosterol inhibits the growth and metastasis of MDA-MB-231 human breast cancer cells grown in SCID mice. Anticancer Res 2000;20:821-824.

38. Bouie PJ, et al., beta-Sitosterol and beta-sitosterol glucoside stimulate human peripheral blood lymphocyte proliferation: implications for their use as an immunomodulatory vitamin combination. Int J Immunopharmacol. 1996 Dec;18(12):693-700.

39. Bouic PJ, Etsebeth S, Liebenberg RW, Albrecht CF, Pegel K, Van Jaarsveld PP. beta-Sitosterol and beta-sitosterol glucoside stimulate human peripheral blood lymphocyte proliferation: implications for their use as an immunomodulatory vitamin combination. Int J Immunopharmacol. 1996 Dec;18(12):693-700.

40. Smith, JE, Rowan NJ, Sullivans R. Medicinal mushrooms: their therapeutic properties and current medical usage with special emphasis on cancer treatments. Cancer Research UK. 2007 monograph. www.icnet.uk

41. Stamets, P and Wu Yao, CD. MycoMedicinals. MycoMedia Productions, division of Fungi Perfecti, LLC. 2002:1-96.

42. Kidd, P. The use of mushroom glucans and proteoglucans in cancer treatment. Alt Med Rev. 2000. 5(1):4-27.

43. Ghoneum, M. NK-Immunomodualtory and anti cancer properties of (MGN-3), a modified xylose from rice bran, in 5 patients with breast cancer. Abstract, 87th Meeting Am. Ass. Cancer Res. (AACR) special conference, "The interface between basic and applied research." Nov 5-8, 1995, Baltimore, MD.

44. Ghoneum, M. Enhancement of human natural killer cell activity by modified arabinoxylane from rice bran (MGN-3). Int Nat. J of Immunotherapy. 1998;2:89-99.

45. Mondoa, E and Kitei, M. Sugars that heal the new healing science of glyconutrients. 2001. Ballantine Publ. Grp. NYC, New York.

46. Ooi, VE and Liu, F. A review of pharmacological activities of mushroom polysaccharides. Int J of Medicinal Mushrooms. 1999. I:195-206.

47. Ooi, VE and Liu, F. Immunomodulation and anticancer activity of polysaccharide protein complexes. Curr Med Chem. 2000. July 7(7);710-729.

48. Koh, JH, Yu KW, suh HJ, choi YM, Ahn TS. Activation of macrophages ant the intestinal immune system by an orally administered decoction from cultured mycelia of Cordyceps sinensis. Biosci biotechnol Biochem. 2002. Feb 66(2):407-11.

49. Zhou S and Gao Y. The immunomodulating effects of Ganoderma lucidum(Curt:Fr) P. Karst (Ling Zhi, Reishi mushroom) Aphyllophoromycetideae. International J of Medicinal Mushrooms. 2002 4;(1);1-12.

50. Sugimachi K, Maehara Y, Ogawa M, Kakegawa T, Tomita M. Dose intensity of uracil and tegafur in postoperative chemotherapy for patients with poorly differentiated gastric cancer. Cancer Chemotherapy and Pharmacology. 1997;40(3):233-38.

51. Fullerton SA, Samadi AA, Tortorelis DG, et al. Induction of apoptosis in human prostatic cancer cells with beta-glucan (Maitake mushroom polysaccharide). Mol Urol 2000;4(1):7-13.

52. Finkelstein MP, Aynehchi S, Samadi AA, Drinis S, Choudhury MS, Tazaki H, Konno S. Chemosensitization of carmustine with maitake ≤-glucan on androgen-independent prostatic cancer cells: involvement of glyoxalase I. J Altern Complement Med. 2002;8:573-80.

53. Cui FJ, Li Y, Xu YY, et al. Induction of apoptosis in SGC-7901 cells by polysaccharide-peptide GFPS1b from the cultured mycelia of Grifola frondosa GF9801. Toxicol In Vitro. 2007 Apr;21(3):417-27.

54. Cui FJ, Tao WY, Xu ZH, et al. Structural analysis of antitumor heteropolysaccharide GFPS1b from the cultured mycelia of Grifola frondosa GF9801. Bioresour Technol. 2007 Jan;98(2):395-401.

PART 3: INTEGRATIVE APPROACHES TO CANCER

INTEGRATING NATUROPATHIC AND CONVENTIONAL THERAPIES

Naturopathic cancer therapies can be integrated very successfully with conventional intervention therapies, namely chemotherapy, radiation therapy, and surgery. The goal of integrating strategies is not to replace conventional therapies or interfere with their effectiveness, but rather to enhance efficacy and decrease side effects. Keep in mind that in doing so we may decrease the effectiveness of conventional therapies by manipulating the Cytochrome P450 interactions, P-Glycoprotein interactions, or any other number of mechanisms of action. In the attempt to decrease side effects, choose a therapy that does not have these interactions.

Drug-Herb Interactions and Complements

When integrating naturopathic with allopathic treatments, bear in mind possible interactions, both adverse and advantageous.

Most known drug interactions are due to changes in the metabolic rate of clearance and the routes related to an altered expression of the functional CYP450 isozymes. Interactions can also take place by the P-glycoprotein, which plays a role in mediating transmembrane transport of chemotherapy.

Common chemotherapeutics are metabolized by the CYP3A4:

Ifosfamide, Paclitaxel, Docetaxel, Abraxane, Vinblastine, Vincristine, Navelbine, Irinotecan, Topotecan, Etoposide, Tamoxifen, Arimidex, Aromasin, Femara, EGFR-TK inhibitors, Iressa, and Tarceva.

Other chemotherapeutics are metabolized through CYP2C19:

Cytoxan and Aromatase inhibitors

Several medicinal herbs interfere with CYP3A4:

Hypericum perforatum (which should be avoided in all chemotherapies because it interferes with CYP2B6, CYP2C9, CYP2C19, CYP2E1, CYP3A4 and P-glycoprotein induction), *Piper methysticum, Hydrastis Canadensis, Uncaria tomentosa, Trifolium pratense, Matricaria chamomilla, Glycyrrhiza glabra*, and grape seed extracts.[1]

Other herbs that interfere with CYP3A4 and CYP2C19: For CYP3A4: *Echinacea sp., Ginseng sp., Ginkgo biloba, Silymarin* (also P-glycoprotein) and Quercitin. For CYP2C19: *Ginkgo a*nd *Valeriana*.[2]

Circumin Caution

Curcumin, a bioflavonoid found in tumeric, has specific indications for many cancer types, but has been contraindicated for Adriamycin and Cytoxan integrative use due to its ability to inhibit chemotherapy-induced apoptosis in human breast cancer cells in conjunction with these chemotherapeutics.[3]

CLINICAL APPLICATION

First, determine the metabolism of the drug: is it metabolized through CYP450 isoenzymes or through P-glycoprotein? If there is a 'yes' to this question, how does the botanical influence the pathway? Here the integrative strategist can determine if it is a caution or a strict avoidance that must be adhered to, and if it is a caution, then at least the half-life interaction with the chemotherapy must be avoided with the administration of the botanical.

Goals of Integrating Naturopathic with Conventional Modalities

- Reduce side effects of treatment
- Maintain quality of life (QOL)
- Prevent mucositis and stomatitis
- Prevent breaks in conventional therapeutics treatment regimen due to side effects or eventual discontinuation of treatment altogether
- Prevent long-term sequelae from conventional interventional treatment protocols
- Maintain good nutritional status
- Prevent the need to interrupt treatment to modify treatment parameters for weight loss because internal organs and structures will shift with weight loss (XRT) and chemotherapy is dosed according to the patients weight and nutritional status.

Integrated Premedications

Premedication Purpose	Conventional Premedication	Naturopathic Complement
To decrease the allergic response to chemotherapy	Dexamethasone Benadryl Ativan	Perilla seed, freeze-dried nettles, NAC, vitamin C[4]
To decrease nausea and vomiting, anxiety, and loss of appetite associated with chemotherapy	Antiemetics: Compazine	Nepeta, chamomilla, cannabis (also combusted) Low dose homeopathics: arsenicum, carbo-veg, nux vomica, ipecac[5]
To counter nausea and vomiting associated with chemotherapy	5HT3 receptor agonists: Zofran Kytril Aloxi Substance P/neurokinin 1 inhibitors (Emend)[6]	
To prevent coagulation	Coumadin: if the patient has a port placed (1 mg dose)	Green leafy vegetables: If patients are already eating green leafy veggies before starting blood thinners, they can continue, but caution should be used if patients are being introduced to green leafy vegetables because they can change bleeding times. Natural blood thinners include vitamin E, C, and *Ginkgo biloba*.[7]
To manage neutropenia, anemia, or thrombocytopenia associated side effects of chemotherapy	Human growth factors: Procrit Aranesp Neupogen Neulasta Leukine Neumega	Medicinal mushrooms: stametes 7, turkey tails Ashwagandha IgG (dairy and colostrum free) Colostrum to increase WBC counts Organic red meats, glandulars, liver fractions to reduce RBC counts Vitamin B-12 Methylated folic acid and vitamin B-6 to help with red blood cell counts[8]

Chemotherapy

Chemotherapy is designed to interrupt the life cycle of cancer cells, stopping them from multiplying, invading, metastasizing, and ultimately creating mortality. Chemotherapies are classified according to their pharmacological action and their specific effect on cellular replication. Cell cycle specific drugs exert an effect within a specific phase of the cell cycle biology. Cell cycle, non-specific drugs exert an effect on all phases of the biological cell cycle, including the resting phase (G0).

PREMEDICATIONS

Most chemotherapies are administered with premedications that are essential for managing the toxicity of some conventional chemotherapies.

Factors that affect the response to chemotherapy
1. The amount of tumor burden the system must endure
2. The therapeutic regimen chosen (combination vs. single agent therapy)
3. The hormone receptor status for some cancers
4. The regimen administration schedule
5. The dose category, either divided fractional dose, which may enhance cancer kill, or long-term infusion, which may minimize side effects
6. The development of drug resistance
7. The inherent nutritional status and psychological health of the patient (*Vis*)

Classes of Chemotherapy Drugs
❖ Alkylating agents
❖ Platinum compounds
❖ Antitumor Antibiotics
❖ Antimetabolites
❖ Topoisomerase Inhibitors
❖ Microtubule Inhibitors
❖ Monoclonal Antibodies
❖ Biological Response Modifiers
❖ Colony Stimulating Factors

ALKYLATING CHEMOTHERAPEUTICS

Pharmaceuticals

Altretamine, BCNU, Busulfan, CCNU, Chlorambucil, Cyclophophamide, Fotumestine, Ifosfamide, Melphalan, Nitrogen Mustard, Pipobroman, Procarbozine, Streptozotocin, Temozolide, Thiotepa, Triethylenemelamine

Pharmacology

Alykylating agents affect the alkylate nucleic acids (DNA and RNA) and will break the DNA helix strand, thus interfering with DNA cancer cell replication. Alkylating agents are cell cycle specific, but not phase specific, and can inflict injury on any part of cell cycle replication. Tumor resistance appears to be related to the capacity of the cells to repair nucleic acid damage and to inactivate the drugs by conjugation with GSH.[9]

Combination Therapies

Most of the regimens that include alkylating agents do so in combination with other chemotherapeutics with a cancer specific indication:
- ❖ Cyclophophamide (Cytoxan) in combination with Adriamycin (AC) in breast cancer
- ❖ Cytoxan with AC, Vincristine, and Prednisone in non Hodgkin's lymphoma (CHOP)
- ❖ Ifosfamide (Ifex) with Carboplatin and Etoposide in NSCLC and metastatic breast cancer (mini ICE)[9]

Toxicity and Side Effects

- ❖ Myelosuppression in a dose-dependent manner with clinical presentations of fatigue
- ❖ Secondary co-infections like candidiasis and slow overall wound healing
- ❖ Hemorrhagic cystitis associated with Cytoxan+Ifex
- ❖ Pan alopecia, mucositis/stomatitis, nausea, and vomiting, neutropenia, and chronic anemia[9]

Naturopathic Complement

These chemotherapies cause multiple side effects, including peripheral neuropathy and neutropenia, and hand and foot syndrome (otherwise known as Palmer plantar erethematosis or PPE). For prevention and treatment of peripheral neuropathy and PPE, apply hexane-free castor oil topically to palms of the hands and soles of the feet one to two times per day. Use thin gloves and socks on top to help the castor oil absorb into the tissues. This can also be used for peripheral neuropathies with the aid of a hot water bottle and castor oil packs.

Also associated with these chemotherapies is mucositis, manifesting as nausea, vomiting, diarrhea, and stomatitis, all leading to cachexia. Use L-glutamine as a preventive and as a treatment for mucositis and stomatitis as well as diarrhea and malabsorption.[10] Catnep tea is very effective for nausea and vomiting, especially before meals. Drink at room temperature (also serve foods warm) with severe mucositis. Use 1 tablespoon of dried herb to one cup of water, cover and steep for 10 minutes. Use with honey if needed to flavor and drink prn. Cannabis is also a great antiemetic and appetite stimulator that can also effect the anxiety associated with cancer diagnosis and treatment.[11] Patients report that the best use of cannabis is for nausea and vomiting[12] It is also an appetite stimulant if administered by combustion. Instead of smoking the herb, a vaporizer can be used, which has a mechanism that burns the cannabis without smoking it and captures the smoke and THC for the patient to inhale.

PLATINUM COMPOUNDS
Pharmaceuticals

Cisplatin (CDDP, Platinol), Carboplatin (Paraplatin), Oxaliplatin (Eloxatin)[9]

Pharmacology

Platinum compounds are an active heavy metal alkylator of DNA, which covalently binds to proteins, RNA, and especially DNA, forming DNA crosslinking.

Combination Therapies

- ❖ Cisplatin in combination with Fluorouaracil (5-FU) in squamous cell carcinoma of the head and neck
- ❖ Cisplatin, Methotrexate, Vinblastine, Doxorubicin in carcinoma of the bladder (MVAC)
- ❖ Cisplatin, Mitomycin-C in an intra-arterial infusion
- ❖ Carboplatin with Taxol in NSCLC and ovarian cancer[9]

Toxicities and Side Effects

- ❖ Myelosuppression, peripheral sensory neuropathy, and pan alopecia

Integrated chemotherapeutic and naturopathic therapies

Chemotherapy Drug	Naturopathic Complement	Therapeutic Dosage (Daily)	Action	Cautions Interactions
Cisplatin Carboplatin	Quercetin[13] Silymarin[14] Curcumin[3] PSK[16] Glutathione[17] Ginkgo biloba[35] Silymarin[14,20] Selenium[21]	100-300 mg qd to tid 250-500 mg qd to tid 200-400 mg qd to tid 1000-3000 mg qd to tid 800-2000 mg qd 120-240 mg qd 600-900 mg qd 400-800mcg qd	To improve effectiveness and decrease chemoresistance To decrease side effects To induce apoptosis	Do not use Quercitin, silymarin, curcumin, glutathione, ginko biloba until chemotherapy is complete
Cytoxan (Cyclophos-phamide)	Folic Acid[8] Vitamin A[23] Glutamine[10,43,45,46] Ashwaganda[25-26]	400-800 mcg 10,000-50,000 IU 10 tid, swish and swallow 500-1000 mg qd to tid	To improve effectiveness To decrease mucositis and cachexia To reduce toxicity, neuro-peria, chemo fatigue	
Cisplatin	Quercitin[13] Silymarin[28] Curcumin[3] Vitamin A[23] Vitamin C[27] Vitamin D[29] Mushrooms[30-31] Silymarin[14] Selenium[34] Ginkgo biloba[35]	100-300 mg qd-tid 250-500 mg qd-tid 200-400 mg qd-tid 10,000-15,000 IU To bowel tolerance (TBT) 1000-5000 IU qd 250-500 mg qd-tid 400-800 mcg qd 120-240 mg qd	To improve effectiveness and chemoresistance To reduce toxicity, chemoresistance	Curcumin interactions Quercitin, silymarin and curcumin on days receiving chemotherapy Do not use regularly, unless chemoresistance until after chemotherapy
Doxorubicin (Adriamycin)	Green tea[36] Quercitin[37] Vitamin A[38-39] Vitamin C[38-39] Vitamin E[38-39] CoQ10[40-41] L-Carnitine[68] Vitamin A[38-39] Vitamin C[38-39] Vitamin E[38-39]	5-10 cups qd 100-300 mg qd-tid 10,000-50,000 IU TBT 10,000-50,000 IU 100 mg qd 100-500 mg qd to tid 10,000-50,000 IU TBT 10,000-50,000 IU	To increase effectiveness, and chemoresistance To reduce toxicity cardiotoxicity To decrease toxicity	Avoid NAC and high- dose vitamin B-6 above 200 mg qd After therapy sequence is complete use high-dose CoQ10, 12 mg qd
Methotrexate	L-Glutamine[10,43,45,46] Vitamin A[44]	10 g, tid, swish and swallow 10,000-50,000 IU	To increase effectiveness To reduce toxicity, mucositis, stomatitis, cachexia	Avoid high doses of folic acid and glutathione

Integrated chemotherapeutic and naturopathic therapies continued

Chemotherapy Drug	Naturopathic Complement	Therapeutic Dosage (Daily)	Action	Cautions Interactions
Fluorouracil (5-FU)	Quercitin[13] Aloe[48] Lentinan[49] Vitamins A[38-39] Vitamins C[38-39] Vitamins E[38-39]	100-300 mg qd-tid 10,000-50,000 IU TBT 10,000-50,000 IU	To increase effectiveness, chemoresistance	Carotenoids L-Glutamine and elevated liver enzymes 3x higher than the normal limits
	CoQ10[50] L-Glutamine[10,51] Vitamin B-6 Castor oil[52]	100 mg qd 10 g, tid, swish/swallow 200 mg qd Topically applied prophy-lactically to palms and plantar surfaces and covered at night for hand/foot syndrome	To reduce toxicity, cardiotoxicity, PPE, peripheral neuropathy	
Vincristine	Vitamin C[53] Vitamin A[54]	10,000-50,000 IU TBT	To increase effectiveness	Iscador
Taxol	Vitamin C[55]	TBT	To increase effectiveness	
	L-Glutamine[56]	10 g, tid swish/swallow	To reduce toxicity	
Interleukin -2	Melatonin[57-60]	20 mg qhs	To increase effectiveness and reduce toxicity	
CPT- 11(Irinotecan or Camptosar)	EPA[85,90,96] (Omega-3, fish oil) Milk thistle[14,20]	2-3 g qd 250-500 mg tid	To reduce side effects	Avoid all laxatives Stop diarrhea early and aggressively with the BRAT(Y) diet and treating mucositis with L-Glutamine
	Green tea[63]	5-10 cups qd	To increase benefit To induce apoptosis	
Oxaliplatin	Glutamine[43] Selenium[34] EPA[85,90,96] (Omega-3, fish oil) Mushrooms[16,31]	10 mg tid swish/swallow, away from food 400-800 mcg qd 2-3 g qd	To reduce side effects and toxicity To prevent PPE and neutropenia	

❖ In Cisplatin, there is a cumulative renal insuffi-ciency, severe mucositis/stomatitis, nausea and vomiting, as well as associated ototoxicity[14,19]

❖ Carboplatin has a lower toxic side effects associ-ated with its use[15]

Naturopathic Complement

Platinum compounds are very toxic with side effects, including peripheral neuropathy.

ANTITUMOR ANTIBIOTICS
Pharmaceuticals

Actinomycin D, Bleomycin, Daunorubicin, Doxoru-bicin (Adriamycin), Doxil (liposomal doxorubicin), Epirubicin, Idarubicin, Mitomycin C, Mitramycin[9]

Pharmacology

Antitumor antibiotics include the related antimicro-bial compounds that produce *Sterptomyces* species in culture and bind with DNA, thus inhibiting DNA and RNA synthesis. This strategy is cell cycle non specific and is only useful in slow growing tumors.

Combination Therapies[9]

* Adriamycin in combination with Cytoxan in breast cancer (AC)
* Mitomycin C with Leucovorin (a folinic acid) and 5-FU with Floxuridine (FUDR) in metastatic colon cancer
* Liposomal Adriamycin (Doxil) used as a single agent in ovarian cancer

Toxicities and Side Effects[9]

* Myelosuppression, pan alopecia, mucostitis/stomatitis, nausea/vomiting, radiation recall, cardiotoxicity, associated especially with Adriamycin
* Hand/Foot syndrome (palmar-plantar erythrodyshesis associated especially with Doxil
* Renal and pulmonary toxicity associated especially with Mitomycin

ANTIMETABOLITES
Pharmaceuticals[9]

Asparaginase, Chlorodeoxyadenosine, Cytosine arabinoside, Deoxycoformycin, Floxuridine (FUDR), Fludarabine phosphate, Capecitabine (Xeloda), Flourouracil (5-FU), Gemcitabine (Gemzar), Hydroxyurea, Mercaptopurine, Methotrexate, Thioguanin.

Pharmacology

Antimetabolites are the structural analogues of normal molecules that are essential for cell growth and replication. They inhibit enzyme production for DNA synthesis, leading to strand breaks and premature chain termination that act in S phase cell cycle and are most effective when cell proliferation is rapid.

Combination Therapies[9]

* 5-FU with Leuocovorin in colon cancer and with Methotrexate
* Cytoxan in breast cancer (CMF)
* Xeloda as a single agent in metastatic breast cancer resistant to anthracyclines and taxanes
* Gemzar as a single agent in pancreatic cancer and metastatic ovarian cancer.

Toxicities and Side Effects[9]

* Myelosuppression, mucositis/stomatitis, nausea and vomiting, diarrhea
* Hand/foot syndrome (palmar-plantar erythrodysthesia) especially associated with Xeloda

* Photosensitivity especially associated with 5-FU and Methotrexate
* Pan alopecia especially with 5-FU

Naturopathic Complement

Myelosuppression is one of the greatest concerns in all patients receiving chemotherapy. This side effect ranges from frank leucopenia to anemias that will interrupt chemotherapy treatment sequences. If the red blood cell or white blood cell counts go to a dangerously low level, treatments will not be administered. This interruption decreases the chemotherapeutic effect and creates the potential for chemoresistance.

Neutropenic Responses to Treatments[30,31]
Use these two medicinal mushrooms:

* Fungiperfecti from Stametes. The Stametes mushroom products are all mycelium instead of mushroom and have an increased biological activity. Stametes 7 is a seven mushroom blend of Royal sun blazeii, cordyceps, reishi, maitake, chaga, lion's mane, and mesima. Each cap is 500 mg of certified organic freeze dried mushroom mycelium. Take 1-2 caps up to t.i.d.
* Trametes versicolus (Turkey tails). Each capsule 500 mg or organic freeze dried mycelium 1-2 caps up to t.i.d.
* If these mushroom blends do not increase the WBC count as desired, add to the mushroom mix Ashwagandha (Withania) organic only, 500 mg-1000 mg up to t.i.d.[25-26]
* Also note that glutamine will also treat and prevent neuropathy but should have been already in use prior to the start of chemotherapy to prevent mucositis.[10]

TOPOISOMERASE INHIBITORS
Pharmaceuticals[9]

Etoposide (VP-16), Teniposide, Irinotecan (CPT-11, Camptosar), Topotecan (Hycamtin).

Pharmacology

Topoisomerase inhibitors are cell cycle inhibitors. Etoposide and Teniposide are podophyllin derivatives from may apple (*Podophyllum spp.*). This action induces an irreversible blockade of cells in premitotic phases of the cell cycle, late G2 and S phases, while also interfering with topoisomerase II function. Camptosar and Topotecan act in S phase by inhibiting topoisomerase and causing double stranded DNA changes. Topotecan can be used a single agent in metastatic ovarian cancer.[9]

Combination Therapies[9]

- Topoisomerase inhibitors with other chemotherapies such as: VP-16 with Ifosfamide, Carboplatin (ICE) in high dose chemotherapy applications with stem cell transplantation
- VP-16, Ifosfamide, Carboplatin in NSCLC and metastatic breast cancer (mini ICE)
- CPT-11 in combination with Leucovorin, 5-FU in metastatic colon cancer

Toxicities and Side Effects[9]

These are dose dependent, and some of the individual drugs have fewer side effects than others. Diarrhea associated mucositis, nausea and vomiting, myelosuppression, pan alopecia, and hypotension associated especially with rapid infusion rates of Etoposide and Teniposide.

Naturopathic Complement

Glutamine, catnip tea (catrepeta), DGL or rhizinate lozenges, cannabis.

MICROTUBULE INHIBITORS
Pharmaceuticals[9]

Docetaxel (Taxotere), Paclitaxel (Taxol), Vinorelbine (Navelbine), Vinblastine sulfate (Velban), Vincristine sulfate (Oncovin)

Pharmacology

Microtubule inhibitors are derived from the vinca alkaloids in periwinkle (*Vinca spp.*). The alkaloids Vincristine and Vinblastine act in G1 and S phase by inhibiting microtubule formation while also inhibiting DNA and RNA formation. The Taxanes (Taxol and Taxotere) are derived from the Pacific Yew tree (*Taxus spp.*) and act in the G2 and M phase to stabilize the microtubule and thus, inhibit cellular division.[9]

Combination Therapies[9]

- Taxol and Carboplatin in ovarian and NSCLC
- Taxotere and Navelbine in metastatic breast cancer or as a single agent in metastatic breast cancer

Toxicities and Side Effects[9]

- Microtubule inhibitors create peripheral neuropathy, which is usually dose limiting
- Transient arthralgia and myalgia, especially with Taxol
- Myelosuppression, pan alopecia, nausea/vomiting and constipation

Naturopathic Complement[9]

Mucositis induced constipation or constipation associated with opiods and other narcotic medications used for pain can be very uncomfortable and chronic. Cherry juice protocol: Use concentrated cherry juice only (no sweeteners or other juices added) to create a peristaltic reflex stimulus. 4-6 oz of cherry juice 3-6 times daily. Use the cherry juice as a bowel training mechanism – 4-6 oz to induce a bowel movement within a few hours – if no bowel movement repeat dose. Try to have the patient train the bowels to move the same time each day. It is usually easier to stimulate after a meal because the act of chewing and swallowing initates peristalsis. Cherry juice is a low glycemic index, high antioxidant, high pynogenal initiator of peristalsis.

Also use EPA 2-3 g q.d., glutamine, medicinal mushrooms, ashwagandha, cannabis.[9,10,25,26,31]

MONOCLONAL ANTIBODIES
Pharmaceuticals[9]

Rituximab (Rituxan), Trastuzumab (Herceptin)

Pharmacology

Monoclonal antibodies are specific. Rituxan is a genetically engineered chimeric (murine and human) monoclonal antibody that is directed against the CD20 antigen on malignant B lymphocytes. Herceptin is a recombinant humanized monoclonal antibody that targets HER2 receptors on some cancer cells, especially indicated for breast cancer + HER2/neu. Chemotherapeutic strategies include the use of Herceptin in metastatic breast cancer that has overexpressed the HER2 protein and can be used in previously treated cases with one or more chemotherapies. Rituxan targets CD20+ B cell non Hodgkin's lymphoma.[9]

Toxicities and Side Effects[9]

The toxicities are also drug specific. Rituxan has hypersensitivity reactions, serious cardiac arrhythmias with global clinical manifestations that include fever with chills, hypotension, bronchospasm with dyspnea, angioedema, headache, nausea and vomiting. Herceptin has dose-limiting cardiomyopathy, fever and chills, nausea, vomiting and diarrhea.

Naturopathic Complement

For cardiomyopathy, CoQ10, L-carnitine, hawthorn berry solid extract ¼-½ tsp q.d. to t.i.d.[68,144,148]

BIOLOGICAL RESPONSE MODIFIERS
Pharmaceuticals[9]

Interferon, Bacillus Calmette-Guerin, Erythropoetin, G-SCF, GM-SCF, Interleukin-2

Pharmacology

The pharmacology of the biological response modifiers

is drug specific: Erythropoetin (Procrit, Epogen, Aranesp, EPO) stimulates the division and differentiation of committed erythroid progenitor cells. G-SCF (Neupagen and Neulasta) do the same thing but stimulate the white blood cell line. GM-SCF (Leukine and Prokine) promote growth and differentiation of myeloid progenitor cells and promote the survival of granulocytes, eosinophils, monocytes and macrophages and induces IL-1 and TNF. These drugs are used as interventions for chemotherapy induced side effects: Procrit for chemotherapy- induced anemia indicated especially in nonmyeloid malignancies; Neupagen/Neulasta and Leukine for granulocytopenia secondary to chemotherapy or from primary bone marrow cancers/metastatic disease.[9]

Toxicities and Side Effects[9]

- Procrit causes associated edema, diarrhea, and hypertension
- Neupogen/Neulasta and Luekine cause long bone pain, musculoskeletal leg cramping, and back pain, as well as general flu-like symptoms

Radiation Therapy

Radiation therapy involves the treatment of cancer cells with ionizing radiation. The aim is to damage the cancerous cells in the target tissue area being treated, while trying to avoid healthy tissue. Although this application damages both cancerous and normal cells, the normal cells have the ability to repair themselves more quickly than the cancer cells.

Radiation Treatments[9]
- External Beam
- Chemosensitizing
- Intensity Modulated Radiation Therapy (IMRT)
- Tomotherapy
- High Dose Rate (HDR) Brachytherapy
- Mammosite

KINDS OF RADIOTHERAPY

External Beam Radiation

This is one of the most common forms of radiation treatment (XRT). External beam XRT uses a linear accelerator to direct radiation into the tumor and tumor bed. This procedure lasts for minutes and is repeated usually 5 days in a row out of a 7 day week over a course of 6 to 8 weeks. It may be used in conjunction with surgery and chemotherapy.

Chemosensitizing XRT

This XRT combines the external beam with low doses of chemotherapy. This strategy is to chemosensitize the tumor cells to the radiation treatment. Side effects tend to be low due to the low doses of chemotherapy used.

Intensity Modulated Radiation Therapy[9]

This procedure changes the size, shape, and intensity of the external beam XRT to coordinate to the size, shape and location of the tumor. A linear accelerator (linac) is a device that uses a number of chambers, each of which adds energy to the electrons, thus accelerating them to higher energies in the megavoltage range. A multileaf collimator (MLC) opens and closes individual leaves to regulate the amount of radiation passing through the patient. IMRT is usually delivered from several different directions (5-13 pinpoint locations). The greater the number of pinpoint locations of the beam, the higher the dose that will be confined to the tumor, thus reducing the risk of side effects. Conventional IMRT requires a lengthy and complicated set up process for each treatment fraction and often the aid of 'tattooing' these locations, or creating wire mesh molds to hold the area still are used. The more beam directions required for the treatment, the more time for each treatment fraction is required.

Tomotherapy[9]

This XRT combines in one system treatment planning, patient positioning, and treatment delivery. This allows a precise treatment delivery and the ability to use doses without increasing radiation exposure to healthy tissues. A CT and planning software are used to establish the precise 3D contours for each tumor area and any regions of risk including organs or surrounding structures. The radiation dose as well as acceptable levels of radiation for these surrounding structures is calculated by the radiation oncologist and a physicist. The planning software calculates the appropriate pattern, position, and intensity of the radiation beam to be delivered in a 360° fashion. The CT scan is done prior to each treatment to verify the position of the tumor and to adjust for changes in the patient's positioning for treatment. The treatment delivery combines IMRT with a helical delivery pattern. The radiation produced by a linear accelerator travels in multiple circles around the gantry ring. The linac moves in unison with a multileaf collimator, which has two sets of interlaced leaves that move quickly to constantly modulate the radiation as it leaves the accelerator. The couch is also moving, guiding the patient slowly through the center of the gantry ring so that each time the linac comes around, it is directing the beam at the target tissue site at a slightly different plane giving a surrounding 3D treatment effect.

Brachytherapy

This procedure uses multiple catheters (up to 30) that are implanted in the tumor and surrounding treatment area.[9] It used in breast, prostate, and lung cancers. After placement of the catheters, radioactive seeds are delivered into each catheter to treat the target area. A seed is delivered into each catheter twice a day for up to 5 days. The total treatment for each session is approximately 20 minutes, and the catheters are removed after each treatment is completed.

Mammosite

A small balloon attached to a thin catheter is placed in the lumpectomy cavity.[9] A radioacative seed is placed within the balloon by a computer controlled machine. Radiation is delivered to a depth of approximately 2 mm. When mammosite XRT is used as a primary treatment, the seed placement is delivered twice a day for up to 5 days. When it is used as a boost therapy and is combined with external beam XRT, it is delivered over 1 to 2 days.

COMMON RADIATION SIDE EFFECTS

Radiation side effects are dependent on the type, amount, and location of the treatment.[9]

- ❖ Radiation- induced fatigue is the most commonly seen side effect regardless of the type of radiation. There is an increased risk in patients who have advanced stage disease, are treated with large radiotherapy fields, have a low pre-radiotherapy hemoglobin level, or poor nutritional status and whose lymphocyte counts are not correlating with the fatigue.
- ❖ Mucositis, stomatitis, and xerostomia are often common and can lead to a poor nutritional status and secondary co-infections, such as candidiasis.
- ❖ Acute diarrhea is not only associated with mucositis reactions, but in radiotherapy directed to the pelvis for prostate or gynecological cancers, it has an increased incidence.
- ❖ Chronic proctitis and dermatitis can be associated with the positioning of the beam application.
- ❖ Radiation-induced cognitive dysfunction

NATUROPATHIC THERAPIES FOR RADIATION SIDE EFFECTS

Radiation-induced fatigue

1. Exercise

It has been shown improving physical function helps combat radiation induced fatigue.[50] Exercise in a randomized controlled breast cancer study showed exercise may mitigate fatigue in breast cancer patients receiving radiation therapy.

30 minutes per day for 3-6 days.[66,67]

2. L-Carnitine

This amino acid has been shown to reduce cancer-related fatigue, not specifically to XRT, with responding clinical improvement.

Divided doses up to 4-6 g q.d.[68]

Radiation-induced mucositis

1. L-Glutamine

This side effect can be treated or prevented with the use of the amino acid L-Glutamine. Glutamine has also been shown to treat radiation-induced hyperpermeability and to protect lymphocytes. It attenuates gut permeability in patients during chemoradiotherapies. Dose: 10 g, t.i.d., swish and swallow.[10,43,69-71]

2. Honey

The use of honey showed a significant reduction in the symptomatic grade 3/4 mucositis in patients treated with honey post radiotherapy, and 55% of the patients treated with topical honey also showed a positive gain in body weight. Radiation-induced xerostomia showed improvements with just a teaspoon of honey daily. The natural bacterial content of honey has shown to decrease *Streptococcus mutans* colonies that are opportunistic in radiation-induced xerostomia patients. Dose: 1 tsp gd-prn.[73-74]

3. Vitamin E

Radiation-induced mucositis treated with natural vitamin E (alpha-tocopherol) as a topical oral rinse before and after radiation treatment showed a reduced risk of acquiring mucositis and also significantly decreased oral pain. Dose: 200-1000 IU.[72]

Radiation-induced diarrhea

1. L-Glutamine

This side effect can be prevented and treated with glutamine.

Dose: 10 g t.i.d., swish and swallow, away from food.[10,43,69-71]

Naturopathic Radiosensitizing Therapies

Naturopathic Therapy	Therapeutic Dose	Cautions/Interactions
Curcumin longa	500-1000 g (activated) qd-tid[93,101,104]	Discontinue during chemotherapy
Quercetin	100-1000 g qd-tid[13,37]	Discontinue during chemotherapy
Proteolytic enzymes	3-5 qd-tid between meals[82]	Discontinue during chemotherapy
Ginkgo biloba	60-120 qd-tid[7,35,115]	Discontinue during chemotherapy
Selenium	200-600 mcg[21]	Discontinue during chemotherapy

2. Probiotics and Prebiotics

Using probiotics aids prebiotic implantation in the treatment of radiation-induced diarrhea and has shown to preserve intestinal integrity and prevent radiation-induced diarrhea.

Dose: 50 billion CFU, b.i.d.[76]

Radiation-induced proctitis

1. Vitamin C and E

This side effect was significantly improved with the use of vitamin E and C; improving symptoms of bleeding, diarrhea and fecal urgency all sustainable in a one year follow up period.

Dose: Vitamin C: TBT, Vitamin E: 400-1200 IU.[77]

Radiation-induced dermatitis

1. Calendula

This side effect was shown to be reduced with *Calendula officinalis succus*. This medicinal herb is highly effective for the prevention of acute radiation-induced dermatitis of grade 2 or higher.

Dose: Topical gel.[78,79]

Radiation-induced cognitive dysfunction

1. Vitamin E

This side effect was shown to be significantly improved with the use of vitamin E (alpha-tocopherol) orally in patients with temporal lobe radionecrosis. Vitamin E at 2000 IU daily for one year resulted in significant improvements in global cognitive ability, memory, verbal and visual skill, but no difference was noted in language or attention.

Dose: 2000 IU q.d.[4,81,110]

2. Melatonin

Melatonin is effective for chemotherapy and radiotherapy co-management use. Oral melatonin is con-sidered at therapeutic dosing at 20 mg nightly. Melatonin has shown to decrease XRT related toxicities with better associated survival curves over a one year period.[80]

Radiation and Antioxidants

Antioxidants are generally recommended if the antioxidants are of an exogenous nature. Endogenous antioxidants are those that are formed naturally in the body's systems, while exogenous are antioxidants that cannot be formed by the body itself. Antioxidants and radiation therapies have shown promise in early clinical trials using green tea (ECGC) and radiation therapies on different cancer cell lines.[63,91]

RADIOSENSITIZATION

Radiosensitization of cancer cells is a therapeutic goal.[9] Oxygenated tissue is the most radiosensitive, while large tumors tend to have hypoxic centers that necrose with continued aberrant growth. Oxygenated tissue saturation increase creates a decrease in hypoxia in the tumor. Radiosensitizers, hyperthermia, and correcting chemo/radio induced anemia helps achieve this state. Hypoxia limits the initiation of cytotoxicity in the tumor, which can lead to radio/chemotherapy resistance; this is also a predisposition to tumor metastases.

Cancer cells are most sensitive to radiation at the M and late G2 phases of cell replication. Cells are less sensitive to radiation in the early S and G1/G0 phases. The strategy is that radiation leads to a mitotic delay in the cell cycle replication, thus effectively reaching cell cycle arrest.[9]

Surgery

Naturopathic therapies can also play a complementary role in surgical treatments for cancer. Surgery precautions include preventive strategies to control bleeding and manage anesthesia effects. There are many foods and herbs that can affect coagulation adversely and should be avoided prior to surgery. Following surgery, anticoagulant effects and clearance of anesthesia are primary concerns. Likewise, there are foods and herbs that can promote coagulation of the blood and detoxification of anesthesia.

INTERACTIONS

There can be many miscellaneous interactions with anticoagulation therapy that can be dangerous. If the integrative therapeutics are helping the patient QOL and outcomes, then the therapeutic levels of anticoagulant effects should be monitored with PT, PTT, and INR so that anticoagulation drugs can be reduced accordingly. It should be noted that some natural substances, such as vitamin E, EPA, and ginkgo, do not affect PT, PTT and INR and must be used cautiously.

Supplementation should be discontinued 3 to 7 days prior to surgery, but this caution does not include homeopathics, which can be used right up until the time of surgery. However, the American Society of Anesthesiologists suggests that all herbal medications be discontinued 2 to 3 weeks before any surgery.

MICROMETASTASIS

Pre- and post surgery protocols have been designed to prevent the spread of the micrometastatic cells of the cancerous tumor, to speed healing and recovery from surgery, and to reduce infections by immuno-nutraceuticals. Surgery has the potential to misplace cancerous cells via biopsy or other surgical procedures. Up to 85% of cancer cell types have a galectin-3 receptor, which plays an active role in cancer cell adhesion and metastasis. Modified citrus pectin has been shown to interfere with cell-to-cell interactions mediated by cell surface carbohydrate binding galectin-3 molecules, thus helping to prevent metastatic disease. Pectasol-C (Econeugenes), 1 scoop, b.i.d.[83,84]

IMMUNOMODULATION

Immunomodulation has been studied mostly in post operative probands with most of the research focused on gastrointestinal tract cancers. The most widely studied substances are glutamine, arginine, EFAs (omega-3, DHA/EPA), and RNA influencing factors. Two 1999 studies show supplementation with all three natural strategies made a significant decrease in pre-albumin and retinol- binding protein, and fewer post operative complications with lowered sepsis scores and a shortened length of hospital stay.[86]

In 2001, these three naturopathic interventions were used again and a lowering of CRP was noted with higher nitric oxide, total lymphocytes (T lymphs, T helper and NK cells), and lower postoperative levels of IL6 and TNF-α.[87] In 2002, it was shown that preoperatively these strategies lowered infection rate and improved significantly gut microperfusion, immune response, and gut oxygenation.[88] Immunonutrients were shown to affect weight loss, postoperative infection rate, and length of hospital stay in another 2002 study.[89] In 2004, further study into the integrative strategy of immunonutrition with omega-3 supplementation alone revealed significantly increased serum protein with active lymphocyte proliferation, and with a relative relation between fat mass and omega-3 to omega-6 ratios.[90]

NATUROPATHIC COMPLEMENTS TO SURGERY COAGULANTS

Several medicinal herbal interactions will actually strengthen the action of anticoagulant therapy by a heterogenous mechanism of action.

Medicinal Herb (Coagulant)[92]
- Danshen (*Salvia miltiorrhiza*)
- Dong quai (*Angelica sinensis*)
- Garlic (*Allium sativim*)
- Ginger (*Zingiber officinalis*)
- Ginkgo (*Ginkgo biloba*)
- Ginseng (*Panax ginseng*)
- Horse Chestnut (*Aesculus hippocastanum*)
- Red Clover (*Trifolium praterse*)
- St John's wort (*Hypericum perforatum*)

Antioxidant Research

The limited information available suggests that endogenously produced antioxidants and thiol-containing compounds may interfere with the effectiveness of some chemoradiotherapies. More than 100 citations of human studies show differing results due to study design, type of malignancy, interventional protocol, and regimen. Inconsistencies preclude a definitive conclusion on using antioxidants conjunctively. However, it is known that total antioxidant status declines with chemotherapies and radiation, and a low antioxidant status may be associated with increased neoplastic activity and subsequent poor quality of life and overall health. In brief, use antioxidants with confidence in their efficacy but with caution for possible adverse interactions.[91,99]

ONCOLOGICAL USE OF ANTIOXIDANTS

Foods and herbs to avoid due to possible interactions with anticoagulant drugs.[2]
These foods and herbs should be avoided for 3 to 7 days prior to surgery and 3-7 days after surgery, if possible.

Alfalfa	Angelica
Bladderwrack	Borage seed
Bromelain	Buchu
Cabbage	Caffeine
Capsicum	Cat's claw
Chlorella	Cod liver oil
Coenzyme Q10	Coffee
Corn silk	Cranberry
Danshen	Devil's claw
DHA	DHEA
DIIM (Diindolylmethane)	Dong Quai
Echinacea	EDTA
EPA	EPO
Fenugreek	Feverfew
Forskolin	GLA
Garlic	Ginger
Ginkgo	Ginseng
Glucosamine sulfate	Goldenseal
Grape fruit	Grape seed
Great Plantain	Green tea
Guarana	Guggul
Holy basil	Horse chestnut
I3C (Indole 3 carbinol)	IP6
Ipriflavone	Kava
Kudzu	L-Carnitine
Licorice	Lycium
Mate	Melatonin
Milk thistle	N-acetyl-cysteine
Nattokinase	Onion
Oolong tea	Pantethine
Papaya	Parsley
Pau D'Arco	Policosanol
Red clover	Reishi
Resveratrol	Saw palmetto
See buckthorn	Soy
Spinach	St. John's wort
Stinging nettles	Tumeric
Valerian	Vanadium
Vinpocetine	Vitamins A,C, E, K
Willow bark	Wine
Yarrow	Activated charcoal
Black walnut	Cascara
Glucomannan	Larch arabinogalactan
Marshmallow	Raspberry leaf
Rice bran	Slippery elm
Sorrel	Sage

Angiogenesis inhibition

The biology of proliferating cancer cells causes cytokines that stimulate increase endothelial cells, which then increases vascular supply to the tumor. Antioxidants inhibit these cytokines: IL-1. IL-8, bFGF (basic fibroblast growth factor), TGF (transforming growth factor, both alpha and beta), PD-EGF (platelet permeability factor), VPF (vascular permeability factor), TNF (tumor necrosis factor).

Vitamin E reduces IL-8 production and angiogenesis; and appears to prevent tumor formation by stimulating a potent immune response to selectively destroy tumor cells. Epigallocatechin is most effective in reducing IL-8 production and angiogenesis. Consumption of green tea catechins or supplemental vitamin E has preventative effects on tumor development.[122]

Cellular membrane integrity

Studies show that lipid peroxidation/protein oxidation in membranes can be prevented by endogenous natural antioxidants. Lycopene could play a role in the recovery of the integrity of biological membranes of the liver after radiation injury.[95] Omega-3 rich diets have beneficial anticancer effects when adding antioxidants such as vitamins E and C.[96]

Exogenous Antioxidants
For radiotherapy side effects, exogenous antioxidants are generally recommended. Endogenous antioxidants are formed naturally in the body's systems, while exogenous are antioxidants that cannot be formed by the body itself. Antioxidants and radiation therapies have shown promise in early clinical trials using green tea (ECGC) and radiation therapies on different cancer cell lines.

Apoptosis

P53 is one of the genetic mediators of apoptosis, and 50% of cancers have abnormal P53 activity.[97] P53 gene mutation was an independent prognostic marker of early relapse and death in breast cancer.[98] A measurement of P53 mutations helps to treat the cancer more effectively. Vitamins can induce differentiation and apoptosis in cancer cells. A mixture of antioxidants and vitamins is more effective than individual vitamins. In contrast to cancer cells, normal cells never undergo apoptosis after conventional tx with vitamins (except retinoids).[99]

N-acetyl-cysteine elevates p53 activity and apoptosis in cancer cells but not in healthy cells;[100] and curcumin induces apoptosis in sarcoma, colon, kidney and hepatocellular cancers but not in normal cells.[101]

CAUTION

Although antioxidant supplementation may reduce the frequency and severity of toxicity associated with chemotherapies and radiation, at the present time it is recommended to avoid endogenously produced antioxidants, such as N-acetyl-cysteine and enzyme CoQ10. The potential mechanism of action for these interactions may lead to greater toxicity or treatment failure. If the treatment sequence is interrupted due to cardiomyopathy, arrythmia, or low ejection fraction, CoQ10 300-1200 mg q.d. can be used during the "break." Once therapy starts again, CoQ10 should be discontinued.

A recent study demonstrated that bladder transitional cancer cell lines treated with silybinin experienced significant growth inhibition and apoptosis. These effects were due to activation of capase-3 and modulation of cyclin cascade.[102]

Astragalus increases the activity of Ag-presenting macrophages and of CD4 T cell activity; theoretically, this could lead to increased ADCC with subsequent tumor cell death.[103] Polysaccharide (PSP) from *Coriolus versicolor* mushroom activates macrophages and stimulates TNF. However, a cytotoxic effect on tumor cell lines is not observed.[105] Curcumin induces apoptosis in a p53-independent manner, and at the higher concentrations, induces capase gene expression.[104] EGCG from *Camellia sinensis*, baicalein from *Scutellaria baicalensis,* and *Cimicifuga racemosa* extracts each increase apoptosis in CLL cells; interrupt VEGF survival signals resulting in capase activation and subsequent cell death.[105,106] *Cimicifuga* induces capases in MCF-7 cells.[107] Quercetin blocks epidermal growth factor receptor-signaling pathways, leading to induction of apoptosis.[108]

General Radioprotection Nutrients
- Antioxidants[109-110]
- Vitamin E[111]
- Zinc[112]
- Selenium[111,114]
- *Ginkgo biloba*[115]
- *Curcuma longa*[116]
- Lentinan[117]
- Adaptogens[119,120,121]

Natural Vitamin E (d-alpha-tocopherol)

Vitamin E induces cell differentiation in cancer cells, inhibits their growth, and causes cell death. Selective inhibition of cancer cell growth is shown with the inhibition of protein kinase C and expression of oncogenes. Vitamin E also inhibits phosphorylation and transactivation of the cancer cell, which is important in cell proliferation of healthy cells. Epidemiological studies link vitamin E use with lower risk of prostate cancer. Long-term supplementation with alpha-toco-

pherol substantially reduced prostate cancer incidence (32%) and mortality from prostate cancer (41%) in Finnish male smokers.[123] Toenail and serum samples from male study subjects showed a fivefold reduction in risk of developing prostate cancer in those with highest levels of gamma-tocopherol compared to those with lowest.[124-126] Pumpkin seeds (*Curcubita pepo*) are a good source of gamma-tocopherol.

Vitamin E has been shown to induce apoptosis and suppress tumor growth by 80%.[127] It inhibits gastric carcinoma cell growth *in vitro* in a dose- and time-dependent fashion.[128] It scavenges ROS tocopherol and ascorbate (vitamin C). α-tocopherol and ascorbate, independently and in combination, decrease the production of reactive oxygen species in human spermatocytes exposed to H_2O_2.[129]

The pretreatment of hepatocytes with tocopherol succinate (TS) dramatically enriched cells and mitochondria with alpha-tocopherol and provided these membranes with complete protection against ethyl methanesulfonate (EMS)-induced oxidative damage. TS pretreatment suppressed EMS-induced cellular ROS production, generated from mitochondrial complex I and III sites.[130] Vitamin C supplementation in chronic hemodialysis patients can reduce the lymphocyte intracellular ROS production, as well as up-regulate hOGG1 gene expression for repair.[131]

Vitamin E and ECGC

One study looked at vitamin E and EGCG with the hypothesis that these antioxidants may be antagonistic during radiation treatment. Tumor growth was 10% slower in EGCG fed mice and 3% slower in vitamin E fed mice. EGCG and vitamin E protected normal tissues from severe XRT related soft tissue reactions. Intramoral apoptosis in the EGCG and vitamin E concentrations were 8.3 fold and 1.3 fold increase as compared to control. Tumor cell invasiveness was decreased by 25% with EGCG and vitamin E compared to control.[122]

Vitamin E and EGCG appear to concentrate in tumors, though the mechansim and significance of this is unkown. EGCG (*in vivo*) and vitamin. E (*in vitro*) significantly slow tumor growth, which is likely due to increased apoptosis and decreased cell proliferation.[132] Anti-angiogenic RNA expression in the

EGCG tumors may explain the slower tumor growth. Vitamin E and EGCG did not reach statistical significance in increasing radiation resistance in implanted tumors. Vitamin E and EGCG significantly decrease radiation reactions in normal tissues.[122]

Retinoids

The orange to red pigments found naturally in fruits and vegetables have been shown to control cancer cell growth, repair precancerous lesions, induce cell differentiation, prevent metastasis, prevent formation of a secondary carcinogenesis, control angiogenesis, and be immunostimulating. Carotenoids induce cellular differentiation, inhibit growth of human melanoma cells, stimulate the level of cAMP induced differentiation and betacarotene in particular, and increase expression of the connexin gene, which

functions to hold normal cells together with each other coding for gap junction in genetic code.[123]

The best activity of retinoids is in squamous cell, cervical, renal cell cancers. They are selective for cancer cells. Organ development is not affected.[124]

Retinoid therapeutic actions[123-124]
- Inhibit growth of protein kinase-C
- Reduce oncogene expression
- Reduce transplanted tumor growth
- Reduce tumor size

Lycopene

Lycopene is the primary red carotenoid found in tomatoes and watermelons. There is an inverse

---

MELATONIN STUDIES

Melatonin has shown to decrease XRT-related toxicities with better associated survival curves over a one-year period. It blocks the mitogenic effects of tumor promoting hormones and growth factors.[134] Concomitant administration of melatonin with TMX induces regression in pts. refractory to TMX alone.[135] It reverses LHRH resistance in cancer, and down regulates 5-lipoxygenase gene expression. Melatonin acts as a biological response modifier in cancer patients.[137] Melatonin, a pineal secretory product with antioxidant properties, protects against cisplatin induced nephrotoxicity in rats.[138]

One study involved 63 patients with histologically proven metastatic NSCLC who did not respond to first line cisplatin chemotherapy. They were randomized to either supportive care alone or melatonin (MLT) at 10 mg at an hour before sleep. There was no therapy-related toxicity in the MLT group, and stabilization of disease was higher in the MLT group (10/31 vs 3/32, p<0.05). Mean survival was greater for those in the MLT group (7.9 vs 4.1, p<0.025). Disease stabilization was most frequent in those without liver mets.[139]

Another study of melatonin involved 50 patients with brain mets from various solid tumors who progressed following radiation and chemotherapy. They were randomized to either supportive care alone (steroids + anticonvulsants) or MLT (20 mg at hour of sleep). Time until progression was significantly longer in the MLT group (5.9 ± 0.8 mo. Vs 2.7 ± 1.06 mo., p<0.05). One year survival was also significantly higher in the MLT group (9/24 vs 3/26, p<0.05). When analyzed by site of primary cancer, only those with a single brain met from lung cancer maintained a significant difference (6/10 vs 2/12).[140]

This study involved 20 previously untreated patients with inoperable lung cancer (16 NSCLC, 4 SCLC). They were randomized to receive either carboplatin (5 AUC on day 1) and etoposide (150 mg/m?/day on days 1-3) or carboplatin-etoposide+MLT (40 mg at hour of sleep) in cross over fashion. No effect wasobserved on depth and duration of toxicity for hemoglobin, ANC, or ANC nadir.[141]

Yet another study involved 250 metastatic solid tumor patients (104 lung cancer) with poor clinical status. They were randomized to receive chemotherapy or chemotherapy + MLT (20 mg at hour of sleep). The lung cancer treatment group received Cisplatin + etoposide or gemcitabine. The 1 year survival rate and the objective tumor regression rate were significantly higher in patients concomittantly treated with MLT than chemotherapy (CT) alone. Tumor response rate 42/124 CT + MLT versus 19/126 CT alone (p<0.001). 1 year survival rate 63/124 CT + MLT versus 29/126 CT alone (p<0.001).[142]

One study looked at post chemoradiation activation of membrane lipid peroxidation and the oxidative modification of proteins.In this trial, 45 patients underwent chemoradiation with concurrent supportive therapy including melatonin 3 mg t.i.d., vitamin A 100,000 IU t.i.d., vitamin E 20% , 1 ml SugQ b.i.d. and Echincacea tincture 20 gtt t.i.d.) as compared to 31 patients who only had chemoradiation. 5-FU and irradiation with wide portals was used on both groups. Irradiation with wide portals causes the activation of lipid peroxidation and oxidative damage of proteins. It also causes suppression of antioxidant defense, causing a decline in glutathione peroxidase, catalase, superoxide dismutase, and reduced glutathione levels. Melatonin and antioxidant complexes cause significant decrease of the oxidative modification of proteins and increase reduced glutathione levels. Melatonin activated the synthesis of the antioxidant enzymes, manifesting an increase in the activity of glutathione peroxidase, glutathione reductase and glutahione-S-transferase.[143]

relationship between dietary intake of lycopene and the risk of developing prostate cancer. The data shows that lycopene supplementation in men before radical prostatectomy, pathology results compared to control subjects:

- 73% vs. 18% had no involvement of surgical margins and/or extra-prostatic tissues
- 84% vs. 45% had tumors <4 ml in size
- PSA levels decreased by 18%[95]

Selenium

The essential trace mineral selenium (Se) has been shown to inhibit intestinal, prostate, lung, and liver tumor development and has been associated with mortality in both experimental animals and humans. Although Se is likely to be one of the most powerful cancer chemopreventive agents in the human diet, its mechanism of action is still under investigation. Low Se status results in a decrease in the expression of genes involved in detoxification, thus reducing the amounts of activated carcinogens.[132]

Melatonin

Melatonin has been studied extensively for chemotherapy and radiotherapy co-management use. Oral melatonin is considered therapeutic at a dosing at 20 mg nightly. Melatonin acts as a powerful antioxidant, especially in combination with classic antioxidants, such as vitamin E and A. The free radical induced oxidative stress caused by radiation can be exacerbated by the decreased efficiency of antioxidant mechanisms.[138]

CoQ10

This enzyme is used with vitamin E to protect patients from chemotherapy-induced cardiomyopathies. CoQ10 is nontoxic, even at high dosages, and has been shown to prevent liver damage from the drugs Mitomycin C and 5-FU. Adriamycin-induced cardiomyopathies have been prevented by concomitant supplementation with CoQ10. It also reduces free radical formation induced by doxorubicin. Research studies with both animals and humans have found that pretreating with coenzyme Q10, at levels of 100 mg per day, reduces cardiac toxicity caused by doxorubicin.[144-148]

Cox-2 Inhibition

Cox-2 substances can inhibit angiogenesis, inhibit cell growth and invasion, inhibit tumor associated inflammation, increase pro-apoptotic effects, and inhibit of Prostaglandin 2 (PGE2) associated aromatase induction.[149-153]

Herbal COX-2 inhibitors

- *Glycyrrhiza uralensis:* Isoliquiritigenin decreases COX-2 expression, resulting in decreased PEG-2 and nitric oxide in mouse and human colon carcinoma cells.[154]
- *Phyllanthus amarus* (used to treat viral hepatitis): In-vitro application of extract inhibits induction of iNOS, COX-2, and TNF-α.[155]
- *Zingiber officinalis:* Traditionally used for pelvic inflammation and congestion. *In-vitro* human synoviocytes obtained during primary knee replacement from OA patients incubated with ginger extract demonstrated significantly suppressed production of TNF-alpha COX-2 expression. NF-kappaB was also suppressed, suggesting that ginger blocks transcription of COX-2.[156]
- *Scutellaria baicalensis:* Traditionally used in traditional Chinese medicine for inflammatory and cancerous conditions. COX-2 is highly expressed in head and neck squamous cell carcinoma cells. Oral administration of *Scutellaria baicalensis* to mice inoculated with these cells caused inhibition of COX-2 expression, whereas celecoxib inhibited COX-2 activity directly. No inhibition was seen in mice inoculated with a nontumorigenic cell line, indicating a selective inhibition of COX-2 in tumor cells. A 66% reduction in tumor mass was also observed in these mice.[157]
- Zyflamend™: Natural Cox-2 inhibition in prostate cancer. Cox-1 and Cox-2 enzyme activities decreased with Zyflamend, respectively, at 45% and 80%. PGE2 production decreased by 91%. Apoptosis was induced in cell lines after a 72-hour treatment period. Suppressed cell line growth occurred after a 72-hour treatment. Activity directly inhibited Cox-2 enzyme activity and decreased signaling through PKCdelta and STAT3. It is potentially a chemopreventative agent and is currently in clinical trial with prostatic intraepithelial neoplasia.[158]

References

1. Hofmann J, Fiebig HH, Winterhalter BR, Berger DP, Grunicke H. Enhancement of the antiproliferative activity of cis-diamminedichloroplatinum(II) by quercetin. Int J Cancer. 1990 Mar 15;45(3):536-39.

2. Najat C, et al.. Renal function after Ifosfamide, Carboplatin, and Etoposide (ICE) chemotherapy, nephrectomy, and radiotherapy in children with Wilms Tumour. Eur J Cancer. 2009 Jan;45(1):99-106. Published online 2008 November 6.

3. Navis I, Sriganth P, Premalatha B. Dietary curcumin with cisplatin administration modulates tumour marker indices in experimental fibrosarcoma. Pharmacol Res. 1999 Mar;39(3):175-79.

4. Kobayashi Y, Kariya K, Saigenji K, Nakamura K. Enhancement of anti-cancer activity of cisdiaminedichloroplatinum by the protein-bound polysaccharide of Coriolus versicolor QUEL (PS-K) in vitro. Cancer Biother. 1994;9(4):351-58. Glutathione reduces the toxicity and improves quality of life of women diagnosed with ovarian cancer treated with cisplatin: results of a double-blind, randomised trial. Ann Oncol. 1997 Jun;8(6):569-73.

5. Cascinu S, Cordella L, Del Ferro E, Fronzoni M, Catalano G. Neuroprotective effect of reduced glutathione on cisplatin-based chemotherapy on advanced gastric cancer: a randomized double-blind placebo-controlled trial. J Clin Oncol. 1995 Jan 13(1); 26-32.

6. Pirotzky E, Guilmard C, Sidoti C, Ivanow F, Principe P, Braquet . Platelet-activating factor antagonist, BN-52021 protects against cis-diamminedichloroplatinum nephrotoxicity in the rat. Ren Fail. 1990;12(3):171-76.

7. Bokemeyer C, Fels LM, Dunn T, Voigt W, Gaedeke J, Schmoll HJ, Stolte H, Lentzen H. Silibinin protects against cisplatin-induced nephrotoxicity without compromising cisplatin or ifosfamide anti-tumour activity. Br J Cancer. 1996 Dec;74(12):2036-41.

8. Gaedeke J, et al. Nephrol Dial Transplant. 1996 Jan;11(1):55-62.

9. Hu YJ, Chen Y, et al. The protective role of selenium on the toxicity of cisplatin-contained chemotherapy regimen in cancer patients. Biol Trace Elem Res. 1997 Mar;56(3):331-41.

10. Branda RF, Nigels E, Lafayette AR, Hacker M. Nutritional folate status influences the efficacy and toxicity of chemotherapy in rats. Blood. 1998 Oct 1;92(7):2471-76.

11. Ghosh J, Das S. Role of vitamin A in prevention and treatment of sarcoma 180 in mice. Chemotherapy. 1987;33:211-18.

12. Gribel' NV, Pashinski_ VG. Antimetastatic properties of aloe juice. Vopr Onkol. 1986;32(12):38-40.

13. Davis L, Kuttan G. Effect of Withania somnifera on cyclophosphamide-induced urotoxicity. Cancer Lett. 2000 Jan 1;148(1):9-17.

14. Agarwal R, Diwanay S, Patki P, Patwardhan B. Studies on immunomodulatory activity of Withania somnifera (Ashwagandha) extracts in experimental immune inflammation. op. cit.

15. Agarwal R, Diwanay S, Patki P, Patwardhan B. J Ethnopharmacol. 1999 Oct;67(1):27-35.

16. Hofmann J, Fiebig HH, Winterhalter BR, Berger DP, Grunicke H. Enhancement of the antiproliferative activity of cis-diamminedichloroplatinum(II) by quercetin.

Int J Cancer. 1990 Mar 15;45(3):536-39.

17. Scambia G, De Vincenzo R, et al.Comparative effect of silybin on gynaecological malignancies: synergism with cisplatin and doxorubicin. Eur J Cancer. 1996 May;32A(5):877-82.

18. Navis I, Sriganth P, Premalatha B. Dietary curcumin with cisplatin administration modulates tumour marker indices in experimental fibrosarcoma. Pharmacol Res. 1999 Mar;39(3):175-79.

19. Kobayashi Y, Kariya K, Saigenji K, Nakamura K. Enhancement of anti-cancer activity of cisdiaminedichloroplatinum by the protein-bound polysaccharide of Coriolus versicolor QUEL (PS-K) in vitro. Cancer Biother. 1994 Winter;9(4):351-58.

20. Smith, JE, Rowan NJ, Sullivans R. Medicinal mushrooms: their therapeutic properties and current medical usage with special emphasis on cancer treatments. Cancer Research UK. 2007 monograph. www.icnet.uk

21. Bokemeyer C, Fels LM, et al. Silibinin protects against cisplatin-induced nephrotoxicity without compromising cisplatin or ifosfamide anti-tumour activity. Br J Cancer. 1996 Dec;74(12):2036-41.

22. Gaedeke J, et al. Nephrol Dial Transplant. 1996 Jan;11(1):55-62;

23. Hu YJ, Chen Y, et al. The protective role of selenium on the toxicity of cisplatin-contained chemotherapy regimen in cancer patients. Biol Trace Elem Res. 1997 Mar;56(3):331-41.

24. Fukaya H, Kanno H. Experimental studies of the protective effect of ginkgo biloba extract (GBE) on cisplatin induced toxicity in rats. Nippon Jibinkoka Gakkai Kaiho. 1999. Jul;102(7):907-17.

25. Sugiyama T, Sadzuka Y, Tanaka K, Sonobe T. Inhibition of glutamate transporter by theanine enhances the therapeutic efficacy of doxorubicin. Toxicol Lett. 2001 Apr 30;121(2):89-96.

26. Scambia G, Ranelletti FO, Panici PB, De Vincenzo R, Bonanno G, Ferrandina G, et al. Quercetin potentiates the effect of adriamycin in a multidrug-resistant MCF-7 human breast-cancer cell line: P-glycoprotein as a possible target. Cancer Chemother Pharmacol. 1994;34(6):459-64.

27. Antunes LM, Takahashi CS. Effects of high doses of vitamins C and E against doxorubicin-induced chromosomal damage in Wistar rat bone marrow cells. Mutat Res. 1998 Nov 9;419(1-3):137-43.

28. Faure H, Coudray C, Mousseau M, Ducros V, Douki T, Bianchini F, Cadet J, Favier A. 5-Hydroxymethyluracil excre-

tion, plasma TBARS and plasma antioxidant vitamins in adriamycin-treated patients.Free Radic Biol Med. 1996;20(7):979-83.

29. Sugiyama S, K Yamada, M Hayakawa, T Ozawa. Approaches that mitigate doxorubicin-induced delayed adverse effects on mitochondrial function. Biochem Mol Biol Int.1995;36:1001-07.

30. Neri B, Neri GC, Bandinelli M. Differences between carnitine derivatives and coenzyme Q10 in preventing in vitro doxorubicin-related cardiac damages. Oncology. 1988;45(3):242-46.

31. Noe, JE. L-Glutamine Use in the treatment and prevention of mucositis and cachexia: a naturopathic perspective. Integrative Cancer Ther. 2010 Jan;8(4): 409-15.

32. Rouse K, Nwokedi E, Woodliff JE, Epstein J, Klimberg VS. Glutamine enhances selectivity of chemotherapy through changes in glutathione metabolism. Ann Surg. 1995 Apr;221(4):420-26.

33. Yamamoto J, Horie T, Awazu S.Amelioration of methotrexate-induced malabsorption by vitamin A. Cancer chemotherapy and pharmacology (impact factor: 2.65). 02/1997;39(3):239-44.

34. Lin CM, Abcouwer SF, Souba WW. Effect of dietary glutamate on chemotherapy-induced immunosuppression. Nutrition.1999 Sep;15(9):687-96.

35. Anderson PM, Schroeder G, Skubitz KM. Oral glutamine reduces the duration and severity of stomatitis after cytotoxic cancer hemotherapy. Cancer. 1998 Oct 1;83(7):1433-39.

36. Nakayama Y, Sakamoto H, Satoh K, Yamamoto T. Tamoxifen and gonadal steroids inhibit colon cancer growth in association with inhibition of thymidylate synthase, survivin and telomerase expression through estrogen receptor beta mediated system. Cancer Lett. 2000 Dec 8;161(1):63-71.

37. Gribel' NV, Pashinski_ VG. Antimetastatic properties of aloe juice. Vopr Onkol. 1986;32(12):38-40.

38. Taguchi T et al, Gan To Kagaku Ryoho;12:366-78. Lentinan (Shiitake) extends randomized study the life of gastric cancer patients in an advanced stage or where the disease has returned, in patients with an advanced form of colon cancer seem beneficial effects of lentinan, but is hard enough and other statistical. Gan To Kagaku Ryoho. 1985; 12:366-78.

39. Okada K, Yamada S, Kawashima Y, et al. Cell injury by antineoplastic agents and influence of coenzyme Q10 on cellular potassium activity and potential difference across the membrane in rat liver cells. Cancer Res. 1980 May;40(5):1663-67.

40. Daniele B, Perrone F, Gallo C, et al. Oral glutamine in the prevention of fluorourcil induced intestinal toxicity: a double blind, placebo controlled, randomized trial. Gut. 2001;48:28-33.

41. Nagore E, Insa A, Sanmartin O. Antineoplastic therapy-induced palmar plantar management. Am J Clin Dermatol 2000; 1(4):225-34.

42. Song EJ et al. Potentiation of growth inhibition due to Vincristine by ascorbic acid in a resistant human non-small cell lung cancer cell line. Eur J Pharmacol 1995; 292:2:119-25.

43. M F Leung, K F Wong,The differentiating effect of retinoic acid and vincristine on acute myeloid leukemia..Journal of hematotherapy.1999;8(3):275-79.

44. Kurbacher CM, Wagner U, Kolster B, Andreotti PE, Krebs D, Bruckner HW.

Ascorbic acid (vitamin C) improves the antineoplastic activity of doxorubicin, cisplatin, and paclitaxel in human breast carcinoma cells in vitro. Cancer Lett. 1996 Jun 5;103(2):183-89.

45. Vahdat L, Papadopoulos K, et al. Reduction of paclitaxel-induced peripheral

neuropathy with glutamine. Clin Cancer Res. 2001 May;7(5):1192-97.

46. Lissoni P. Modulation of anticancer cytokines IL-2 and IL-12 by melatonin and the other pineal indoles 5-methoxytryptamine and 5-methoxytryptophol in the treatment of human neoplasms. .Ann N Y Acad Sci. 2000;917:560-67.

47. Lissoni P, Bolis S, Brivio F, Fumagalli L. A phase II study of neuroimmunotherapy with subcutaneous low-dose IL-2 plus the pineal hormone melatonin in untreatable advanced hematologic malignancies. Anticancer Res. 2000 May-Jun;20(3B):2103-05.

48. Lissoni P, Barni S, Cazzaniga M, Ardizzoia A, Rovelli F, Brivio F, Tancini G. Efficacy of the concomitant administration of the pineal hormone melatonin in cancer immunotherapy with low-dose IL-2 in patients with advanced solid tumors who had progressed on IL-2 alone. Oncology. 1994 Jul-Aug;51(4):344-47.

49. Lissoni P, Fumagalli L, Paolorossi F, Rovelli F, Roselli MG, Maestroni GJ. Anticancer neuroimmunomodulation by pineal hormones other than melatonin: preliminary phase II study of the pineal indole 5-methoxytryptophol in association with low-dose IL-2 and melatonin. J Biol Regul Homeost Agents. 1997 Jul-Sep;11(3):119-22.

50. Windsor PM, Nicol KF, Potter J. A randomized, controlled trial of aerobic exercise for treatment-related fatigue in men receiving radical external beam radiotherapy for localized prostate carcinoma. Cancer. 2004 Aug 1;101(3):550-57.

51. Victoria Mock, Constantine Frangakis, et al. Exercise manages fatigue during breast cancer treatment: A randomized controlled trial. Psycho-Oncology. 2005 June;14: 464-77.

52. Cruciani RA, Dvorkin E, et al. L-carnitine supplementation for the treatment of fatigue and depressed mood in cancer patients with carnitine deficiency: a preliminary analysis.Ann NY Acad Sci. 2004;1033:168-76.

53. Cheng, JC. Appropriate endpoint of mucositis and correct statistical method for the drug effect interpretation. Int J Radiat Oncol Biol Phys. 2000 Oct1;48(3):909-10.

54. Yoshida S, Matsui M, Shirouzu Y, Fujita H, Yamana H, Shirouzu K. Effects of glutamine supplements and radiochemotherapy on systemic immune and gut barrier

function in patients with advanced esophageal cancer. Ann Surg. 1998 Apr;227(4):485-91.

55. Huang EY, Leung SW, Wang CJ, Chen HC, Sun LM, Fang FM, Yeh SA, Hsu HC, Hsiung CY. Oral glutamine to alleviate radiation-induced oral mucositis: a pilot randomized trial. Int J Radiat Oncol Biol Phys. 2000 Feb 1;46(3):535-39.

56. Ferreira PR, Fleck JF, Diehl A, Barletta D, Braga-Filho A, Barletta A, Ilha L. Protective effect of alpha-tocopherol in head and neck cancer radiation-induced mucositis: a double-blind randomized trial. Head Neck. 2004 Apr;26(4):313-21.

57. Sela MO, Shapira L, Grizim I, Lewinstein I, Steinberg D, Gedalia I, Grobler SR. Effects of honey consumption on enamel microhardness in normal versus xerostomic patients.J Oral Rehabil. 1998 Aug;25(8):630-34.

58. Sela M, Maroz D, Gedalia I. Streptococcus mutans in saliva of normal subjects and neck and head irradiated cancer subjects after consumption of honey. J Oral Rehabil. 2000 Mar;27(3):269-70.

59. Hanna N, Shepherd FA, et al. Randomized phase III trial of pemetrexed versus docetaxel in patients with non-small-cell lung cancer previously treated with chemotherapy. J Clin Oncol. 2004 May 1;22(9):1589-97.

60. Salminen E, Elomaa I, Minkkinen J, Vapaatalo H, Salminen S. Preservation of intestinal integrity during radiotherapy using live Lactobacillus acidophilus cultures.Clin Radiol. 1988 Jul;39(4):435-37.

61. Kennedy M, Bruninga K, Mutlu EA, Losurdo J, Choudhary S, Keshavarzian A. Successful and sustained treatment of chronic radiation proctitis with antioxidant vitamins E and C. Am J Gastroenterol. 2001 Apr;96(4):1080-84.

62. Pommier P, Gomez F, Sunyach MP, D'Hombres A, Carrie C, Montbarbon X. Phase III randomized trial of Calendula officinalis compared with trolamine for the prevention of acute dermatitis during irradiation for breast cancer. J Clin Oncol. 2004 Apr 15;22(8):1447-53.

63. Pommier P, Gomez F, Sunyach MP, D'Hombres A, Carrie C, Montbarbon X. Phase III randomized trial of Calendula officinalis compared with trolamine for the prevention of acute dermatitis during irradiation for breast cancer. J Clin Oncol. 2004 Apr 15;22(8):1447-53.

64. Lissoni P, Meregalli S, Nosetto L, Barni S, Tancini G, Fossati V, Maestroni G. Increased survival time in brain glioblastomas by a radioneuroendocrine strategy with radiotherapy plus melatonin compared to radiotherapy alone. Oncology. 1996 Jan-Feb;53(1):43-46.

65. Prasad KN. Rationale for using high-dose multiple dietary antioxidants as an adjunct to radiation therapy and chemotherapy.J Nutr. 2004 Nov;134(11):3182S-3S.

66. Lund EL, Quistorff B, Spang-Thomsen M, Kristjansen PE. Effect of radiation therapy on small-cell lung cancer is reduced by ubiquinone intake. Folia Microbiol (Praha). 1998;43(5):505-06.

67. Lund EL, Quistorff B, Spang-Thomsen M, Kristjansen PE. Effect of radiation therapy on small-cell lung cancer is reduced by ubiquinone intake.Folia Microbiol (Praha). 1998;43(5):505-06.

68. Argento A, Tiraferri E, Marzaloni M. [Oral anticoagulants and medicinal plants. An emerging interaction.] [Article in Italian]. Ann Ital Med Int. 2000 Apr-Jun;15(2):139-43.

69. Izzo AA, Ernst E. Interactions between herbal medicines and prescribed drugs: a systematic review. Drugs 2001;61(15):2163-75.

70. Fugh-Berman A. Herb-drug interactions. Lancet. 2000 Jan 8;355(9198):134-38.

71. Anna Rita Bilia, Sandra Gallori, Franco F Vincieri.St. John's wort and depression: efficacy, safety and tolerability-an update. Life Sci. 2002 May 17;70 (26):3077-96.

72. Pienta KJ, Naik H, Akhtar A, Yamazaki K, Replogle TS, Lehr J, Donat TL, Tait L, Hogan V, Raz A. Inhibition of spontaneous metastasis in a rat prostate cancer model by oral administration of modified citrus pectin. J Natl Cancer Inst. 1995 Mar 1;87(5):348-53.

73. Nangia-Makker P, Hogan V, Honjo Y, Baccarini S, Tait L, Bresalier R, Raz A. Inhibition of human cancer cell growth and metastasis in nude mice by oral intake of modified citrus pectin. J Natl Cancer Inst. 2002 Dec 18;94(24):1854-62.

74. Gianotti L, Braga M, Fortis C, Soldini L, Vignali A, Colombo S, Radaelli G, Di Carlo V. A prospective, randomized clinical trial on perioperative feeding with an arginine-, omega-3 fatty acid-, and RNA-enriched enteral diet: effect on host response and nutritional status. JPEN J Parenter Enteral Nutr. 1999 Nov-Dec;23(6):314-20.

75. Di Carlo V, Gianotti L, Balzano G, Zerbi A, Braga M. Complications of pancreatic surgery and the role of perioperative nutrition. Dig Surg.1999;16(4):320-26.

76. Wu GH, Zhang YW, Wu ZH. Modulation of postoperative immune and inflammatory response by immune-enhancing enteral diet in gastrointestinal cancer patients. World J Gastroenterol. 2001 Jun;7(3):357-62.

77. Braga M, Gianotti L, Vignali A, Carlo VD. Preoperative oral arginine and n-3 fatty acid supplementation improves the immunometabolic host response and outcome after colorectal resection for cancer. Surgery. 2002 Nov;132(5):805-14.

78. Gianotti L, Braga M, Nespoli L, Radaelli G, Beneduce A, Di Carlo V. A randomized controlled trial of preoperative oral supplementation with a specialized diet in patients with gastrointestinal cancer. Gastroenterology. 2002 Jun;122(7):1763-70.

79. de Luis DA, Izaola O, Aller R, González-Sagrado M, Cuéllar L, Terroba MC. [Utility of a omega 3 fatty acids oral enhanced formula in biochemical parameters of head and neck cancer patients].Med Clin (Barc). 2004 Oct 16;123(13):499-500.

80. Elena J. Ladas, Judith S. Jacobson, Deborah D. Kennedy, Katherine Teel, Aaron Fleischauer and Kara M. Kelly. Antioxidants and cancer therapy: a systemic review. J Clin Oncol. 2004;22:517-28.

81. Zhou S, Lim LY, Chowbay B. Herbal modulation of P-glycoprotein.Drug Metab Rev. 2004 Feb;36(1):57-104.

82. Sivagurunathan S, et al. Dietary curcumin inhibits chemotherapy-induced apoptosis in models of human breast cancer. Cancer Res. 2002;62:3868.

83. Kamat JP, Devasagayam TP, Priyadarsini KI, Mohan H. Reactive oxygen species mediated membrane damage induced by fullerene derivatives and its possible biological implications. Toxicology. 2000 Nov 30;155(1-3):55-61.

84. Saada Helen N, Azab Khaled S. Role of lycopene in recovery of radiation induced injury to mammalian cellular organelles. Pharmazie. 2001 Mar;56(3):239-41.

Yam D et al. Suppression of tumor growth and metastasis by dietary fish oil combined with vitamins E and C and cis-platin. Cancer Chemother Pharmacol 2001; 47:1:34-40.

85. Hunter T, Pines J. Cyclins and cancer II: cyclin D and CDK inhibitors come of age. Cell 1994; 79:573-82.

86. Nicole Falette, Marie-Pierre Paperin, Iet al.Prognostic Value of P53 Gene Mutations in a Large Series of Node-negative Breast Cancer Patients Cancer Res. 1998 April 1; 58:1451-55.

87. Cole WC, Prasad KN. Contrasting effects of vitamins as modulators of apoptosis in cancer cells and normal cells: a review. Nutr Cancer. 1997;29(2):97-103.

88. Donnerstag B., Ohlenschlager G, Cinatl J, Amrani M, Hofmann D, Flindt S, Treusch G, Trager L. Reduced glutathione and S-acetylglutathione as selective apoptosis-inducing agents in cancer therapy. Cancer Lett. 1996;110:63-70.

89. Jiang MC, Yang-Yen HF, Yen JJY, Lin JK. Curcumin induces apoptosis in immortalized NIH 3T3 and malignant cancer cell lines. Nutr Cancer. 1996;26:111-20.

90. Tyagi A, Agarwal C, Harrison G, Glode LM, Agarwal R. Silibinin causes cell cycle arrest and apoptosis in human bladder transitional cell carcinoma cells by regulating CDKI-CDK-cyclin cascade, and caspase 3 and PARP cleavages. Carcinogenesis. 2004 Sep;25(9):1711-20.

91. Zhao KS, Mancini C, Doria G. Enhancement of the immuneresponse in mice by Astragalus membranaceus extracts. Immunopharmacology. 1990;20:225-33.

92. Liu WK, Ng TB, Sze SF, Tsui KW. Activation of peritoneal macrophages by polysaccharopeptide from the mushroom Coriolus versicolor. Immunopharmacology 1993;26:139-46.

93. Radhakrishna Pillai G, Srivastava AS, Hassanein TI, Chauhan DP, Carrier E.Induction of apoptosis in human lung cancer cells by curcumin. Cancer Lett. 2004;208:163e70.

94. Yean K L, Bone ND, et al. VEGF receptor phosphorylation status and apoptosis is modulated by green tea component, epigallocatechin-3-gallate (EGCG), in B-cell chronic lymphocytic leukemia. Blood. 2004;104:788-94.

95. Lan He Amelioration of anti-cancer agent adriamycin-induced nephrotic syndrome in rats by Wulingsan (Gorei-San), a blended traditional Chinese herbal medicine.School of Pharmaceutical Sciences, Sun Yat Sen University, China Food Chem Toxicol. 2008;46:1452-60.

96. Hostanska K, et al. Cimicifuga racemosa extract inhibits proliferation of estrogens receptor-positive and negative human breast carcinoma cell lines by induction of apoptosis. Breast Cancer Res Treat 84:151-60.

97. Lee LT, Huang YT, Hwang JJ, Lee PP, Ke FC, Nair MP, Kanadaswam C, Lee MT. Blockade of the epidermal growth factor receptor tyrosine kinase activity by quercetin and lute-olin leads to growth inhibition and apoptosis of pancreatic tumor cells Anticancer Res. 2002 May-Jun;22(3):1615-27.

98. Belkacemi Y, Touboul E, Meric JB, Rat P, Warnet JM. Radi-ation-induced cataract: physiopathologic, radiobiologic and clinical aspects. Cancer Radiother. Aug 2001;5(4):397-412.

99. Weiss JF, Landauer MR Radioprotection by antioxidants. Ann N Y Acad Sci. 2000;899:44-60.

100. Lamson DW, Brignall MS.Antioxidants in cancer therapy; their actions and interactions with oncologic therapies. Altern Med Rev 1999 Oct;4(5):304-29.

101. Mutlu-Türko_lu U, Erbil Y, Oztezcan S, Olgaç V, Toker G, Uysal M. The effect of selenium and/or vitamin E treatments on radiation-induced intestinal injury in rats. Life Sci. 2000 Apr 7;66(20):1905-13.

102. Cai L, Cherian MG, Iskander S, Leblanc M, Hammond RR. Metallothionein induction in human CNS in vitro: neuroprotection from ionizing radiation. Int J Radiat Biol. 2000 Jul;76(7):1009-17.

103. Nagler RM, Eichen Y, Nagler A. Redox metal chelation ameliorates radiation-induced bone marrow toxicity in a mouse model. Radiat Res. 2001 Aug;156(2):205-09.

104. Büntzel J. [Experiences with sodium selenite in treatment of acute and late adverse effects of radiochemother-apy of head-neck carcinomas. Cytoprotection Working Group in AK Supportive Measures in Oncology Within the scope of MASCC and DKG. Med Klin (Munich). 1999 Oct 15;94 Suppl 3:49-53.

105. Lamproglou I, Boisserie G, Mazeron JJ, Bok B, Baillet F, Drieu K. Effect of Ginkgo biloba extract (EGb 761) on rats in an experimental model of acute encephalopathy after total body irradiation. Cancer Radiother. 2000 May-Jun;4(3):202-06.

106. Inano H, Onoda M, Inafuku N, Kubota M, Kamada Y, Osawa T, Kobayashi H, Wakabayashi K. Potent preventive action of curcumin on radiation-induced initiation of mammary tumorigenesis in rats. Carcinogenesis. 2000 Oct;21(10):1835-41.

107. Varadkar P, Dubey P, Krishna M, Verma N. Modulation of radiation-induced protein kinase C activity by phenolics.J Radiol Prot. 2001 Dec;21(4):361-70.

108. Lamproglou I, Boisserie G, Mazeron JJ, Bok B, Baillet F, Drieu K.[Effect of Ginkgo biloba extract (EGb 761) on rats in an experimental model of acute encephalopathy after total body irradiation].Cancer Radiother. 2000 May-Jun;4(3):202-6. French.

109. Gong SL, Li XM, Lü Z, Liu SZ. [Protective effect of panaxatriols on function of reproductive endocrine axis in radiation-injured rats]. [Chinese] Zhongguo Yao Li Xue Bao 1993 Jul;14(4):358-60.

110. Kim SH, Jeong KS, Ryu SY, Kim TH. Panax ginseng prevents apoptosis in hair follicles and accelerates recovery of hair medullary cells in irradiated mice. In Vivo. 1998 Mar-Apr;12(2):219-22.

111. Miyanomae T, Frindel E. Radioprotection of hemopoiesis conferred by Acanthopanax senticosus Harms (Shigoka) administered before or after irradiation. Exp Hematol. 1988 Oct;16(9):801-06.

112. Lawenda, BD, Smith, D, Xu, L., Niemierko, A., Silverstein, J., Held, K.,Jain, R., Loeffler, J., Blumberg, J. Dietary Antioxidant Supplementation During Radiation Therapy: Potential for Radiation Protection of Tumors. Department of Radiation Oncology, Naval Medical Center, San Diego, CA; 2004.

113. Gundimeda U, Hara S, Anderson WB, Gopalakrishna R: Retinoids inhibit the oxidation modification of protein kinase C induced by oxidant tumor protmotors. Arch Biochem Biophys. 1993;300:576-630.

114. Prasad KN, et al. Vitamins regulate gene expression and induce differentiation and growth inhibition in cancer cells their relevance in cancer. Prevention Arch Otolaryngol Head Neck Surg. 1993;119(10):1133-40.

115. Cole WC, Prasad KN. Contrasting effects of vitamins as modulators of apoptosis in cancer cells and normal cells: A review. Nutr. Cancer 1997;29:97-103.

116. Norton L. Introduction to clinical aspects of preneoplasia. A mathematical relationship between stromal paracrine autonomy and population size. In: Marks PA, Turler H, Weil R, editors. Challenges of modern medicine Vol 1. Precancersous lesions. A multidisciplinary approach. Milan (Italy): Ares-Serono Symposia;1993,269-75.

117. Neuzil J, Weber T, Schröder A, Lu M, Ostermann G, Gellert N, Mayne GC, Olejnicka B, Negre-Salvayre A, Sticha M, Coffey RJ, Weber C. Induction of cancer cell apoptosis by {alpha}-tocopheryl succinate: molecular pathways and structural requirements. op.`cit. Journal. 2001;15(2):403-15.

118. Rose AT, McFadden DW. Alpha-tocopherol succinate inhibits growth of gastric cancer cells in vitro. J Surg Res 2001;95:19-22.

119. Donnelly ET, McClure N, Lewis SE The effect of ascorbate and alpha-tocopherol supplementation in vitro on DNA integrity and hydrogen peroxide-induced DNA damage in human spermatozoa. Mutagenesis 1999;14:505-12.

120. Zhang JG, Nicholls-Grzemski FA, Tirmenstein MA, et al. Vitamin E succinate protects hepatocytes against the toxic effect of reactive oxygen species generated at mitochondrial complexes I and III by alkylating agents. Chem Biol Interact 2001 Dec 21;138(3) :267-84.

121. Tarng DC, Liu TY, Huang TP. Protective effect of vitamin C on 8-hydroxy-2'-deoxyguanosine level in peripheral blood lymphocytes of chronic hemodialysis patients. Kidney Int. 2004 Aug;66(2):820-31.

122. Rao L, Puschner B, Prolla TA. Gene expression profiling of low selenium status in the mouse intestine: transcriptional activation of genes linked to DNA damage, cell cycle control and oxidative stress. J Nutr 2001;131:3175-81.

123. A Lemus-Wilson, PA Kelly and DE Blask. Melatonin blocks the stimulatory effects of prolactin on human breast cancer cell growth in culture. British Journal of Cancer. 1995;72:1435-40.

124. Lissoni P, Barni S, Meregalli S, et al. Modulation of cancer endocrine therapy by melatonin: A phase II study of tamoxifen plus melatonin in metastatic breast cancer patients progression under tamoxifen alone. Br J Cancer 1995;71:854-56.

125. Lissoni P, et al. No Title. Eur. Urol. 1997;31(2):178.

126. Kepler CR, Hirons KP, et al. Intermediates and products of the biohydrogenation of linoleic acid by Butyrinvibrio fibrisolvens. J. Biol. Chem. 1966;241:1350-54.

127. Neri B, De Leonardis V, Gemelli MT, et al. Melatonin as biological response modifier in cancer patients. Anticancer Res, 1998;18:1329-32.

128. Hara M, Yoshida M, Nishijima H, Yokosuka M, Iigo M, Ohtani-Kaneko R, et al. Melatonin, a pineal secretory product with antioxidant properties, protects againstcisplatin-induced nephrotoxicity in rats. J Pineal Res 2001;30:129-38.

129. Lynch EM. First-line chemotherapy containing cisplatin. Oncology. 1992;49:336-39.

130. Lissoni P, Barni S, Ardizzoia A, Tancini G, Conti A, Maestroni G. A randomized study with the pineal hormone melatonin versus supportive care alone in patients with brain metastases due to solid neoplasms. Cancer. 1994;73:699-701.

131. Ghielmini M, Pagani O, de Jong J, et al. Double-blind randomized study on the myeloprotective effect of melatonin in combination with carboplatin and etoposide in advanced lung cancer. Br J Cancer. 1999;80:1058-61.

132. Lissoni P, Barni S, Mandalà M, Ardizzoia A, Paolorossi F, Vaghi M, Longarini R, Malugani F, Tancini G. Decreased toxicity and increased efficacy of cancer chemotherapy using the pineal hormone melatonin in metastatic solid tumour patients with poor clinical status. Eur J Cancer. 1999 Nov;35(12):1688-92.

133. Oliynk, EV. The supporting treatment with antioxidant complexes and melatonin in patients with stomach cancer undergoing chemoradiation. Bukovinian State Medical Academy. Chernivtsi, Ukraine;2004.

134. Langsjoen Per.H., Vadhanavikit S., Folkers K. Response of patients in classes III and IV of cardiomyopathy to therapy in a blind and crossover trial with coenzyme Q10. In: Proc. Natl. Acad. of Sci., 1985; 82:4240-44.

135. Gaby, AR.1987; Judy WV, et al. No Title.1984:231-41; Ogura R, et al. No Title. J Appl Biochem. 1979;1:325.

136. Anonymous. Nutr Rev 1988;46:1367; Beyer RE. Biochem Cell Biol 1992;70(6):390-403.

137. Judy WV, Hall JH, Dugan W, et al. Coenzyme Q10 reduction of Adriamycin® cardiotoxicity. In: Biomedical and clinical aspects of coenzyme Q. Vol. 4. Amsterdam: Elsevier/North Holland Biomedical Press, 1984;231-41.

138. Ogura R, Toyama H, Shimada T, Murakami M. The role of ubiquinone (coenzyme Q10) in preventing Adriamycin®-induced mitochondrial disorders in rat heart. J Appl Biochem .1979;1:325.

139. Albena T, et al. Relation of structure of curcumin analogs to their potencies as inducers of Phase 2 detoxification Carcinogenesis. 1999;20 (5):911-14.

140. Chendil D, Ranga RS, Meigooni D, Sathishkumar S, Ahmed MM. Curcumin confers radiosensitizing effect in prostate cancer cell line PC-3.Oncogene. 2004 Feb 26;23(8):1599-607.

141. Adams BK, Cai J, Armstrong J, Herold M, Lu YJ, Sun A, Snyder JP, Liotta DC, Jones DP, Shoji M. EF24, a novel synthetic curcumin analog, induces apoptosis in cancer cells via a redox-dependent mechanism. Anticancer Drugs. 2005 Mar;16(3):263-75.

142. Karunagaran D, Rashmi R, Kumar TR. Induction of apoptosis by curcumin and its implications for cancer therapy.Curr Cancer Drug Targets. 2005 Mar;5(2):117-29.

143. Manson MM, Farmer PB, Gescher A, Steward WP Innovative agents in cancer prevention.Recent Results Cancer Res. 2005;166:257-75.

144. Corpet DE, Pierre F. Point: From animal models to prevention of colon cancer. Systematic review of chemoprevention in min mice and choice of the model system.Cancer Epidemiol Biomarkers Prev. 2003 May;12(5):391-400.

145. Takahashi T, Takasuka N, Iigo M, et al. Isoliquiritigenin, a flavonoid from licorice, reduces prostaglandin E2 and nitric oxide, causes apoptosis, and suppresses aberrant crypt foci development. Cancer Sci. May 2004;95(5):448-53.

146. Kiemer AK, Hartung T, Huber C, Vollmar AM. Phyllanthus amarus has anti-inflammatory potential by inhibition of iNOS, COX-2, and cytokines via the NF-kappaB pathway.J Hepatol. 2003 Mar;38(3):289-97.

147. Frondoza CG, Sohrabi A, Polotsky A, Phan PV, Hungerford DS, Lindmark L. An in vitro screening assay for inhibitors of proinflammatory mediators in herbal extracts using human synoviocyte cultures. In Vitro Cell Dev Biol Anim. 2004;40:95-101.

148. Zhang DY, Wu J, Ye F et al. Inhibition of cancer cell proliferation and Scutellaria baicalensis. Cancer Res. 2003;63:4037-3043.

149. Capodice, JL, Bemis, DL, Buttyan, R., Katz, AE. Zyflamend, a Unique Herbal Preparation Inhibits Arachidonic Acid Metabolism and Suppresses Prostate Cancer Cells, In Vitro. Columbia University Medical Center, New York, NY;2004.

150. Weisburger JH. Tea and health: the underlying mechanisms. Proc Soc Exp Biol Med 1999;220:271-75.

151. Seely D, Mills EJ, Wu P, Verma S, Guyatt GH. The effects of green tea consumption on incidence of breast cancer and recurrence of breast cancer: a systematic review and meta-analysis. Integr Cancer Ther. 2005;4:144-55.

152. Kuroda Y, Hara Y. (1999) Antimutagenic and anticarcinogenic activity of tea polyphenols. Mutation Research 1999;436:69-97.

153. Weisburger JH, Rivenson A, Kingston DG, Wilkins TD, Van Tassell RL, Nagao M, et al. Dietary modulation of the carcinogenicity of the heterocyclic amines. Princess Takamatsu Symp.1995;23:240-50.

154. Ebata J, Fukagai N, Furukawa H. Mechanisms of antimutagenesis by catechins towards N-nitrosodimethylamine. Environ Mutagen Res. 1998;20:45-50.

155. Klaunig JE, Xu Y, Han C, et al. The effect of tea consumption on oxidative stress in smokers and nonsmokers. Proc Soc Exp Biol Med 1999;220:249-54.

156. Einbond LS, Shimizu M, Xiao MD, et al. Growth inhibitory activity of extracts and purified components of black cohosh on human breast cancer cells. Breast Cancer Res. Treat. 2004;83:221-31.

157. Agarwal R, Agarwal C, Ichikawa H, et al. Anticancer potential of silymarin: from bench to bed side. Anticancer Res. 2006;26:4457-98.

158. Bhatia N, et al. Inhibition of human carcinoma cell growth and DNA synthesis by silibinin, an active constituent of milk thistle: comparison with silymarin. Cancer Letters. 1999;147:77-84.

159. Scambia G, De Vincenzo R, Ranelletti FO, et al. Antiproliferative effect of silybin on gynaecological malignancies: synergism with cisplatin and doxorubicin. Eur J Cancer 1996;32A:877-82.

160. Maggiolini M, Bonofiglio D, Marsico S, Panno ML, Cenni B, Picard D, Andò S. Estrogen receptor alpha mediates the proliferative but not the cytotoxic dose-dependent effects of two major phytoestrogens on human breast cancer cells. Mol Pharmacol. 2001 Sep;60(3):595-602.

161. Jones JL, et al. Genistein inhibits tamoxifen effects on cell proliferation and cell cycle arrest in T47D breast cancer cells. American Surgeon. 2002;68(6):575-77.

162. Fazlul H S, et al. Soy isoflavones and cancer prevention. Clinical Science Review. Cancer Invest. 2003; 21(5):744-57.

163. Upadhyay S, Neburi M, Chinni SR, et al. Differential sensitivity of normal and malignant breast epithelial cells to genistein is partly mediated by p21(WAF1). Clin Cancer Res 2001;7:1782-89.

164. Oh SM, Chung KH Estrogenic activities of Ginkgo biloba extracts. Life Sci. 2004 Jan 30;74(11):1325-35.

165. Mori H, Niwa K, Zheng Q, et al. Cell proliferation in cancer prevention; effects of preventive agents on estrogen-related endometrial carcinogenesis model and on an in

vitro model in human colorectal cells. Mutat Res. Sep2001;480-81:201-07.

166. Auborn KJ, et al. Indole-3-Carbinol is a Negative Regulator of Estrogen. J Nutr. 2003;133:2470S.

167. Hsieh TC, Lu X, Chea J, Wu JM.Prevention and management of prostate cancer using PC-SPES: a scientific perspective. J Nutr. 2002 Nov;132(11 Suppl):3513S-3517S.

168. Jiang J, et al. Ganoderma lucidum inhibits proliferation and induces apoptosis in human prostate cancer cells PC-3. Int.Journal of Oncology. 2004;24:1093-99.

169. Zi XL, Zhang J, Agarwal R, Pollak M. Silibinin up-regulates insulin like growth factor binding protein 3 expression and inhibits proliferation of androgen independent prostate cancer cells. Cancer Research. 60:5617-20.

170. Bemis DL, Capodice JL, Buttyan R, Katz AE. Botanicals in the Treatment of Prostate Cancer: Pre-clinical research. New York, NY: Columbia University Medical Center;2004.

171. Kumar NB. The Specific Role of Isoflavones in Reducing Prostate Cancer Risk. H. Lee Moffitt Cancer Center and Res. Inst., Tampa, FL;2004.

PART 4:
SPECIFIC CANCERS

reast cancer is a malignant proliferation of epithelial cells that line the ducts and lobules of the breast. These epithelial malignancies of the breast are a clonal disease, which means a single transformed cell becomes aberrant. This transformation is through a series of somatic or germline point mutations that eventually lead to a full malignancy of the aberrant cell progeny. This means that breast cancer can exist in a non-invasive (in situ) form or even in an invasive (infiltrating) form, but in a non-metastatic disease state for a long period of time. The non-invasive form is thought to be antecedent to the development of a more invasive form of the cancer.

Breast cancer usually consists of a mass or lesion that is not tender, firm, or hard, with poorly delineated margins (caused by local infiltration). Very small (1-2 mm) erosions of the nipple epithelium may be the only manifestation of Paget's carcinoma. Watery, serous, or bloody discharge from the nipple is an occasional early sign, but this is more often associated with benign disease.[1]

Epidemiology

INCIDENCE

In the United States in 2007, there were about 180,510 cases of invasive breast cancer with approximately 41,000 deaths from the disease. Breast cancer is the most common cause of cancer in women, but with improved early detection and treatment options, mortality from the disease has begun to decrease. Breast cancer is the major cause of morbidity and mortality in elderly women, with about 50% of the 180,000 new cases occurring in women over 65 years old. Statistics show that 6.53% of white women and 4.70% of black women over the age of 65 develop breast cancer, but only about 1.5% die of it.[1]

PREVALENCE

The most aggressive cell type of all breast cancers, the inflammatory carcinoma of the breast, has equal prevalence in women pre- and post-menopausally. The most common cause of cancer among postmenopausal women is intraductal carcinoma (ductal carcinoma in situ, or DCIS). It is generally a multicentric growth that

has less than 25% recurrence rate locally after partial mastectomy. In less than 2% of these cases, the axillary lymph nodes are involved. Lobular carcinoma in situ often involves both breasts but is rare in the postmenopausal population. Paget's disease of the nipple reflects the spread of cancer through the skin of the nipple. Paget's is usually associated with ductal or intraductal carcinoma and less so with more invasive cancer types. These cancers are thought to be of the less invasive in nature.[1]

Of the invasive carcinomas, invasive ductal carcinoma comprises approximately 70% of all cases among women of all ages. Some cancers risk increase with age, while other types decrease. The mucinous (colloid) carcinoma has an increased risk of occurrence with age, but is a slow growing tumor in elderly women. The risk of medullary carcinoma, usually a cancer that affects both breasts, decreases with age.[1]

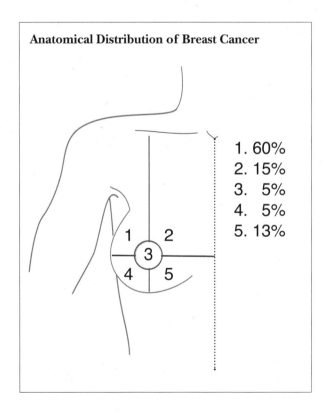

Anatomical Distribution of Breast Cancer

1. 60%
2. 15%
3. 5%
4. 5%
5. 13%

Anatomy of the Breast

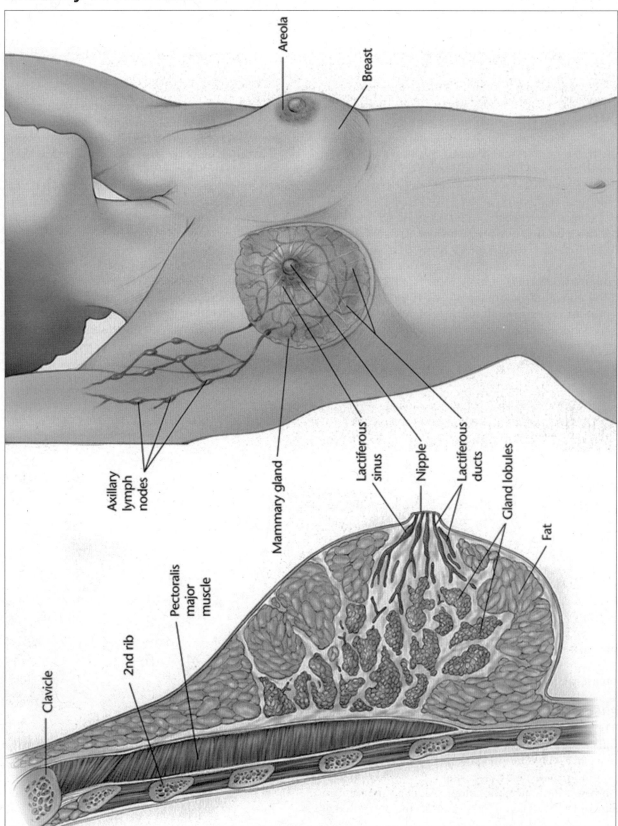

Histopathology

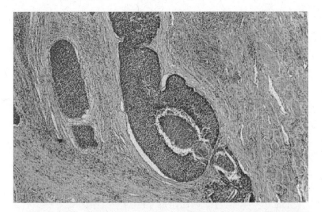

Ductal Carcinoma in Situ (DCIS)
Shows cellular changes with inflammatory artifacts and excited estrogen (E2) receptors.

In the continual presence of inflammation, these receptor sites multiply and create even more inflammatory changes. The atypical cell (atypia) progresses to the dysplastic cell (dysplasia) and further to the metaplastic cellular changes (metaplasia). Each cellular changing event causes cascading inflammatory washings leading to a more progressive disease.

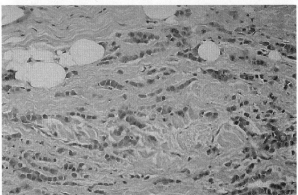

Invasive Carcinoma
Shows aberrant cellular changes in the inflammatory tissue changes that are chronic.

Aberrant cellular changes create mutations leading to receptor site mutation/creation of aberrant cells. This is seen in the slide with the increased metaplastic changes noted by increased cellular nuclei; these tissue changes are initiated, maintained, and mutated into the aberrant cell that is invasive carcinoma.

Woman's Risk of Developing or Dying from Breast Cancer[2]

Age	Risk of Developing Breast Cancer %		Risk of Developing Invasive Breast Cancer %		Risk of Dying of Breast Cancer %	
	White	*Black*	*White*	*Black*	*White*	*Black*
Birth -110	10.2	7.5	9.8	7.3	3.6	3
20-30	.04	.07	.04	.07	0	.02
20-40	.49	.61	.47	.61	.09	.15
20-110	10.34	7.72	9.94	7.42	3.05	3.11
35-45	.88	.8	.83	.75	.14	.21
35-55	2.53	2.32	2.37	2.16	.56	2.98
35-110	10.27	7.74	9.82	7.33	3.56	2.98
50-60	1.95	1.74	1.86	1.68	.33	.35
50-70	4.67	3.34	4.48	3.38	1.04	.93
50-110	8.96	6.42	8.66	6.25	2.75	.26
65-75	3.17	2.1	3.08	1.99	.43	.78
65-85	5.48	3.81	5.29	3.66	1.01	.78
65-110	6.53	4.7	6.29	4.53	1.53	1.14

(Adapted from information from CA: A Cancer Journals for Clinicians.)

> **Risk factors for developing breast cancer[3]**
> - Increasing age
> - Personal or family history of breast cancer
> - History of colon or endometrial cancer in first-degree relatives
> - Reproductive history: early menarche, late menopause, no pregnancies or late first pregnancy at age > 31
> - Diet: regular consumption of alcohol, high-fat diet (inconclusive evidence)
> - Body size: abdominal obesity
> - Estrogen replacement therapy
> - Exposure to high doses of ionizing radiation
> - History of atypical hyperplasia on biopsy for benign breast disease

Causal Factors

Like any major disease, the cause of breast cancer has attracted immense speculation, some based on fact, some on myth.

MENSTRUAL CYCLE

The biggest risk factor for developing breast cancer is age-related to the menstrual cycle. Women who have early menarche and late menopause and are nulliparous are at the greatest risk. When evaluating a patient with breast cancer, the three dates that must be ascertained are onset of menarche, age at first full-term pregnancy, and age at onset of menopause. The variance of 70% to 80% in breast cancer found globally can be accounted for by these three factors.

- Breast cancer is thought to be a hormone-dependent disease because women without functioning ovaries (who have not received hormone replacement therapy) do not develop breast cancer. The female to male ratio is about 150:1.
- Data show that women who have menarche at the age of 16 have half the risk of developing breast cancer compared to women who have menarche at the age of 12.
- Menopause that occurs 10 years before the median age of 52 reduces the lifetime risk of breast cancer by 35%.
- Women who have their first full term pregnancy by age 18 lower their risk of breast cancer by 30% to 40% when compared to nulliparous women.
- Women who have an identical twin sister with breast cancer are at least three times more likely than average to develop cancer. If the twin was diagnosed before age 40 years, 25% of the remaining siblings developed cancer over the next 20 years.

- Regardless of parity or age at first full-term pregnancy, the duration of breast-feeding can significantly reduce the risk of development of breast cancer.[4]

Hormone Replacement Therapy

Exogenous hormonal use and its association with the incidence of occurrence in breast cancer is still a controversial topic among research scientists and allopathic practitioners. North American women, until the 21st century, used hormone replacement therapy (HRT) in postmenopause to curtail the hormonal deficiency side effects of menopause. The use of oral contraceptives in this culture can also be considered a form of HRT. The Women's Health Initiative (WHI) trial sponsored by the National Institutes of Health (NHI) showed data that changed these medical practices in relation to hormone therapies. HRT prescriptive use in postmenopausal women was a standard of care not only to manage normal menopausal symptoms, but also supposedly protective against the development of osteoporosis and heart disease.[5]

However, data from the WHI trial showed that conjugated equine estrogens plus synthetic progestins increased the risk of breast cancer in post menopausal women. This data also reflected that there is an adverse effect on cardiovascular event, while offerings some benefit with the decrease in bone fractures and colorectal cancer occurrence rates.[5]

HRT is an area of rapid reevaluation, but it would appear (at least from breast cancer and cardiovascular disease vantage points) that there are serious concerns about long-term HRT use. HRT in women previously diagnosed with breast cancer increases recurrence rates.

RADIATION EXPOSURE

Radiation is also an associated risk factor for younger women developing breast cancer. Women who have been exposed to radiation before the age of 30 either in the form of multiple fluoroscopies (200-300 cGy) or treatment for Hodgkin disease (>3600 cGy) have shown a substantial increase in the risk for developing breast cancer. Radiation exposure in women after the age of 30 appears to have a minimal association with the development of breast cancer.[6]

ETHNIC BACKGROUND

North American elderly women have a 1 in 9 chance of developing invasive breast cancer, while Asian women have a 1 in 5 to 1 in 10 chance of developing breast cancer compared to North American women. Biologically, Asian women have relatively lower amounts of estrogens and progesterone, which is not genetically explained. Asian women who move to a Western civilization have sex steroid levels comparable to other women in that environment. Notable is that the daughters of these immigrant women often differ remarkably in height, weight, and hormone levels from Asian women living in Asia.[7]

STATURE

Height and weight affect the onset of menarche, as well as the plasma levels of estrogens. Dietary factors have been postulated to be an influence in the difference between these populations of women, although the standard body of scientific literature still considers this postulate controversial. There is an associated link between total caloric fat intake and an increase in breast cancer risk that has been accepted by the scientific community.[8]

Increased calories has been shown to contribute to breast cancer risk by affecting earlier menarche, later age of menopause, and increased levels of postmenopausal estrogen concentrations enhanced from peripheral aromatase activity in fatty tissues. Could this be from the factory farming practices of the industrialized world, which includes the use of bovine growth hormone? Could the development of breat cancer be influenced by a diet of fast foods that are high in calories, with a high glycemic index and load, but low in whole grain fibers and nutrients. Could the environment of the cell, of the woman, of the planet have a contributory effect?

GENETIC MARKERS

Only about 10% of breast cancers can be directly linked to genetic mutations in the germ cell line. Several of these genes have been implicated in familial cases of breast cancer. Inherited mutations of the p53 tumor suppressor gene (the Li-Fraumeni syndrome) lead directly to an increased incidence in not only breast cancer but other malignancies. Inherited mutations in the PTEN have also been associated with breast cancer development. By far the best known of these germ cell line mutations is the BRCA tumor suppressor gene mutations. These mutations account for 5% to 10% of all breast cancers.[9]

BRCA-1

The BRCA-1 is found on the chromosomal locus 17q21 and encodes for a zinc finger protein that is thought to function as a transcription factor. BRCA-1 gene is involved in gene repair, and women who inherit this mutation (from either parent) have a 60% to 80% lifetime risk of developing breast cancer, with

BRCA-1 and BRCA-2 Facts

- Genes codes along one pathway protect cells from the effects of DNA damage
- Carriers have a 50% to 85% chance of developing breast cancer by age 70
- Carriers diagnosed with breast cancer have a higher risk of recurrence
- Risk of developing ovarian cancer increases from 16% to 60%
- Carriers of BRCA mutations who have children appear to be at higher risk for developing breast cancer by age 40 years than carriers who are nulliparous-in contrast to the usual risk factors for sporadic breast cancer. Interestingly-and despite the association of BRCA1 with an increased risk of hormone receptor-negative breast tumors-recent data confirm that oophorectomy in women with either mutation before the age of 40 years significantly reduces the risk of breast cancer (up to 75%).[1]

an associated 33% risk of developing ovarian cancer. Men who carry the mutant allele have an associated risk of prostate cancer, as well as breast cancer. The BRCA-1 gene mutation also carries an increased risk for colon, pancreatic, gastric, and fallopian tube cancer development.

More than 100 mutations have been found on the BRCA-1, which makes it difficult to identify high-risk patients. Women of Ashkenazi Jewish descent have a specific BRCA-1 mutation as a deletion of adenine and guanine at position 185. Population studies have shown that up to 20% of Jewish women with breast cancer diagnosed at 40 years of age or less have a BRCA-1 mutation.[10]

BRCA-2

BRCA-2, found on chromosomal locus 13q12, is also associated with a greater risk of breast cancer in both women and men. For women under the age of 40 at the time of diagnosis, the likelihood of a BRCA-1 mutation is as high as 27% if her tumor is hormone receptor negative and of a high nuclear grade. Most women who are BRCA-1 carriers tend to develop hormone receptor negative forms of breast cancer, while the BRCA-2 carriers tend to develop hormone positive forms. BRCA-2 gene mutation also carries an increased risk of prostate, pancreatic, gall bladder, bile duct, stomach, and malignant melanoma cancers. In sporadic cases of breast cancer, tumor suppressor activity may have become inactivated by the loss of heterozygosity of BRCA 1&2 genes.[10]

PROPHYLACTIC CHEMOTHERAPY

The BRCA1/2 significance in the literature and vernacular of cancer treatment is related to treatment options associated with this gene mutation. Detection of these gene mutations and post diagnoses offers the same conventional treatment recommendations, but with the option of bilateral radical mastectomies and an aggressive long-term and naturopathic protocol. Detection of these gene mutations in non breast cancer patients offers the option of prophylactic mastectomy and chemotherapy.

In the Breast Cancer Prevention Trial, a 49% decrease in risk of invasive breast cancer was seen with the use of prophylactic Tamoxifen in the high risk population of women with the BRCA 1/2 gene mutation(s). There was also an associated increased risk of developing endometrial cancer, uterine sarcoma, pulmonary embolism, deep vein thrombosis, and stroke (Fisher). The data with regards of BRCA 1 vs. BRCA 2 shows that the risk factor in healthy women who carry the BRCA 2 gene mutation was reduced by 62% when these women used the Tamoxifen prophylactically. In the healthy women with the BRCA 1 mutation, no reduction of risk was found with the use of prophylactic drugs.[11]

HER 2

By far the most interesting of all statistics is that an increased expression of a dominant oncogene, human epidermal growth factor receptor 2 (HER 2), has been found in 25% of all breast cancer cases.[16] The product of this gene is the HER-2/neu (erbB2), a member of the epidermal growth factor receptor family, which is overexpressed in breast cancers due to gene amplification. This overexpression is thought to contribute to the transformation of the breast epithelium in order to create a cancer growth. It has been found to be positive in 20% to 30% of breast cancers.[12]

The HER-2 overexpression does correlate with several negative prognostic features, including estrogen receptor negative status, a high S phase fraction, positive nodal involvement, mutated p53, and a high nuclear grade at the time of diagnosis.[18] A positive HER-2/neu has also been associated with an increase in vascular endothelial growth factor (VEGF) mRNA expression, which results in the induction and enhancement of VEGF secretion. This was also found to correlate closely with a shortened disease-free survival rate and a shortened overall survival rate in node positive patients.[12]

HER-2/neu overexpression suggests that there is a resistance to cyclophosphamide, methotrexate, and 5-flourouracil chemotherapy strategies. This overexpression of HER-2/neu has now been used as a target for systemic chemotherapy used in adjuvant and metastatic disease.[13]

Trastuzumab (Herceptin) is a monoclonal antibody therapy directed at the receptor site of HER-2/neu. There is a cautionary cardiotoxicity associated with the treatment. Flourescence in situ hybridization (FISH) test is more accurate than the HercepTest (HER-2) test for immunohistochemical assay. The HercepTest is considered negative if only weakly positive at 1+ or 2+, while a 3+ is considered strongly positive. The standard now is to confirm all 2+ HercepTests with a FISH. The FISH is a cost effective evaluation that shows an increase in cost effectiveness using FISH alone or as a confirmation for all positive HercepTest rather than only the weakly positive. This was correlated with the HercepTest and adjusted for quality of adjusted life in years, lifetime cost, and incremental cost effectiveness.[14,15]

OTHER GENETIC FACTORS

Many other genes have been found to contribute to the risk and development of breast cancer. Many more have not yet been identified and studied. These acquired defects creating an aberrant cell line are not only seen in familial breast cancer, but also in sporadic breast cancer.

- p53 mutation is an acquired defect that is seen in almost 40% of all breast cancers and 1% of all breast cancer in women under the age of 40.[16]
- PTEN acquired mutations occur in approximately 10% of all breast cancers.[17]
- Ataxia-telangiectasia mutation is responsible for a rare childhood neurological disorder, but female carriers are at five times the risk for developing breast cancer.[18]

DNA Flow Cytometry

Other markers to consider are found through DNA flow cytometry. It has been found that normal diploid or tetraploid DNA content has a better prognosis than aneuploid tumors (non ploidy). Using DNA flow cytometry adjunctively to sentinel lymph node biopsy in the presence of lymph node metastases can be a helpful predictor in prognosis and treatment options.[19]

- **S-phase fraction** in the cell cycle shows that >5% indicates a higher risk of recurrence and is even more predictive in diploid tumors.
- **Ki-67 protein** is a marker for proliferation that

> **ONCOTYPE DX BREAST CANCER ASSAY**
>
> A recent study evaluated the use of a 21 gene expression assay (Oncotype Dx Breast Cancer Assay) to predict a patient's individual risk of recurrent breast cancer 10 years after initial diagnosis. All of the women in the study had received 5 years of adjuvant Tamoxifen; the test was performed on the original tumor block. A "recurrence score" from 0 to 100 was reported, and defines the level of risk of distant disease recurrence as low, intermediate, or high. This score could help in determining the appropriate treatment for these relatively good risk cancers.[21]
>
> The assay has been validated in two studies, and specifically in women with cancers that are hormone receptor positive and in women who have received adjuvant tamoxifen. One additional trial suggested that the primary benefit of adjuvant chemotherapy with CMF was in the high-risk groups with rapidly proliferating disease, whereas the primary benefit of hormonal therapy was in the low-risk group with slow growing cells. Although the test is now approved for use, it is very expensive and is not routinely covered by most insurers.[22]

should be absent from resting cells (G(0)) phase, but present during all active phases of the cell cycle.[20]

❖ **Mucin glycoprotein gene** (MUC-1) is associated with breast cancer development also and is better known for the specific fractions that are tested for using antibodies for different antigenic sites: CA 27.29, CA 15.3, CEA. These three markers may all be elevated in the breast cancer patient, especially in pretreatment diagnosis.

❖ **CA 27.29** is the most common and most accurate tumor marker used with breast cancer. There is an increased discrimination between primary breast cancer and healthy patients, which makes this marker not only sensitive but specific, when compared to CA 15.3 marker. The CA 27.29 was found to be more reliably elevated in advanced stage disease versus early stage disease, useful in the indication of increased or decreased tumor burden, while being an excellent indicator of the patient's response to treatment (response marker). CEA is a non specific antigen that may be elevated in breast cancer but is usually associated with colorectal and gastric cancers.

Oncotype DX Test

This test has been recently approved by the FDA as a multigene diagnostic assay, specifically indicated for breast cancer. This test looks for the presence of gene mutations in sets of genes associated with response to chemotherapeutic treatment options, as well as the likelihood of recurrence. It must be run on the original tumor sample. It is used in conjunction with the standard staging, grading, and tumor marker assays.

Studies indicate that it is most promising for the newly-diagnosed breast cancer patient who is estrogen receptor positive with stage 1-2 disease and will be treated with Tamoxifen. It has currently been accepted for use with breast cancer, for insurance reimbursement in the United States, but still is not used adjunctively for other cancer diagnoses.[21,22]

Assessment

Diagnosis of breast cancer follows a standard three-part protocol. The first diagnostic technique is a breast self-examination (BSE), followed by a physical exam conducted by a clinician who determines whether a biopsy (aspiration) or ultrasound is needed to determine a diagnosis.[23]

The breasts are a common site for a potentially fatal malignancy that can be detected early with a simple physical exam. The presenting feature in approximately 70% of patients is a painless breast lump. More than 90% of these breast lumps are discovered by the patient. The prognostic association between early detection of a small lesion and overall improved outcome is direct. Other symptoms of a mass are less frequent in their presentation: breast pain, nipple discharge, redness, swelling, induration and hardness, even enlargement or shrinking of the breast itself. Symptoms that indicate a suspected tumor with metastatic advancement would include jaundice, enlarged axillary lymph nodes, lymphedema or swelling in the arm, back pain, weight loss, lack of appetite and fatigue. These can all indicate late discovery of the lesion and are rarely seen in early diagnosis.[1,23]

Triple diagnostic technique for early diagnosis of breast cancer

↓

1. Breast self-examination

↓

2. Physical examination

↓

3. Aspiration or ultrasound

Breast Self-Examination Guidelines

Breast self-examination visual inspection

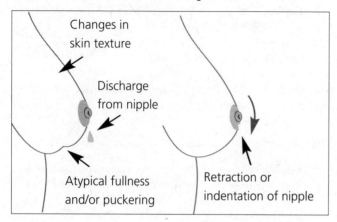

Changes in skin texture

Discharge from nipple

Atypical fullness and/or puckering

Retraction or indentation of nipple

Breast self-examination manual inspection standing

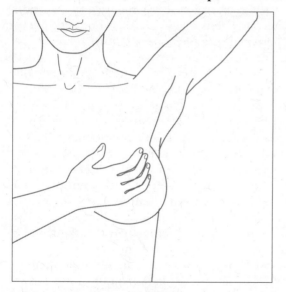

With fingertips close together, gently probe each breast in one of these three patterns.

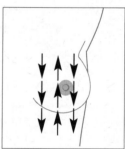

Breast self-examination manual inspection reclining

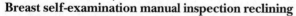

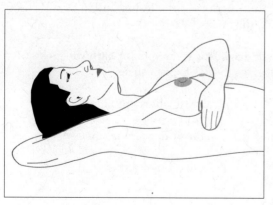

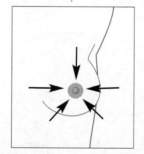

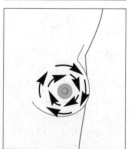

Menstruating women

In menstruating women, both BSE and clinical breast examinations should be done in the follicular phase, preferably days 5 to 7of the cycle. If the lesions are not suspicious or equivocal and the mass persists through a menstrual cycle, further examination and diagnostics should be performed.[23]

BREAST SELF-EXAMINATION

Breast self examination (BSE) is a controversial topic where outcome data suggests the BSE does not change the survival statistics in breast cancer. However, "women should be strongly encouraged to examine their breasts monthly. A potentially flawed study from China has suggested that BSE does not alter survival, but given its safety, the procedure should still be encouraged."[23] A palpable breast lump is present in 50% of all breast cancer cases, so BSE is still highly recommended by clinicians and may be the first line in the detection of a cancerous growth.[23]

Teaching the patient the proper technique increases BSE's effectiveness in early detection of a lesion. These physical maneuvers help to detect the asymmetry of the breasts and dimpling of the skin. With contraction of the pectoralis muscles, occult lesions can be visualized.

Premenopausal women should perform the examination 7 to 8 days after the start of the menstrual period when the breast tissue is less fibrously dense. Postmenopausal women should pick one day a month as the designated BSE date.

Breast Self-Examination Guidelines[24]

1. First, there should be a visual inspection in front of a mirror with the hands in different positions – by the sides, overhead, and pressed firmly on the hips or palm to palm.
2. Second, there should be a manual inspection while standing. While standing, raise the arm of the breast that is to be inspected and, and with the opposite hand's finger pads carefully palpate the breast in a methodical pattern side to side, up and down, and in a circle.
3. Third, there should be a manual inspection while reclining. In a supine position, place the hand under the head and follow the steps for the standing position.

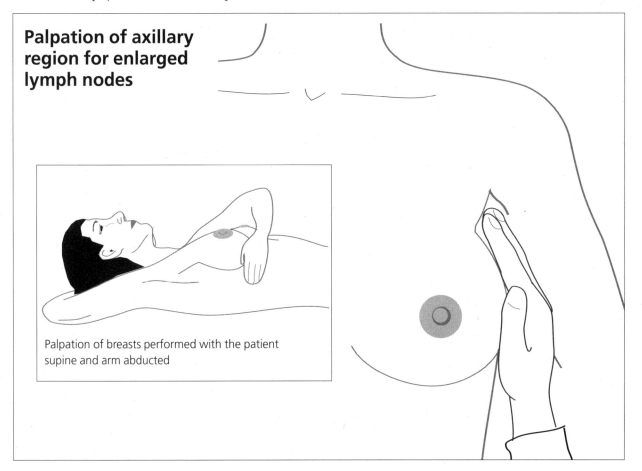

Palpation of axillary region for enlarged lymph nodes

Palpation of breasts performed with the patient supine and arm abducted

PHYSICAL EXAMINATION

The clinician's physical examination is the second arm of the triple diagnostic technique in early detection of breast cancer.[23,24] Clinicians use the same techniques as the BSE. The examination should include all the breast material that extends from the tail of the breast into the axillary and down the inner upper arm. If a woman is large breasted, the clinician should take more care to ensure all the breast material has been examined.

- Conduct the examination in a well-lit area so that skin changes, retraction, or dimpling can be easily seen.
- Inspect the breast with the patient sitting, arms at her sides, and then overhead.
- Identify any abnormal variations in breast size and contour, minimal nipple retraction, slight edema, redness, or retraction of the skin. These may be a positive sign of an occult lesion.
- Continue the examination if you suspect a lesion. Retraction or dimpling of the skin can often be accentuated by having the patient raise her arms overhead or press her hands on her hips or palm to palm to contract the pectoralis muscles.
- Palpate thoroughly the axillary and supraclavicular areas for enlarged nodes with the patient sitting and lying supine.
- Palpate the breast for masses or other changes with the patient both seated and supine with the arm abducted with the palm placed under her head.
- Palpate with a rotary motion of your fingerpads. A horizontal stripping motion has also been recommended.

Palpation

Physical examination alone cannot exclude malignancy. Lesions with certain features are more likely to be cancerous (hard, irregular, tethered or fixed, or painless lesions). A negative mammogram in the presence of a persistent lump in the breast does not exclude malignancy. Palpable lesions require additional diagnostic procedures, including biopsy. A lesion palpated in a postmenopausal woman should always be followed up with further diagnostics.[23]

CLINICAL EXAMINATION ANOMALIES

- A small lesion, less than 1 cm in diameter, may be difficult or even impossible for the examiner to feel, but may be discovered by the patient. She should always be asked to demonstrate the location of the mass; if the practitioner fails to confirm the patient's suspicions and imaging studies are normal, the examination should be repeated in 2 to 3 months, preferably 1 to 2 weeks after the onset of menses. Ultrasound is often valuable and mammography essential when an area is felt by the patient to be abnormal, but the physician feels no mass. MRI may also be considered, but the lack of specificity should be discussed by the practitioner with the patient.[1]
- During the premenstrual phase of the cycle, increased innocuous nodularity may suggest neoplasm or may obscure an underlying lesion.
- If there is any question regarding the nature of an abnormality under these circumstances, the patient should be asked to return after her period.

BIOPSY

Virtually all breast cancer is diagnosed from a biopsy of a lesion that was detected either by palpation or mammography. Aspiration by fine needle biopsy (FNA) or ultrasonography (US) can be used to determine whether a lesion is fluid filled (cystic) or solid. Not all solid masses can be detected by ultrasound; thus, a palpable mass that is not visualized on ultrasound can be presumed to be a solid mass. Mammography has a higher sensitivity and specificity for small solid tumor formation, and is still a gold standard in screening and diagnostic testing. MRI of the breast has a high sensitivity, higher than that of mammography, but it has a lower specificity. MRI of the breast is a great diagnostic tool once a patient has been diagnosed with breast cancer and should be considered in follow up care.[25]

The best test is ultimately the histopathology examination that looks at tissue or cells removed via biopsy or surgery. Proceeding further into treatment options should never be undertaken without a definitive histopathology to direct the treatment protocol. Biopsy is the safest examination of a suspicious lesion found on clinical/physical exams but should follow imaging studies to guide and indicate whether biopsy is needed. Mammography and follow up ultrasound are the standards of care in imaging the breast and ruling in or out, suspicious findings for biopsy. "About 60% of lesions clinically thought to be cancer prove on biopsy to be benign, while about 30% of clinically benign lesions are found to be malignant. These findings demonstrate the fallibility of clinical judgment and the necessity for biopsy."[1]

Needle Biopsy

A needle biopsy is the simplest method. It can involve either a fine needle aspiration of the suspected cells (FNA) or a core sampling of tissue with a hollow needle

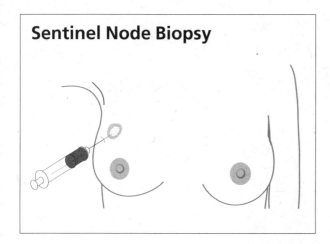

Sentinel Node Biopsy

(core needle biopsy). FNA is because as cells are aspirated with a small needle, they can be examined cytologically for aberration. This technique is the least expensive of all and has no associated morbidity.[26]

There are some issues with sampling, especially if the lesions are deep in the breast tissue, and a FNA does require a skilled pathologist in cytologic diagnosis to examine the sample. With this sampling, it is hard to tell noninvasive cancers from invasive forms of cancer, and there are fairly high false negative rates at around 10%. The false positive rates are extremely low at 1% to 2%. Therefore, if the clinical examination and breast imaging studies are positive but the FNA is negative, a suspicious dominant mass would not be left in the breast regardless of the FNA results.[27]

SENTINEL NODE BIOPSY

- ❖ Cytologic examination of nipple discharge or cyst fluid may be helpful on rare occasions.
- ❖ As a rule, mammography (or ductography) and breast biopsy are required when nipple discharge or cyst fluid is bloody or cytologically questionable.
- ❖ Ductal lavage, a technique that washes individual duct systems with saline and loosens epithelial cells for cytologic evaluation, is being evaluated as a risk assessment tool but appears to be of little value[28]

METASTASES

Metastases tend to spread regionally to lymph nodes, which may be palpable. Frequently, several movable, nontender, partially firm axillary lymph nodes that are <5 mm in diameter are found. These generally are not significant. Firm or hard nodules that are >1cm are typical sites of metastasis. If the axillary lymph nodes are firm, matted, and affixed to the skin or other structures, this usually indicates advanced metastatic disease (stage III). In 85% of cases where the clinician thinks axillary lymph nodes are involved, pathohistology proves the clinician true. When there are positive axillary lymph nodes involved, these cancers would not be considered in situ. Noninvasive cancers do not metastasize (invade). Metastases have been found in about 30% of the patients with negative lymph node involvement.[26]

ULTRASONOGRAPHY

An ultrasound (US) is used primarily to differentiate a solid lesion from cystic forms. US is not thought of as a diagnostic imaging tool on its own, but can show revealing features that would be highly suggestive of a cancerous growth. Irregular margins, new solid masses, or an irregular mass within a cyst all can be salient features of a growing breast cancer. Often a US is ordered after a mammography to further investigate a finding on the mammogram and determine whether that lesion is cystic or solid. An ultrasound needle biopsy is often used for non palpable mammographic densities that are found with the imaging study. If a cyst is aspirated, there will be a nonbloody fluid, and this indicates that it is a cyst and no further cytology is required.[29]

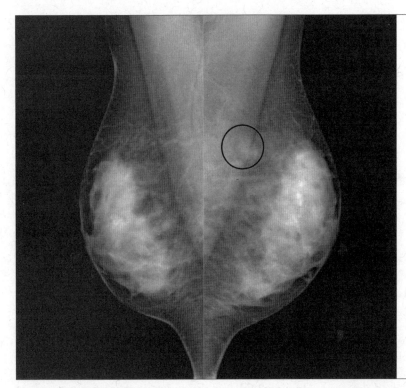

Mammography

Hard to spot on mammography: area indicated within the ring, multiple speculated calcifications are highly suspect findings and usually indicative of a breast cancer.

BREAST IMAGING

While a breast self-examination, clinical physical, biopsy, and ultrasound are adequate in most cases for diagnosing this cancer, other imaging techniques can be helpful, if not conclusive.

Mammography

Mammography is currently the standard of care in screening diagnostics for breast cancer. When an abnormality is found on mammography alone and is non palpable clinically, an ultrasound and biopsy are usually indicated next.

A computerized sterotactic core needle biopsy guided by mammography is often indicated to retrieve a core sampling of tissue. Vacuuming the core sample increases the amount of tissue retrieved, which improves the histological exam and, ultimately, diagnosis.[28]

Positive Findings on Mammography

Tiny microcalcifications are the easiest to recognize on mammography as an abnormal finding. The most common findings associated with breast cancer are these clustered microcalcifications that are polymorphic in character. Usually in these clusters there are at least five to eight in number and aggregated in one area of the breast tissue. Often times they are arranged in a V or Y shaped configuration that may be associated with a mammographic mass density.

Usually these densities have irregular borders and architectural distortion that may be subtle and very difficult to detect.

Mammography is limited in its sensitivity and correctly identifies malignancies in only 20% to 30% of suspicious lesions. Dense, fibrous breast tissue (usually associated with a younger age of the female at the time of the test) makes accurate identification of tumors and abnormal structures difficult, and it is impossible for mammography to image areas surrounding the breasts or to look for tumors that may have migrated from the breast tissue to adjacent areas of tissue, lymph, and bone. Other imaging techniques have been developed to help overcome this limitation of mammography, although each has its own limitations.[29]

Better mammographic technology, including digitized mammography, routine use of magnified views, and greater skill in mammographic interpretation, combined with newer diagnostic techniques (MRI, magnetic resonance spectroscopy, positron emission tomography) may make it possible to identify breast cancers even more reliably and earlier. Screening by any technique other than mammography is not indicated; however, younger women who are BRCA-1 or BRCA-2 carriers may benefit from MRI screening where the higher sensitivity may outweigh the loss of specificity.[29]

Miraluma Test Results

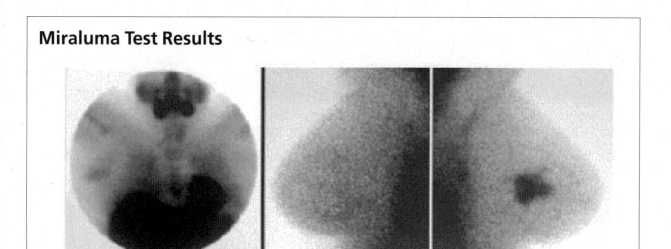

Miraluma

Miraluma, also called scintimammography or sestamibi breast imaging, is a nuclear medicine test used for breast imaging. It is used by a radiologist in adjunct to mammography when trying to locate suspicious lesions. It is particularly beneficial in dense breast tissue in identifying these suspicious lesions. Using the miraluma a reduction in the number of biopsies performed in women with dense and fibrous breast tissue has been noted as well as the ability to find some malignancies that would otherwise have been missed in these tissue types. Miraluma can produce some striking pictures of these inconspicuous lesions, even in the midst of the dense tissue. Miraluma is highly sensitive with a low specificity, which makes it not a good candidate for a first-line diagnostic tool. It is effective when used adjunctively with mammography in women with dense breast tissues.

However, the miraluma test uses radioactive drugs that are thought to accumulate in areas of increased metabolic activity associated with malignant cells. The patient receives a small amount of technetium 99, a radiopharmaceutical, by injection and then the breasts are imaged with a Gamma camera. In vitro studies show that the concentration of the drug is up to 9x higher in malignant than in normal cells.[30]

Positive findings on Miraluma test
- Patient Hx: Asymmetric density within the UOQ of the right breast corresponding to palpable abnormality. Density questionable due to scarring from previous surgery. Mammogram finds suspect mass. Ultrasound revealed multiple cysts.
- Miraluma findings: Abnormal uptake in the right breast corresponding with mass seen on mammography.
- Histopathology results: Intraductal carcinoma, comedocarcinoma features

Breast Thermography

In thermography, a heat-sensing infared camera is used to record the surface temperature or heat produced by the different parts of the body being examined. Abnormal tissue growth can cause temperature changes on the surface of the skin, which will show up positive on the thermogram. Thermography is not a good screening device – it is highly sensitive with a very low specificity. It can be used adjunctively, especially to detect tumors that may not be palpable. It does not adequately detect DCIS and is only approved for adjunct evaluation in conjunction with mammography.[31]

Grading and Staging

Grading and staging of breast cancer patients is of the upmost importance in making an accurate prognosis as well as indicating the conventional therapeutic protocol route. Most of the therapeutic decision making will be based on the TNM status: T stands for the primary tumor, N for the regional nodes, and M for metastasis. The classification of staging in breast cancer has changed several times over the last two decades in order to perfect a tool that tends to be more complex, but the results are significant in the changes of outcomes.[32]

Conventional Therapies for Breast Cancer

Surgery, radiation, chemotherapy, and hormone therapy are deployed separately or in various combinations to arrest and eradicate breast cancer. Naturopathic medicine has been integrated with these

Staging of Breast Cancer

Primary Tumor (T)

T0	No evidence of primary tumor
TIS	Carcinoma in situ
T1	Tumor 2 cm
T1a	Tumor >0.1 cm but 0.5 cm
T1b	Tumor >0.5 but 1 cm
T1c	Tumor >1 cm but 2 cm
T2	Tumor >2 cm but 5 cm
T3	Tumor >5 cm
T4	Extension to chest wall, inflammation, satellite lesions, ulcerations

Regional Lymph Nodes (N)

PN0(i-)	No regional lymph node metastasis histologically, negative IHC
PN0(i+)	No regional lymph node metastasis histologically, positive IHC, no IHC cluster greater than 0.2 mm
PN0(mol-)	No regional lymph node metastasis histologically, negative molecular findings (RT-PCR)a
PN0(mol+)	No regional lymph node metastasis histologically, positive molecular findings (RT-PCR)a
PN1	Metastasis in one to three axillary lymph nodes, or in internal mammary nodes with microscopic disease detected by sentinal lymph node dissection but not clinically apparent
PN1mi	Micrometastasis (>0.2mm, none >2.0 mm)
PN1a	Metastasis in one to three axillary lymph nodes
PN1b	Metastasis in internal mammary nodes with microscopic disease detected by sentinel lymph node dissection but not clinically apparentb
PN1c	Metastasis in one to three axillary lymph nodes and in internal mammary lymph nodes with microscopic disease detected by sentinel lymph node dissection but not clinically apparent. b (If associated with greater than three positive axillary lymph nodes, the internal mammary nodes are classified as pN3b to reflect increased tumor burden.)
pN2	Metastasis in four to nine axillary lymph nodes, or in clinically apparent internal mammary lymph nodes in the absence of axillary lymph node metastasis
pN3	Metastasis in ten or more axillary lymph nodes, or in infraclavicular lymph nodes, or in clinically apparent c ipsilateral internal mammary lymph nodes in the presence of 1 or more positive axillary lymph nodes; or in more than 3 axillary lymph nodes with clinically negative microscopic metastasis in internal mammary lymph nodes; or in ipsilateral SCLNs

Distant Metastasis (M)

M0	No distant metastasis

M1	Distant metastasis (includes spread to ipsilateral supraclavicular nodes)

Stage Grouping

Stage 0	TIS	N0	M0
Stage I	T1	N0	M0
Stage IIA	T0	N1	M0
	T1	N1	M0
	T2	N0	M0
Stage IIB	T2	N1	M0
	T3	N0	M0
Stage IIIA	T0	N2	M0
	T1	N2	M0
	T2	N2	M0
	T3	N1, N2	M0
Stage IIIB	T4	Any N	M0
	Any T	N3	M0
Stage IIIC	Any T	N3	M0
Stage IV	Any T	Any N	M1

Adapted from the American Joint Committee on Cancer (AJCC), Chicago, Illinois. AJCC Cancer Staging Manual, 6th ed. New York, NY: Springer, 2002.[32]

conventional treatments to enhance their efficacy and reduce adverse side effects.

SURGERY AND RADIATION

Conventional treatment is guided by disease grading and staging, the patient's physical condition, and the patient's preferences. The biopsy and sentinel lymph node biopsy (a sentinel node is the first node that receives drainage from the tumor site) direct the disease grading and staging. The sentinel node and biopsy can reduce the need for axillary lymph node dissection. The sentinel node can be identified in over 90% of patients and has a positive predictive value in almost 100% of the cases.[33]

Staging

Stage 0:

DCIS, regardless of tumor size, is cured in 98% of cases with a surgical intervention of partial or total mastectomy followed by radiation therapy; axillary dissection and systemic adjuvant chemotherapy are not deemed necessary.[32]

Stage I and II:

Localized breast cancer management includes local and systemic (adjuvant) treatment strategies. Local treatment includes surgical intervention of mastectomy (partial or total) and axillary lymph node dissection. Mastectomy is followed by radiation therapies to prevent local recurrence and microscopic metastasis from occurring. This is the typical conventional protocol for women who have an invasive form of breast cancer with axillary lymph node involvement, invasive ductal or lobular carcinoma that is greater than 1cm in largest diameter, or with favorable histological findings invasive carcinoma greater than 3 cm in largest diameter because of the high risk associated with recurrence after localized therapies. Tamoxifen has been shown to increase disease-free survival rates and overall survival rates in postmenopausal women, although there

---

BREAST-CONSERVING THERAPY

Large randomized studies have shown that disease-free survival rates are similar for those patients treated with partial mastectomy plus axillary dissection followed by radiation therapy as compared to those treated with modified radical mastectomy.[26] The NSABP trial (The National Surgical Adjuvant Breast and Bowel Project) randomized patients into three groups:

1. Lumpectomy with tumor free margins (1 mm circumference) plus whole breast radiation
2. Lumpectomy alone
3. Total mastectomy

All the patients had axillary lymph node dissection and some had tumors as large as 4 cm with or without palpable lymph nodes. Twenty years of follow up showed the lowest local recurrence rate among those patients treated with lumpectomy and post operative radiation. Overall survival rates and disease-free survival rates were similar among the three treatment groups, showing that lumpectomy with axillary lymph node dissection followed by adjuvant radiation therapy is as effective as modified radical mastectomy for the management of patients with stage I and II breast cancer.

Tumor size is a major consideration in determining whether breast conservation surgery is warranted. The larger sized tumor and subareolar tumors are difficult to excise without deformity but are not necessarily contraindications. The NSABP trial did accept tumors as large as 4 cm, which makes the achievement of acceptable cosmetic results dependant on the patient having a sufficiently sized breast to enable an excision of a 4 cm tumor without deformity.[26]

The Breast Cancer Prevention Trial (BCPT) revealed a > 49% reduction in breast cancer among women with a risk of at least 1.66% taking the drug for 5 years. Raloxifene has shown similar breast cancer prevention potency but may have different effects on bone and heart. The two agents have been compared in a prospective randomized prevention trial (the STAR trial). The agents are approximately equivalent in preventing breast cancer with fewer thromboembolic events and endometrial cancers with raloxifene; however, raloxifene did not reduce noninvasive cancers as effectively as tamoxifen, so no clear winner has emerged.[11]

Contraindications to breast conserving surgery would include multifocal lesions, fixation of the tumor to the chest wall or skin, cancer involved in the nipple or overlying skin, and metastatic disease upon initial diagnosis. Modified radical mastectomy is the standard therapy for these patients. A modified radical mastectomy includes the removal of the entire breast, overlying skin, nipple, and aerolar complex, as well as the underlying pectoralis fascia and axillary lymph nodes. The advantage is that radiation therapy may not be necessary, although if multiple lymph nodes are involved, radiation is still indicated. The cosmetic and psychological impact of mastectomy can have a detrimental impact on the patient, so the patient should always be well informed and a part of the decision making for this interventional therapy.[31]

is no advantage and some increase in detrimental side effects to continuing Tamoxifen therapy beyond 5 years. Women with ER- breast cancer do not generally benefit from Tamoxifen, although Tamoxifen has shown a reducing effect in the incidence of contralateral breast cancer development in women with both ER- and ER+ breast cancer. Primary treatment with tamoxifen is only recommended in those patients who cannot undergo interventional surgery.[34]

Stage III:

Locally advanced breast cancer is managed with a combination of systemic and local therapies. Often preoperative systemic chemotherapy regimens that contain doxorubicin or mitoxantrone is the first intervention to reduce the tumor size (burden). After this reduction is obtained, then surgical intervention with mastectomy followed by radiation may be used. With this strategy about 50% of patients are alive and disease free 5 years post treatment. "It is unclear whether adjuvant chemotherapy and hormonal therapy after preoperative chemotherapy and regional treatment in locally advanced breast cancer decrease further recurrence or prolong life. In the case of inflammatory breast cancer, hormonal therapy by itself is seldom effective; a combination of chemotherapy and hormonal therapy is advisable."[35]

Stage IV:

In women who are postmenopausal with ER+ tumors or tumors whose receptor status in unknown, hormonal therapy is indicated as the best treatment with a long disease-free survival rate. Antiestrogens are the first line therapeutic strategies followed by aromataste inhibitors and progestins. "In about 15% of patients with bone metastases, tamoxifen causes tumor flare-up resulting in hypercalcemia. This transient complication can be managed with IV fluids and furosemide and does not warrant stopping the drug. Patients sometimes respond to a second hormonal treatment after the first becomes ineffective."[36] In patients who are hormone receptor negative (or unresponsive) or who have a life-threatening disease (metastatic spread to the liver or lungs), chemotherapy is the indicated first-line therapy. Combinations of chemotherapeutics are now the conventional treatment regimen used for better long-term outcomes.[37]

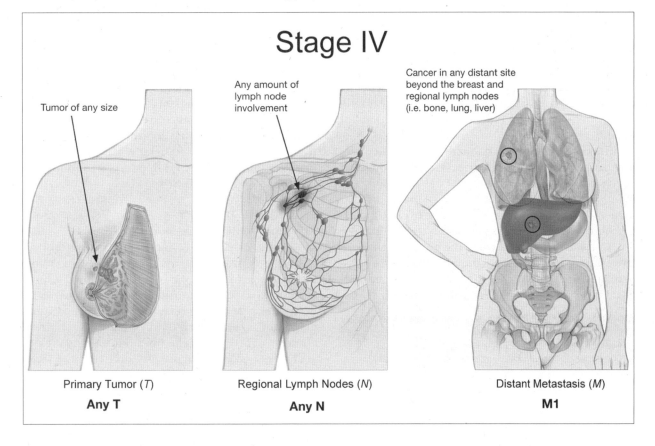

Stage IV

Tumor of any size

Any amount of lymph node involvement

Cancer in any distant site beyond the breast and regional lymph nodes (i.e. bone, lung, liver)

Primary Tumor (*T*)
Any T

Regional Lymph Nodes (*N*)
Any N

Distant Metastasis (*M*)
M1

CHEMOTHERAPY

Breast cancer responds well to a many different chemotherapeutic agents, especially taxanes, anthrocyclines, alkylating agents, and antimetabolites. Using these agents in multiple combinations has been found to improve response rates. The choice of using a multidrug combination depends on whether or what type of adjuvant chemotherapy was administered.

More than half the patients treated for localized breast cancer develop metastatic disease, which is the overall cause of mortality in breast cancer patients. Soft tissue, bone, and visceral (liver and lung) metastatic disease accounts for approximately one third of breast cancer relapse. Recurrences can appear anytime after the first-line therapies are completed, with half of all recurrences occurring more than 5 years after initial therapy.[38]

Diagnosis of metastatic disease changes the treatment strategies for both the patient and her clinician, and is considered palliative, though not curative. The choice of the therapeutics takes into consideration the overall condition of the patient, the hormone receptor status of the tumor, and the clinical judgment of the practioner. Endocrine therapy is indicated for positive receptor status, while patients with rapidly progressing disease, especially in the viscera, do not seem to benefit from endocrine therapies.[39]

Local therapies, such as surgery and radiation, may be able to manage a patient's disease, relieving symptoms of metastatic disease, especially in bony sites. In patients with only bony metastatic disease, systemic chemotherapy has a very modest effect, whereas radiation therapy may be effective for long periods of time.[40]

Bisphosphonates are a standard of allopathic oncological care in metastatic disease to the bones, in order to increase bone density and maintain well being for as long as possible. New back pain in patients with cancer should always be explored diagnostically on an emergent basis due to the affinity of breast cancer to metastasize to the bone. When there is metastatic involvement to the endocrine organs, systemic dysfunctions can occur and are managed with local therapies instead of a systemic approach.[41]

CMF Regimen

The most common adjuvant chemotherapy protocol is the CMF regimen. Patients may also respond to this protocol in metastatic disease:

- Cyclophosphamide
- Methotrexate
- Fluorouracil. Patients.

Chemotherapy Protocol Options

Single agent: In progressive disease, it is common practice to use a single chemotherapeutic agent. The use of a single agent reduces toxicity while still having a therapeutic effect. The previous discussion of Onco-Typing the aberrant cell for future use in therapeutic strategies comes into play at this point. Most oncologists use either paclitaxel or anthracycline when the initial regimen of chemotherapy fails.[43]

Combinations: The standard combination of cyclophosphamide, methotrexate, and fluorouracil has been substituted in some cases with docetaxel, Herceptin, and carboplatin. A randomized study has suggested that docetaxel may be superior to paclitaxel. Herceptin (trastuzumab) is a humanized antibody to erbB2, and when this receptor is positive, the use of Herceptin with paclitaxel has shown increased survival rates in women with metastatic disease. Avastin (bevacizumab) has shown promising data in the improvement of response rates and duration to paclitaxel. Other tertiary chemotherapeutic strategies include gemcitabine, capecitabine, Navelbine, and oral etoposide.[38,43]

Neoadjuvant strategies: In stage III and IV breast cancer the use of neoadjuvant chemotherapies has gained widespread use. In 90% of patients with locally advanced disease that is not optimum for surgical excision, the use of multidrug chemotherapy that includes anthracycline has shown to reduce the bulk of the tumor burden and make the patient a candidate for surgery and radiation therapy. The best outcomes for these patients are seen in integrative multimodality clinics that coordinate surgery, radiation, and systemic chemotherapy. These approaches produce long-term disease-free survival in one-third to one-half of the patients.[43]

ENDOCRINE THERAPY

The status of ER/PR hormonal receptors is not only significant in diagnosis and prognosis but also in choosing conventional treatment strategies. While breast cancer is thought of as a hormonal cancer because normal breast tissue is estrogen dependant, this phenotype may be retained in both primary and metastatic breast cancer. The best way to determine if any form of breast cancer is hormone dependant is by analysis of estrogen and progesterone receptor levels on the cancer cell surface itself.[42]

The role of endogenous and exogenous hormones in the treatment of breast cancer has been widely studied by cancer researchers and the results remain controversial.

Endogenous estrogen formation may be blocked by using analogues of luteinizing hormone releasing hormone (LHRH) in premenopausal women. It has also been shown through outcomes data that 50% of women who respond to one hormonal therapy will respond to other hormonal therapies. "It is not uncommon for patients to respond to two or three sequential endocrine therapies; however, combination endocrine therapies do not appear to be superior to individual agents, and combinations of chemotherapy with endocrine therapy are not useful. The median survival of patients with metastatic disease is approximately 2 years, and many patients, particularly older persons and those with hormone-dependent disease, may respond to endocrine therapy for 3 to 5 years or longer."[44]

Tumors that are positive for the estrogen receptor and negative for the progesterone receptor have a response rate of ~30%. Tumors that have both receptors have a response rate approaching 70%. If neither receptor is present, the objective response rates are <10%. "Tumors that are positive for the estrogen receptor and negative for the progesterone receptor have a response rate of ~30%. Tumors that have both receptors have a response rate approaching 70%. If neither receptor is present, the objective response rates are <10%."[23] Tumors that lack either or both of these receptors are more likely to recur than tumors that have one or both of them.

Endocrine therapy protocols

Receptor analyses of this kind provide information as to the correct ordering of endocrine therapies. By analyzing the estrogen and progesterone receptor levels of a tumor, information is provided that then can direct the choice of the correct endocrine therapy.

Hormone modulation therapies
- Aromatase inhibitors
- Selective estrogen receptor modulators (SERMs)
- Hormone blockade strategies:
  - LHRH agonists (Lupron)
  - Surgical oophorectomy in premenopausal women

Endocrine therapy should start with an aromatase inhibitor rather than tamoxifen (SERM) modulation. For the small group of women who are ER+ and HER-2/neu +, response rates to aromatase inhibitors are substantially higher than to tamoxifen. Estrogen receptors are considered positive if expressed in 10% of nuclei.[45]

There may be a false positive status associated with

women who are concomitantly taking tamoxifen or high levels of estrogen replacement therapy (ERT). Progesterone receptors may be a false positive if sampled during the luteal phase of a menstruating female. The positive receptor status of ER/PR is associated with an increased overall disease-free survival rate; and it is more likely to be well differentiated and have a low grade of diploidy. A slower proliferation rate may be the associated biochemical difference in this group of women.[46]

ER+/PR+ status

Studies have shown how this status directs conventional hormonal modulation therapies in early stage diagnoses with the 5-year use of Tamoxifen (SERM):[34]
- Reduces recurrence by 50% and mortality by 28%
- High ER expression: decreased recurrence by 60%
- Low ER expression: decreased recurrence by 43%

In advanced stage breast cancer, 70% of all ER+/PR+ cases studied responded to hormone modulation with response rates higher than 45%:[47]
- 35% to 45% response rates with ER-/PR+ or ER+/PR- receptors
  - Higher response with PR+/ER-
  - PR thought to indicate intact endocrine response pathway
- 10% ER-/PR- cases responded

Antiestrogens

In the BCPT trials, tamoxifen was shown to be a promising SERM for preventing breast cancer in women who are at an increased risk of developing the disease.[11] This data spurred the creation of more oncogenic pharmaceuticals to target cancer cell biology. Aromatase inhibitors were developed that showed increase effect with better long-term survival statistics when used as an initial endocrine therapeutic. In one study of women who were ER+ and also HER-2/neu+, response rates to aromatase inhibitors were significantly higher than to tamoxifen. Pharmaceutical research into newer more "pure" anti-estrogens that are free from clinical side effects are currently in clinical trial.[48] The theory is that decreasing estrogen will in turn shrink the tumor. This idea is seen at work in the use of LHRH hormone blockade with analogues of luteinizing hormone releasing hormone in women who are premenopausal. Metastatic hormone dependent patients may respond to endocrine therapy for 3 to 5 yrs longer than those with hormone independent metastatic disease showing a mortality rate of approximately 2 years.[48]

5-Year Survival Rate for Breast Cancer by Stage

Stage	5-Year Survival, %
0	99
I	92
IIA	82
IIB	65
IIIA	47
IIIB	44
IV	14

Adapted from from data of the National Cancer Institute-Surveillance, Epidemiology, and End Results (SEER).[31]

Naturopathic Approaches

The naturopathic approach to treating breast cancer and supporting conventional breast cancer treatments is fourfold, grounded in our knowledge of cell biology and inflammatory pathways.

> **Naturopathic therapeutic goals and order**
> 1. Decrease inflammation
> 2. Control growth factors
> 3. Suppress proliferation
> 4. Enhance chemoprevention

To achieve these therapeutic goals, naturopathic medicine employs the modalities of clinical nutrition, botanical medicine, and immunotherapy (psychoneuroendoimmunology).

DECREASE INFLAMMATION

Inflammation is the 'hot bed' where a cell can denature, become aberrant, and transform itself into a cancer cell. Decreasing inflammation and modulating inflammatory interleukins and cytokines is fundamental for treating breast cancer successfully. This involves countering the generation of free radicals that contribute to inflammation.

Free Radicals

Free radicals are highly reactive molecules that not only create and maintain inflammation, but also perpetuate the inflammation response by direct oxidative damage to cells. These same free radicals also excite, or increase, the activity of the different enzymes (proteins) that perpetuate the inflammatory response. Free radicals cause oxidative stress on the system, and once they reach a threshold of out numbering the antioxidants to counter balance, then the free radicals are creating a chronic inflammation dysfunction.

At this point in the system, the free radicals are damaging and denaturing cellular DNA, orchestrating cellular mutations, and reducing apoptosis. All of the strategies that a cancer cell needs for co-creation and progression are met by the state of chronic inflammation. Antioxidants can circumvent this by 'scavenging' the free radicals and preventing the inflammatory cycle from expression. Antioxidants then are preventing damage to DNA, turning off inflammation by reducing oxidative damage to the cell, thus preventing cancer expression.[50]

Antioxidant treatment

Antioxidants enhance cancer therapies by increasing tumor response and decreasing toxicity. Studies have shown that high doses of antioxidants will induce cell differentiation, growth inhibition, and apoptosis in human cancer cells both *in vitro* and *in vivo*, although one study of lung cancer has shown an increase in the incidence of this cancer in male Finnish cigarette smokers administered betacarotene.

Antioxidant Anticancer Action of Nutraceutical and Botanical Medicines

Nutraceutical and Botanical Medicine	Therapeutic Dose	Antioxidant Action
Vitamin E d-alpha-tocopherol	400-500 IU qd	Shown to reduce IL-8 production and angiogenesis while preventing tumor formation by stimulating a potent immune response that selectively destroys tumor cells[51]
		Can induce apoptosis and suppresses tumor growth by 80%[55]
		Inhibits gastric carcinoma cell growth in vitro in a dose and time dependent fashion[56]
		α-tocopherol and ascorbate independently, and in combination, decrease the production of reactive oxygen species in human spermatocytes exposed to H2O2[57]
		The pretreatment of hepatocytes with tocopherol succinate (TS) dramatically enriched cells and mitochondria with alpha-tocopherol and provided these membranes with complete protection against ethyl methanesulfonate (EMS)-induced oxidative damage. TS pretreatment suppressed EMS-induced cellular ROS production, generated from mitochondrial complex I and III sites[58]
Green tea	50-85% polyphenols 100-300 mg qd-tid	EGCG from green tea is very effective in reducing IL-8 production and angiogenesis. Green tea catechins, supplemented with vitamin E, have a synergistic preventive effect on tumor development. Antioxidants have shown to affect cellular membrane integrity by preventing lipid peroxidation[49]
Lycopene	10-50 mg qd-tid	Specific carotenoid antioxidant that could play a role in the recovery of the integrity of cell membrane of the liver after radiation injury[52]
Omega-3 fatty acids	2-3 g EPA qqd EPA/DHA in a 2:1	Omega-3 rich diets with vitamins E and C have shown to have beneficial anticancer effects[53]
Astragalus	100-300 mg qd-tid	Increases the activity of Ag-presenting macrophages and of CD4 T cell activity. Theoretically, this could lead to increased ADCC with subsequent tumor cell death[54]
Melatonin	20 mg qhs	Blocks the mitogenic effects of tumor promoting hormones and growth factors. Increases P53 activity and cancer cell apoptosis[59]
		Concomitant administration of melatonin with TMX induces regression in patients refractory to TMX alone[60]
		Reverses LHRH resistance in Ca[61]

Nutraceutical and Botanical Medicine	Therapeutic Dose	Antioxidant Action
Melatonin (continued)	20 mg qhs	Melatonin acts as a biological response modifier in cancer patients[62]
		Melatonin, a pineal secretory product with antioxidant properties, protects against cisplatin induced nephrotoxicity in rats[63]
		50 patients with brain mets from various solid tumors who progressed following radiation and chemotherapy[64]
		Randomized to either supportive care alone (steroids + anticonvulsants) or progression significantly longer in MLT group (5.9 ± 0.8 mo. Vs 2.7 ± 1.06 mo., p<0.05)
		One year survival significantly higher in the MLT group (9/24 vs 3/26, p<0.05)
		When analyzed by site of primary cancer, only those with a single brain met from lung cancer maintained a significant difference (6/10 vs 2/12MLT (20 mg/day qhs)
		20 previously untreated patients with inoperable lung cancer (16 NSCLC, 4 SCLC)[65]
		Randomized to receive either carboplatin (5 AUC on day 1) and etoposide (150 mg/m_/day on days 1-3) or carboplatin-etoposide+MLT (40 mg qhs) No effect observed on depth and duration of toxicity for hemoglobin, ANC, or ANC nadir in cross over fashion
		250 metastatic solid tumor patients (104 lung) with poor clinical status
		Randomized to receive chemotherapy or chemotherapy + MLT (20 mg qhs)
		Lung Cancer[66] Cisplatin + etoposide gemcitabine The 1 year survival rate and the objective tumor regression rate were significantly higher in patients concomittantly treated with MLT than chemotherapy (CT) alone
		Tumor response rate 42/124 CT + MLT versus 19/126 CT alone (p<0.001)
Zinc	15-30 mg qd	Apoptosis[67,68]
Selenium	200 mcg qd	The essential trace mineral selenium (Se) has been shown to inhibit intestinal, prostate, lung, and liver tumor development and associated mortality in both experimental animals and humans[69]

Nutraceutical and Botanical Medicine	Therapeutic Dose	Antioxidant Action
Selenium (continued)		Although Se is likely to be one of the most powerful cancer chemopreventive agents in the human diet, its mechanism of action is still under investigation
		Low Se status results in a decrease in the expression of genes involved in detoxification, thus reducing the amounts of activated carcinogens[69]
Ginkgo biloba	120-240 mg qd	Chemosensitization[70]
Curcumin	200-400 mg qd-tid	Chemosensitization[72]
Adaptogens		Growth inhibition of protein kinase-C[73-75]
		Reduces oncogene expression
		Reduce transplanted tumor growth
		Reduction in tumor size
Vitamin C	1-3 grams qd up to (TBT) bowel tolerance	No reduction in cytotoxicity of chemotherapy[76]
		Stabilizes P53[77]
		Decreased lipid accumulation post CMF treatment[78]
		Vitamin C supplementation in chronic hemodialysis patients can reduce the lymphocyte intracellular ROS production, as well as up-regulate hOGG1 gene expression for repair[79]
CoQ10	100-300 mg qd-qid	CoQ10 is used with vitamin E to protect patients from chemotherapy-induced cardiomyopathies. CoQ10 is nontoxic even at high dosages and has been shown to prevent liver damage from the drugs Mitomycin C and 5-FU Adriamycin-induced cardiomyopathies have been prevented by concomitant supplementation with CoQ10[80]
		Doxorubicin (Adriamycin®) mechanism: CoQ10 reduces free radical formation induced by doxorubicin[81]
		Studies with both animals and humans have found that pretreating with Coenzyme Q10, at levels of 100 mg per day, reduces cardiac toxicity caused by doxorubicin[81]

Antioxidant Combinations for Breast Cancer Therapy

1. CoQ10
2. Curcumin
3. Vitamin E
4. Vitamin D3
5. Vitamin C

Antioxidants in combinations are far more potent than single antioxidant agents.[49] They optimize activity at different oxygen tensions and are more effective against clones of cancer cells with differing metabolic patterns.

In one study, they were shown to potentiate one another. A mixture of four antioxidants, including omega-3 fatty acids, markedly inhibited the growth of human melanoma cells in vitro.[82] Omega-3 fatty acids are safe and effective antioxidants that are not contraindicated with many of the chemo/radio treatment strategies.[53]

Antioxidants inhibit angiogenesis.[83] Proliferating cancer cells cause cytokines that stimulate an increase in endothelial cells, which then increases vascular supply to the tumor. Antioxidants inhibit these cytokines: IL-1. IL-8, bFGF (basic fibroblast growth factor), TGF (transforming growth factor, both alpha and beta), PD-EGF (platelet permeability factor), VPF (vascular permeability factor), and TNF (tumor necrosis factor).[84]

Antioxidants also have indicated apoptotic effects by inducing differentiation and apoptosis. A mixture of antioxidants with vitamins is even more effective than individual vitamins in creating this effect. This effect was seen in cancer cells that were evading apoptosis after conventional treatment until treated with vitamins.[87]

COX-2

The role of inflammation in breast cancer has been directly linked to an overexpression of COX-2. The overexpression of this proinflammatory pathway has been linked to DIC as well as established breast cancer. Overexpression of COX-2 causes an autocrine stimulation of an aromatase gene by tumor cells. This stimulation is due to the conversion of arachidonic acid (AA) to prostaglandin 2 (PGE2) series by the COX-2 enzyme.

PGE2 is then considered a proinflammatory state because it stimulates the aromatase enzyme. The increased aromatase enzyme leads to an increased estrogen (ER) formation at the site of the cancer. The continued progression of breast cancer is associated with the increased expression of ER. This combined result is a stimulation of the tumor to both grow and invade surrounding healthy tissues.

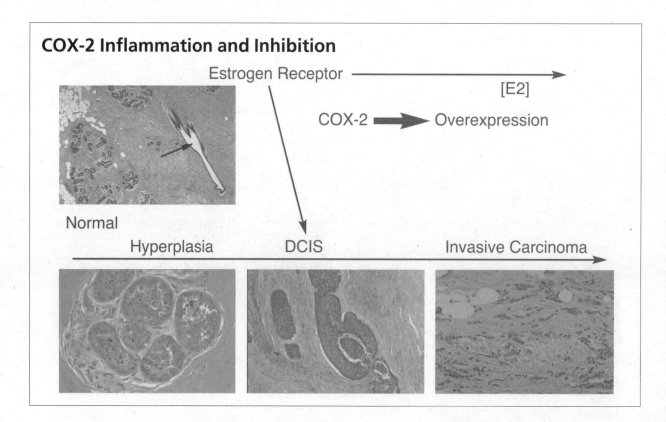

COX-2 Inflammation and Inhibition

Estrogen Receptor

[E2]

COX-2 ➡ Overexpression

Normal

Hyperplasia   DCIS   Invasive Carcinoma

The therapeutic goal is to inhibit the COX-2, thus preventing the PGE2 series to turn on aromatase and stimulate ER production. COX-2 inhibition is an exciting new area of cancer treatment and research. COX-2 inhibition in breast cancer pathogenesis results in:

- Inhibition of angiogenesis
- Inhibition of cell growth and invasion
- Inhibition of tumor associated inflammation
- Pro-apoptotic effects
- Inhibition of PGE2 associated aromatase induction

Herbal COX-2 Inhibitors

Many herbs have specific anti-inflammatory action and can be used as effective anti-cancer agents. These medicinal herbs have been used in traditional indigenous cultures for thousands of years. Their ability to affect the cyclooxygenase (COX-1 and COX-2) pathway of inflammation is a 'hot bed' for current clinical research when it comes to cancer prevention and treatment.

Glycyrrhiza glabra

Licorice been shown to be a great COX-2 inhibitor, but because it is highly phytoestrogenic,, it is not appropriate as a first-line naturopathic therapy in the treatment of breast cancer. This herb will be discussed in other integrative naturopathic oncology protocols for other cancers.[85]
Dose: Solid extract. ¼ tsp. q.d.-t.i.d.

Phyllanthus amarus

The in vitro application of the extract of this Ayurvedic herb has shown that it does inhibit the induction of iNOS, COX-2, and TNF-alpha.[86]
Dose: 100-500 mg q.d.-t.i.d.

Zingiber officinalis

Ginger has been shown to have a positive effect on nausea and dyspepsia associated with chemo/radio therapies. Traditionally, this herb has a long-standing use for pelvic stagnation or inflammation. In vitro studies on human synoviocytes that were obtained during primary knee replacement from osteoarthritis patients were incubated with ginger extract. A significant demonstration of ginger's ability to suppress production of TNF-alpha as well as COX-2 expression was found. Also associated in this study was the suppression of NF-kappa B, which suggests that ginger blocks the transcription of COX-2.[87]
Dose: 50-1000 mg q.d.

Scutellaria baicalensis

This herb and other species of this genera have been used traditionally to treat inflammatory and cancerous conditions. An in vitro study was done on mice inoculated with head and neck squamous cell carcinoma comparing Scutellaria baicalensis to celecoxib (celebrex™). Head and neck squamous cell cancer has a high expression of COX-2. This study revealed that the herb administered orally to the inoculated mice caused inhibition of COX-2 expression, while the celebrex inhibited COX-2 activity directly. No inhibition was seen in mice inoculated with a non tumorgenic cell line, which indicates that a selective activity of COX-2 inhibition is happening in the tumor cells. There was a 66% reduction of the tumor mass observed in the herbally treated verum group of mice.[88]
Dose: 100-300 mg q.d.-t.i.d.

Curcuma longa

The root of this herb has been used historically as an anti-inflammatory that promotes wound healing and enhances longevity. The root contains curcumin, a herbal constituent under clinical trial in relation to cancer and chemoprevention. An identified mechanism of action of curcumin is that it does induce Phase 2 detoxification enzymes, especially glutathione transferases and quinine reductase. Curcumin has also been found to inhibit the procarcinogenic activation of Phase 1 enzymes, such as cP4501 A1 in vitro.[89] This finding induced many researchers to look at curcumin as a chemopreventitive as well as in the use of overcoming chemoresistance.[37]
Dose: 500-1000 mg q.d.-t.i.d.

CONTROL CELL GROWTH FACTORS

Controlling the factors that stimulate or inhibit cell growth is another naturopathic approach to be integrated with conventional treatment strategies. In many cases, stimulation will increase aberrant cell growth and thus needs to be controlled, while inhibition of the inflammatory process can be stimulated by cell receptor site ignition.

Manipulation of estrogen and progesterone receptors is key to controlling cell growth. Foods high in phytoestrogens, as well as phytoestrogen supplements, can play an important role in inhibiting aberrant cell growth in ER+ cancers.

Soy Foods

Using soy phytoestrogens therapeutically continues to be a controversial topic among oncologists and integrative naturopaths. The concept of phytoestrogen filling ER+ receptor sites and deferring the estradiol biochemical pathway has received positive and negative support in animal model research.[45] Further investigation is warranted before the safety and efficacy can be fully determined.

The active flavonoids in soy that have the most activity are genistein and daizden. Genistein has been studied exclusively in breast cancer models and has been found to bind to ERα on MCF-7 (ER+ breast cancer cells) and stimulate transcription and proliferation of MCF-7 cells.[45] This was found to be concentration dependent: at levels up to 1 μM, genistein is a full ERα agonist. Long-term exposure has been postulated to promote breast cancer development and stimulate the progression of ER+ tumors.

Genistein blood levels in humans on high soy diets are reported between 1 μM - 6 μM and the maximum concentration that can be reached physiologically is reported to be 18.5 μM.[90] At concentrations above 10 μM, other mechanisms may cause cytotoxic effects on breast cancer cells, as well as modulate inflammation. At high concentrations that are largely unachievable through diet, at 50 μM - 100 μM, most of these cytotoxic effects are found.[91] At these high concentrations, genistein will up-regulate heat shock protein mRNA, which is involved in apoptotic signaling, and at the same time down-regulate mRNA expression of ERa. Other decreases in downstream regulators were found by effecting tyrosine kinase expression, which causes a cell cycle arrest in G0-G1 and G2-M by up-regulating p21. P21 is a protein that acts as a molecular switch that triggers telomere initiated senescence.[92]

Ginkgo biloba

This medicinal herb is strongly phytoestrogenic by the actions of its flavonoid constituents. *Ginkgo biloba* extract (GBE) contains 24% phytoestrogens (PE), identified in one study as kaempferol, quercitin, and isorhamnetin. GBE and its PEs bind to both ERα and ERβ, with a higher affinity for the ERβ. In this same study, the GBE and PEs both induced cell proliferation in ER+ MCF=7 cells.[39,103]

Glycyrrhiza glabra

Licorice also contains phytoestrogenic flavonoids. It is used in classical herbal medicine as a phytoestrogen precursor and adaptogen. However, in animal studies investigating estrogen dependent endometrial carcinoma cells, licorice extracts have demonstrated anti-estrogen effects when given with estradiol. It was postulated by the investigators that the mechanism of action is the suppression of estrogen induced c-fos/jun mRNA expression and the expression of corresponding proto-oncogene proteins in the uterine tissue studied. It is conceivable that this effect overshadows the phytoestrogenic effect of the licorice extract, or that the phytoestrogenic effect is minimal in whole herb extracts.[46]

Indole-3-carbinol and 3-3'-diindolylmethane

These compounds affect antiproliferative signaling pathways and show control in cell-cycle gene transcription in human breast cancer cells by regulating promoter-Sp1 transcription factor interactions. These compounds are found naturally in the Brassica or cruciferous vegetables, but you would need to eat approximately 20 lbs of these vegetables a day to receive a therapeutic dose. I3C and DIM convert estrone to the 2-hydroxyestrone metabolite, which is the proper pathway of estrogen excretion. This coupled with antiproliferative and apoptotic effects, while inhibiting transcription of genes driven by ERα binding. These data show that I3C induces apoptotic genes in breast cancer and theoretically can have synergistic effect with aromatase inhibitors.[93]

Silybum marianum

Milk thistle inhibits EGFR receptor sites through the plant constituents silymarin and especially silibinin. Inhibition of receptor and non receptor tyrosine kinase signaling pathways showed positive inhibition of TNF-α and mRNA expression. These actions resulted in decreased cell growth and DNA synthesis in human prostate, breast, and cervical cancer cells. Silybin inhibits the growth of ovarian cells in a dose-dependent manner. The growth of these cells was arrested in the G1 phase of cell division.[94]

SUPPRESS PROLIFERATION

Medicinal herbs can help suppress aberrant cell proliferation by and promote apoptosis.

Cimicifuga racemosa

Extracts of black cohosh were found to induce cell cycle arrest at G1 by decreasing cyclin D1. Cyclin D1 promotes transition from G1 to S in the cell cycle and is overexpressed in 50% to 60% of primary human breast cancers. The constituent actein has this particular effect by decreasing cyclin D1. This growth inhibition was demonstrated with alcoholic extract of the plant for both ER+ and ER- cells. The effect in human probands has not been explored, and the required dose to create this effect in humans is unknown.[95] It is still unclear if black cohosh is safe for use in women with active breast cancer or a history of breast cancer, although there is no convincing data demonstrating harm or risk. Although *Cimicifuga* is not considered a phytoestrogen, it may have other tumor promoting actions.

> **Apoptosis-promoting Herbs**
> Induction of p53 cell-mediated apoptosis activity was shown by phytochemicals genistein from soy, EGCG from green tea, curcumin from turmeric, and silibinin from milk thistle.[96-99]

PROMOTING CHEMOPREVENTION

Specific medicinal herbs and nutrients help promote chemoprevention.

Green tea

Clinical trials show that green tea has inhibitory actions on almost all steps of carcinogenesis. The pooled relative risk for the highest levels of green tea consumption on the risk of developing breast cancer was 0.79 (95% CI, 0.62-1.01; p=0.064). The highest levels of green tea consumption (typically >5 cups daily) showed a pooled relative risk of 0.56 (95% CI, 0.38-0.83; p = 0.0041) for stage I and II disease.[100]

Curcumin

When DES-fed rats were supplemented with curcumin, the incidence of mammary tumors was 28% as opposed to 84.6% in DES only rats.[71]

Glycyrrhiza glabra

Early in-vitro research demonstrated inhibition of human breast cancer cell (MCF-7) proliferation by *Glycyrrhiza uralensis* extract.[85]

Quercetin

In-vitro research has demonstrated that quercetin binds to ERα, but impairs activation of signal transduction pathways.[101]

Chemotherapy-Specific Integrated Therapies

Several naturopathic therapies increase the effectiveness of standard chemotherapies and reduce side effects. Among the most common naturopathic therapies are silymarin (milk thistle), which supports detoxification of the chemotherapeutic, and CoQ10 (ubiquinone), which supports antioxidation mechanisms.

SILYMARIN MARIANUM

Adriamycin (doxorubicin), Cytoxan (cyclophosphamide), Taxotere (docetaxel), Femara (letrozole), and Taxol (paclitaxel) are the most common chemotherapeutics used in the treatment of breast cancer, and all are cleared through the CYP3A4 isoenzyme pathway of the cytochrome p450 monooxygenase system in the liver. This pathway is very sensitive to drug/herb/nutrient interaction and clearance,

Highly Recommended Integrative Therapies

Therapy	Dose
Silymarin	250-500 mg qd-tid[105]
CoQ10	100-400 mg qd-tid[24,80-81,102,104]
Melatonin	20 mg at bedtime[59-66]
Medicinal mushrooms: *Coriolus versicolor* (turkey tails), *Grifola frondosa* (maitake), *Ganoderma lucidum* (reishi)	Extracted by an aqueous cold water extraction method and then can be used at levels up to 3000 mg qd in divided doses long term or as freeze-dried Mycellium (fruiting bodies)[106]
EGCG from green tea	5-10 cups daily with 50-100% polyphenolics per cup of tea or the equivalent of 600-1800 mg daily in divided doses (not decaffeinated because then the polyphenols are removed and these are the active cancer fighters[100]

Chemotherapeutic and Naturopathic Integrated Therapies

Chemotherapeutic	Naturopathic	Daily Dose	Caution
Cytoxan (cyclophosphamide) Taxotere (docetaxel) Femara (letrozole) Taxol (paclitaxel)	*To increase effectiveness:* Silymarin	250 mg	Fixates CYP 450 Avoid Quercitin
	To reduce toxicity: Glutamine	10 g tid, swish & swallow	
Adriamycin (Doxorubicin)	*To increase effectiveness:* Green tea Quercitin Vitamin A Vitamin C Vitamin E	5-10 cups qd 100-300 mg qd-tid 10,000-50,000 IU qd 1000-3000 mg qd 400-1000 IU qd	Avoid use of NAC, glutathione, and curcumin
	To reduce toxicity: CoQ10 L-Carnitine Vitamin A Vitamin C Vitamin E	100 mg qd 500-1000 qd 10,000-50,000 IU qd 1000-3000 mg qd 400-1000 IU qd	
Cisplatin/Carboplatin	*To increase effectiveness:* Glutathione	800-2000 mg	Do not use with chemotherapies
	To reduce toxicity: Glutamine	10 g tid, swish and swallow	
Cisplatin	*To increase effectiveness:* Quercitin Silymarin Curcumin Vitamin A Vitamin C Vitamin D Medicinal Mushrooms (Stamets 7, Turkey tails)	100-300 mg qd-tid 250 mg qd 200-400 mg qd-tid 10,000-50,000 IU qd 1000-3000 mg qd 2000-5000 IU qd	Avoid quercitin, silymarin, and curcumin on days receiving chemotherapy 3-day Rule: discontinue natural therapies three days before and after chemotherapy
	To reduce toxicity: Selenium	400-800 mcg qd	Avoid NAC and high-dose vitamin B-6 above 200 mg q.d.
Taxol / Taxotere	*To increase effectiveness:* Glutamine Vitamin C Selenium	10 g tid, swish & swallow TBT 4-6 mcg	Avoid Berberine, Quercitin. Should not be taken with taxanes, dacarbazine, tamoxifen, anastrozole, exemestane, letrozole, or eriotinib
	To reduce toxicity: Glutamine	10 g tid, swish & swallow	

Chemotherapeutic and Naturopathic Integrated Therapies

Chemotherapeutic	Naturopathic	Daily Dose	Caution
Tamoxifen	*To increase effectiveness:* Melatonin	20 mg qhs	Avoid I3C with Tamoxifen. May have harmful estrogenic effects and can increase the speed at which the tamoxifen is metabolized as well as some studies showing that it may increase estrogen metabolism toward carcinogenic and anticarcinogenic metabolites
	To reduce side effects: Hot flushes are a side effect of Tamoxifen-reducing estrogens:		
	Sage (*Salvia officinalis*) Within a few weeks, patients report a decrease in night sweats as well	1-3 cups	Consider use of DIM alternatively. Avoid Quercitin.

and may metabolize the chemotherapies inappropriately with these interactions. *Silymarin* (milk thistle) affects the clearance of the cyp450 pathway and may actually speed up clearance and decrease the side effects of chemotherapy; grapefruit juice has been postulated to have the same effect. Disease of the liver, CHF, polypharmacy with prescriptive antidepressants, antihistamines, and antibiotics may slow the metabolism of chemotherapeutics and cause an increase risk for toxicity.

COQ10

The effect of CoQ10 on Adriamycin, one of the oldest chemotherapeutics used in breast cancer treatment, has been studied extensively. The mechanism of action for Adriamycin has been shown to deplete mitochondrial CoQ10, and this is the working postulate for its cardiotoxic effect. It is now considered a standard of care to use CoQ10 with Adriamycin therapy up to 300 mg daily.[80-81] CoQ10 is a fat soluble compound that must cross the biphosphate cell membrane layer in order to be used for mitochondrial ATP production and cellular repair. It was found that decreased plasma levels were found in women with breast cancer and the lowest levels found in women with the worst outcomes.[24] CoQ10 acts as a powerful antioxidant that inhibits tumor-associated growth in relation to kinase activity, while also promoting apoptosis through the down-regulation of Bcl-2.[102] It has a great safety profile with no reports of toxicity or clinical side effects. It has been shown to potentiate anticoagulant therapies, while in one study with warfarin actually indicated that it decreased the anticoagulant effect of this drug.[104] Contraindications include the use of quercitin, turmeric, and other bioflavonoids,

as well as N-acetyl-cysteine and glutathione during the use of chemotherapy. B vitamins, especially riboflavin, vitamins E and C, and l-carnitine.

References

1. McPhee SJ, Papadakis MA, eds. Gonzales R, Z Roni. Online eds. 2009. CURRENT Medical Diagnosis & Treatment.48th ed. 2009.

2. Seidam H, Musghinski MH, Geib SK, Silverberg E. Probabilites of eventually developing of dying of cancer-United States. CA-A Cancer Journal for Clinicians. 1985;35(1):36-56.

3. Singletory SE. Rating the risk of factors for breast cancer. Ann Surg 2003;237(4):474-82.

4. Wallace RB, Sherman BM, Bean JA, Leeper JP, Treloar AE. Menstrual cycle patterns and breast cancer risk factors. Cancer Res. 1978 Nov;38(11 pt.2):4021-24.

5. Writing Group for the Women's Health Initiative Investigators. Risk and Benefits of estrogen plus progestin in healthy menopausal women. JAMA. 2002;288:221-32.

6. Boyce JD. Fact Sheet, http://envirocancer.cornell.edu/factsheet/physical/fs52.radiation.cmf 2010:Breast Cancer and Environmental Risk Factors; Ionizing Radiation and Breast Cancer. Cornell University and The Program on Breast Cancer and Environmental Risk Factors in New York State.

7. http://www.cdc.gov/cancer/breast/statistics/race.htm. 2012.

8. Van der Brandt P, Spielgelman D, Yuan SS, Adami HO, et al. Pooled analysis of prospective cohort studies on height, weight and breast cancer. Am J Epid. 2000;152(6):514-27.

9. http://cgems.cancer.gov. 2012 NCI Cohort Consortium.

10. http://www.cancer.gov/cancertopics/BRCA. 2006.

11. National Cancer Institute (NCI) USA National Institutes

of Health, The Breast Cancer Prevention Trial (BCPT) 2005; http://www.cancer.gov/clinicaltrials/digetspage/BCPT

12. Slamon DJ, Godolphin W, Jones LA, et al. Studies of the HER-2/neu proto-oncogene in human breast and ovarian cancer. Science 1999;244:707-12.

13. King MC, Wieand S, Hale K. Tamoxifen and breast cancer incidence among women with inherited mutations in BRCA1 and BRCA2. JAMA. 2001;286(18):2251-56.

14. http://www.cancer.gov/contraceptives/factsheet/herceptin. 2006.

15. Elkin EB, Weinstein MC, Winer EP. HER-2 Testint and trastuzumab therapy for metastatic breast cancer: a cost effectiveness analysis. J Clin Onc 2004;22(5):854-63.

16. Gasco M, Shrami S, Crook T. The p53 pathway in Breast Cancer. Breast CA Res 2002;4:70-76.

17. Petrocelli T, Slingerland JM. PTEN deficiency: a role in mammary carcinogenesis. Breast CA Res 2001;3:356-60.

18. Hall J. The ataxia-telangiectasis mutated gene and breast cancer: gene expression profiles and sequence variants. CA Lett. 2005;227(2):105-14.

19. Mannweiler S, Tsybrovskyy O, Regauer S. The flow cyotmetric DNA index can predict the presence of lymph node metastasis in invasive ductal breast carcinoma. APMIS. 2002;110(7-8):580-86.

20. Gion M, Mione R, Leon AE. Comparison of the diagnostic accuracy of CA 27.29 and CA 15.3 in primary breast cancer. Clin Chem. 1999;45(5):630-37.

21. www.oncotypedx.com/breast. 2012.

22. www.genomichealth.com/en-us/oncotypedx.aspx. 2012.

23. Lippman ME. Harrison's Online, Chapter 86, Breast Cancer. Harrison's Principles of Internal Medicine, 17th ed. New York, NY: McGraw Hill Co., 2009.

24. MacDonald B, Jennings K. The Breast Cancer Companion. Self Published by authors, 2009. Contact bmacdnd@yahoo.com.

25. Harris J, et al (eds). Diseases of the Breast. 3rd ed. Philadelphia, PA: Lippincott-Raven; 2004.

26. Lamb J, Anderson TJ, Dixon MJ, Levack PA. Role of fine needle aspiration cytology in breast cancer screening. J Clin Path. 1987;40(7):705-09.

27. Ishikawa T, Hamaguchi Y, Tanabe M, et al. False positive and false negative cases of fine needle aspiration for palpable breast lesions. Breast CA 2007;14(4):388-92.

28. www.s.komen.org/breastcancer . 2012.

29. Berg WA, Zhang Z, Lehrer D, et al. Detection of breast cancer with addition of annual screening ultrasound or a single screening MRI to mammography in women with elevated breast cancer risk. JAMA. 2012;307(13):1394-1404.

30. National Cancer Institute: USA National Institutes of Health, The Breast Cancer Prevention Trial (BCPT). www.cancer.gov/clinicaltrials/diegestpage/BCPT. 2005.

31. National Cancer Institute: USA National Institutes of Health, Surveillance Epidemiology and End Results

(SEER). www.seer.cancer.gov 2007. Parisky YR, Sardi A, et al. Efficacy of computerized imaging analysis to evaluate mammographically suspicious lesions. Am J Roentgenol. 2003;180:263-69.

32. American Joint Committee on Cancer (AJCC) Staging Manual. 6th ed. New York, NY: Springer; 2002. www.springeronline.com

33. Frumovitz M, Pedro T, Levenback C. Lymphatic mapping and sentinel node detection in gynecologic malignancies of the lower genital tract. Curr Onco Reports. 2005;17(6):435-43.

34. Fisher B, Costantino JP, Wickerham DL. Tamoxifen for prevention of breast cancer: Report of the National Surgical Adjuvant Breast and Bowel Project P-1 Study. J Natl cancer Inst. 1998:90(18):1371-88.

35. www.cancer.gov/cancertopics/pdq/treatment/breast/ ...allpages. 2011.

36. www.6z1.org/stages-i-and-h-breastcancer.html .2010.

37. Karunagaran D, Rashmi R, Kumar TR. Curr Cancer Drug Targets. 2005;5(2):117-29.

38. Sjogren S, Inganas M, Lindgren A, et al. Prognostic and predictive value of c-erbB-2 overexpression in primary breast cancer, alone and in combination with other prognostic markers. J Clin Onco. 1998;16(2):462-69.

39. Oh DS, et al. Estrogen regulated genes predict survival in hormone receptor positive breast cancers. J clin Onco. 2006;24:1656.

40. Ragaz J, et al. Locoregional radiation therapy in patients with high risk breast cancer receiving adjuvant chemotherapy:20 year results of the British Columbia Randomized Trial. J Natl Cancer Inst. 2005;97:116.

41. Lipton A. Bisphosphates and metastatic breast cancrcinoma. Cancer. 2003;97(3 suppl):848-53.

42. Roussouw JE, et al. Risks and benefits of estrogen plus progestin in healthy postmenopausal women. JAMA. 2002;288:321.

43. Carrick S, Parker S, Thornton CE, et al. Single agent versus combination chemotherapy for metastatic breast cancer. Cochrane Database system review. 2009 April;15(2).

44. Wilken N. Chemotherapy alone versus endocrine therapy in metastatic breast cancer. 2010 Cochrane Database. www.thecochranelibrary.com/details/metastaticbreast-cancer.html

45. Maggiolini M, Bonofiglio D, et al. Estrogen receptor alpha mediates the proliferative but not the cytotoxic dose dependent effects of two major phytoestrogens on human breast cancer cells. Mol Pharmacol. 2001;60(3):595-602.

46. Mori H, Niwa K, Zheng Q, Yamada Y, et al. Cell proliferation in cancer prevention; effects or preventive agents on estrogen related endometrial carcinogenesis model and on an in vitro model in human colorectal cells. Mutt Res. 2001 Sept 1;480-481:201-07.

47. Schwartz LH, Koerner FL, Edgenton SM, et al. pS2 expression and response to hormonal therapy in patients with advanced breast cancer. Cancer Res. 1991;51:624-28.

48. Kimmick GG, Muss HB. Endocrine therapy in metastatic breast cancer. Cancer Res and Treat. 1997;94:231-54.

49. Hanninen O, Kaartinen K, Rauma AL, et al. Antioxidants in vegan diet and rheumatic disorders. Toxicol. 2000;30(1-3):45-53.

50. Frei B. Efficacy of dietary antioxidants to prevent oxidative damage and inhibit chronic disease. The J of Nut 2004;Nov 1;134(11).

51. Hsieh TC, Elangovan S, Wu JM. Differential suppression of proliferation in MCF-7 and MDA-MB-231 breast cancer cells exposed to alpha, gamma and omega-tocotrienols is accompanied by altered expression of oxidative stress modulatory enzymes. Anti Cancer Res. 2012;30(10):4169-76.

52. Saada HN, Khaled A. Role of lycopene in recovery of radiation induced injury to mammalian cellular organelles. Pharmazie. 2001;56(3):239-41.

53. Heaney ML, et al. Vitamin c antagonizes the cytotoxic effects of neoplastic drugs. Cancer Res. 2008;68(19):8031-38.

54. Zhao KS, Mancini C, Doria G. Enhancement of immune response in mice by Astragulus membranaceus extracts. Immunopharmacology. 1990;20:225-34.

55. Neuzil J, Weber T, Schroder A, Lu M, et al. Induction of cancelled apoptosis by alpha-tocopheryl succinate: molecular pathways and structural requirements. Faeseb J. 2001;15(2):403-15.

56. Rose AT, McFadden DW. Alpha tocopheryl succinate inhibits growth of gastric cancer cells in vitro. J Surg Res. 2001;95(1):19-22.

57. Donnelly ET, McClure N, Lewis S EM. The effect of ascorbate and alpha tocopherol supplementation in vitro on DND integrity and hydrogen peroxide induced DNA damage in human spermatozoa. Mutageneisis 1999;14(5):505-12.

58. Zhang JG, Nicholls-Grzemski FA, Tirmenstein MA, et al. Vitamin E succinate protects hepatocytes against the toxic effect of reactive oxygen species generated at mitochondrial complexes I and III by alkylating agents. Chem Biol Interact.

59. Lemus-Wilson AL, Kelly PA, Blask DE. Melatonin blocks the stimulating effects of prolactin on human breast cancer cell growth in culture. Br J CA. 1995;72(16):1435-40.

60. Lissoni P, Barni S, Meregallis S, et al. Modulation of cancer endocrine therapy by melatonin: a phase II study of tamoxifen plus melatonin in metastatic breast cancer patients progressing under tamoxifen use alone. Br J CA. 1995;71:854-56.

61. Lissoni P, et al. Reversal of clinical resistance to LHRH analogue in metastatic prostate cancer by the pineal hormone melatonin: efficacy of LHRH analogue plue melatonin in patients progressing on LHRH analogue alone. Eur Urol. 1997;31(2):178-81.

62. Neri B, De Leonardis V, Gemelli MT, et al. Melatonin as a biological response modifier in cancer patients. Anticancer Res 1998;18(2B):1329-32.

63. Hara M, Yoshida M, Nishijima H, et al. Melatonin a pineal secreting product with antioxidant properties protects against cisplatin induced nephortoxicity in rats. J Pineal Res. 2001;30(3):129-38.

64. Lissoni P, Barni S, Ardizzola A, et al. A randomized study with the pineal hormone melatonin versus supportive care alone in patients with brain metastasis due to solid neoplasms. Cancer. 1994;73(3):699-701.

65. Ghielmini M, Pagani O, de Jong J, et al. Double blind randomized study on the myeloprotective effect of melatonin in combination with carboplatin and etoposide in advanced lung cancer. Br J Ca. 1999;80:1058-1061.

66. Lissoni P, Barni S, Mandala M, et al. Decreased toxicity and increased efficacy of cancer chemotherapy using the pineal hormone melatonin in metastatic solid tumour patients with poor clinical status. Eur J CA. 1999;35(12):1688-92.

67. Cai L, Cherian MG, Iskander S, et al. Metallothionein induction in human CNS in vitro: neuroprotection from ionizing radiation. Int J Radiat Biol. 2000;76(7):1009-17.

68. Nagler RM, Eichen Y, Nagler A. Redox metal chelation ameliorates radiation induced bone marrow toxicity in a mouse model. Radiat Res 2001;156(2):205-09.

69. Buntzel J. Experiences with sodium selenite in treatment of acute and late adverse effects of radio chemotherapy of head and neck carcinomas. Cytoprotection Working Group in AK Supportive Measures in Ocnolcoy withing the Scope of MASCC and DKG. Med Klin. 1999;94(3 suppl):49-53.

70. Lamproqlou I, Boisserie G, Mazeron JJ, et al. Effect of Ginkgo biloba extract (EGB 761) on rats in an experimental model of acute encephalopathy after total body irradiation. CA Radiat 2000;4(3):202-06.

71. Inano HI, Onoda M, et al. Chemoprevention by curcumin during the promotion stage of tumorgenesis of mammary gland in rats irradiated with rays. Carcinogenesis. 1999;20(6):1011-18.

72. Varadkar P, Dubey P, Krishna M, Verma N. Modulation of radiation induced protein kinase C activity by phenolics. J Radiat Prot. 2001;21(4):361-70.

73. Gong SL, Li XM, Lu Z, Liu SZ. Protective effect of panaxatriols on function of reproductive endocrine axis in radiation injured rats. Zhonoqqujo Yao Li Xue Bao. 1993;14(4):358-60.

74. Kim SH, Jeong KS, Ryu SY, Kim TH. Panax ginseng prevents apoptosis in hair follicles and accelerates recovery of hair medullary cells in irradiated mice. In Vivo. 1998;12(2):219-22.

75. Miyanomae T, Frindel E. Radioprotection of hemopoiesis conferred by Acanthopanax senticosus (Shigoka) administerd before and after irradiation. Exp Hemotol. 1988;16(9):801-6.

76. Elsedorn TJ, Weiji NI, Mithoe S, et al. Chemotherapy induced chromosomal damage in peripheral blood lymphocytes of cancet patients supplemented with antioxidants or placebo. Mutt Res. 2001;498(1-2):145-58.

77. Reddy VG, Khanna N, Singh N. Vitamin C augments

chemotherapeutic response of cervical carcinoma HeLa cells by stabilizing p53. Biochem Biophys Res Commun. 2001;282(2):409-15.

78. Muralikrishnan G, Stanely AV, Pillai SK. Dual role of vitamin C on lipid profile and combined application of cyclophosphamide, methotrexate and 5-fluorouracil treatment in fibrosarcoma bearing rats. Cancer Lett. 2001;169(2):115-20.

79. Tarny DC, Liu TY, Huang TP. Protective effect of vitamin C on 8-hydroxy-2'-deoxyguanosine level in peripheral blood lymphocytes of chronic hemodialysis patients. Kid Int. 2004;66:820-31.

80. Conklin KA. Coenzyme Q10 for prevention of anthracycline induced cardiotoxicity. Int CA Ther 2005;4(2):110-30. Saltiel E. Doxirubicin (Adriamycin) cardiomyopathy-a critical review. West J Med1983;139(3):332-41.

81. Albini A. Cardiotoxicity of anti-cancer drugs: the need for cardio-oncology and cardio oncological prevention. J NCI J Natl CA Inst 102(1):14-25.J Am Coll Nut 2002;21(5):416-21.

82. Pathak AK, Singh N, et al. Potentiation of the effect of paclitaxel and carboplatin by antioxidant mixture on human lung cancer H520 cells.

83. Polytarchou C, Papdimitriou E. Antioxidants inhibit angiogenesis in vivo through down regulation of nitric oxide synthase expression and activity. Free Rad Res. 2004;38(5):501-8.

84. Blanchard JA, Barve S, Joshi-Barve S, et al. Antioxidants inhibit cytokine production and suppress NF-kappaB activation in CAPAN-1 and CAPAN-2 cell lines. Dig Dis Sci 2001;46(12):2768-72.

85. Jo EH, Hong HD, Ahn NC, et al. Modulations of the Bcl-2/Bax family were involved in chemopreventive effects of licorice root (Glycyrrhiza uralensis Fisch) in MCF-7 human breast cancer cell. J Agric Food Chem 2004;52(6):1715-19.

86. Kiemer AK, Hartung T, Huber C, Vollmar AM. Phyllanthus amarus has anti-inflammatory potential by inhibition of iNOS, COX-2, and cytokines via the NG-kappaB pathway. J Hepatol 2003;38:289-97.

87. Frondoza CG, Sohrabi A, Polotsky A, Phan PV, Hunberford DS, Lindmark L. An in vivo screening assay for inhibitors of proinflammatory mediators in herbal extracts using human synoviocyte cultures. In Vivo Cell Dev Biol Anim. 2004;40(3-4):95-101.

88. Zhang KS, Mancini C, Doria G. Enhancement of immune response in mice by Astragulus membranaceus extracts. Immunopharm. 1990;20:225-34.

89. Dinkova-Kostova A, Talay P. Relation of structure of curcumin analogs to their potencies as inducers of Phase 2 detoxification enzymes. Carcinogenesis. 1999;20(5):911-14.

90. Jones JL, Daley BJ, et al. Genistein inhibits tamoxifen effects on cell proliferation and cell cycle arrest in T47D breast cancer cells. Am Surg. 2002;68(6):575-7;discussion 577-78.

91. Sarkar FH, Li Y. Soy isoflavones and cancer prevention. Cancer Invest. 20003;21(5):744-57.

92. Upadhyay S, Neburi M, Chinni SR, Alhasan S, Miller F, Sarkar FH. Differential sensitivity of naromal and malignant breast epithelial cells to genistein is partly mediated by p21(WAF1). Clin CA Res. 2001;7(6):1782-89.

93. Auborn KJ, Fan S, Rosen EM, Goodwin L, Chandraskaren A, William DE, et al. Indole-3-carbinol is a negative regulator of estrogen. J Nutr. 2003;133(7 suppl):2470S-2475S.

94. Scambia B, DeVincenzo R, et al. Antiproliferative effect of silybin on gynaecological malignancies: synergism with cisplatin and doxorubincin. Eur J CA. 1996;32A(5):877-82.

95. Einbond LS, Shimizu M, Xiao D, et al. Growth inhibitory activity of extracts and purified components of black cohosh on human breast cancer cells. Breast CA Res Treat .2004;83(3):221-31.

96. Yi Ching Hsieh YC, Santell RC, et al. Estrogenic effects of genistein on the growth of estrogen receptor positive human breast cancer (MCF-7) cells in vitro and in vivo. CA Res. 1998;58:3833-38.

97. Sah JF, Balasubramanian S, Eckert RI, Rorke EA. Epigallocatechin-3-gallate inhbits epidermal growth factor receptor signaling pathway: evidence for direct inhibiton of ERK1/2 and AKT kinases. J Biol Chem. 2004;279:12755-76.

98. Tseng CR, Shiu HC, Kuo ML. Curcumin induces p53 dependent apoptosis in human basal cell carcinoma cells. J Invest Derm. 1998;111(4):565-61.

99. Dhanalakshmi S, Mallikarjuna GU, et al. silibinin prevents ultraviolet radiation caused skin damages in SKH-1 hairless mice via a decrease in thymine dimer positive cells and an up regulation of p53-p21/Cip1 in epidermis. Carcinogenesis. 2004;25(8):1459-65.

100. Seely D, Mills EJ, Wu P, Verma S, Guyatt GH. The effects of green tea consumption on incidence of breast cancer and recurrence of breast cancer: a systematic review and meta analysis. Int CA Ther. 2005;4(2):144-55.

101. Virgili F, Acconcia F, Ambra R, Rinna A, Totta P, Mariano M. Nutritional flavonoids modulate estrogen receptor alpha signaling. IUMB Life 2004;56(3):145-51.

102. Bahar M, Khaghani S, Pasalar P, et al. Exogenous coenzyme Q10 modulates MMP-2 activity in MCF-7 cell line as a breast cancer cellular model. Nut J. 2010;9:62.

103. Oh SM, Chung KH. Estrogenic activities of Ginkgo biloba extracts. Life Sci. 2004;74(11):1325-35.

104. Ravid A, Rocker D, Machlenkin A, et al. 1,25-Dihydroxyvitamin D3 enhances the susceptibility of breast cancer cells to doxorubicin induced oxidative damage. Cancer Res. 1999;59(4):862-7.

105. Bhatia N, Zhao J, Wolf DM, Agarwal R. Inhibition of human carcinoma cell growth and DNA synthesis by silibinin, an active constituent of milk thistle: comparison with silymarin. CA Lett. 1999;47(1-2):77-84.

106. Standish LJ, Wenner C, Sweet E, et al. Trametes versicolor mushroom immune therapy in breast cancer. J Soc Integ Onco. 2008;6(3):122-28.

Pathophysiology

Colon cancer begins in the colon; rectal cancer begins in the rectum. Colorectal cancer is a more general term that encompasses cancers that begin in either the colon or the rectum. Although colon and rectal cancers are similar, there are some differences in how they develop and are treated.[1,2]

- Almost all colorectal cancers are adenocarcinomas, which develop from the lining of the large intestine (colon) and rectum.
- Colorectal cancer usually begins as a button-like swelling on the surface of the intestinal or rectal lining or on a polyp.
- As the cancer grows, it begins to invade the wall of the intestine or rectum. Nearby lymph nodes also may be invaded.
- Because blood from the wall of the intestine and much of the rectum is carried to the liver, colorectal cancer usually spreads (metastasizes) to the liver soon after spreading to nearby lymph nodes.

COLORECTAL POLYPS

Tumors of the colon and rectum arise from the inner wall of the large intestine. Benign tumors of the large intestine are called polyps and malignant tumors of the large intestine are called cancers. Benign polyps do not invade nearby tissue or spread to other parts of the body, and can be easily removed during colonoscopy.[3] They are not life-threatening. If benign polyps are not removed from the large intestine, they can become malignant, and it is thought that most of the cancers of the large intestine are believed to have developed from polyps.[4]

A polyp is a growth of tissue from the intestinal or rectal wall that protrudes into the intestine or rectum and may be noncancerous or cancerous. Polyps vary considerably in size; the bigger the polyp, the greater the risk that it is cancerous or precancerous. Polyps may grow with or without a stalk; those without a stalk are more likely to be cancerous than those with a stalk. Adenomatous polyps, which consist primarily of glandular cells that line the inside of the large intestine, are likely to become cancerous; in other words, they are considered precancerous.[4]

Some polyps are the result of hereditary conditions, such as familial polyposis, Gardner's syndrome, and Peutz-Jeghers syndrome.[5] In familial polyposis, 100 or more precancerous polyps develop throughout the large intestine and rectum during childhood or adolescence. In nearly all untreated people, the polyps develop into cancer of the large intestine or rectum (colorectal cancer) before age 40.[3-5] In Gardner's syndrome, various types of noncancerous tumors develop elsewhere in the body (for example, on the skin, skull, or jaw) in addition to the precancerous polyps that develop in the large intestine and rectum.[3-5]

Colon polyps develop by the same mechanism as all cancers: unbound rapid cellular dysplastic growth that results in masses of extra tissue (polyps) being formed. Colon polyps are initially benign. Over years, benign colon polyps can acquire additional chromosome damage via the same strategies as all cancer growth, promotion, and progression strategies that ensure a cancerous growth.[3,4]

Colon polyps may be classified pathologically as a nonneoplastic hamartoma (juvenile polyp), a hyperplastic mucosal proliferation (hyperplastic polyp), or an adenomatous polyp. Only adenomas are clearly premalignant, and only a minority of such lesions becomes cancer. Adenomatous polyps may be found in the colons of ~30% of middle-aged and ~50% of elderly people; however, <1% of polyps ever become malignant.[4,5]

MOLECULAR PATHOGENESIS

Almost all colorectal cancers arise from adenomatous polyps. Only adenomas are clearly precancerous with only a small percentage actually developing into a cancerous lesion. Most polyps produce no symptoms and remain clinically undetected. Occult blood in the stool is found in <5% of patients with polyps.[3-5] A number of molecular changes are noted in adenomatous polyps, dysplastic lesions, and polyps containing microscopic foci of tumor cells (carcinoma in situ), which are thought to reflect a multistep process in the evolution of normal colonic mucosa to life-threatening invasive carcinoma.[1-2] These developmental steps toward carcinogenesis include, but are not restricted to, point mutations in the K-*ras* protooncogene; hypomethylation of DNA, leading to gene activation;

Anatomy of the Colon and Rectum

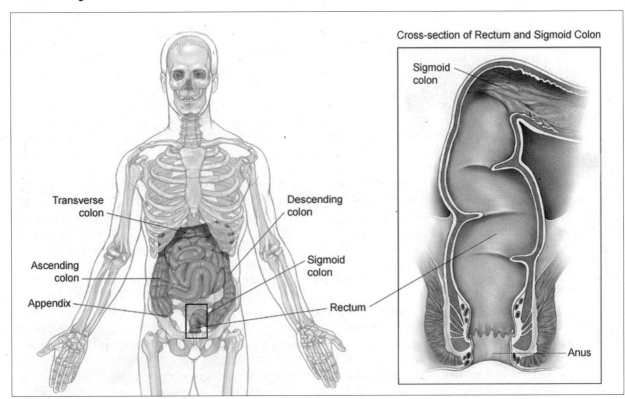

Colorectal Adenomatous Polyps

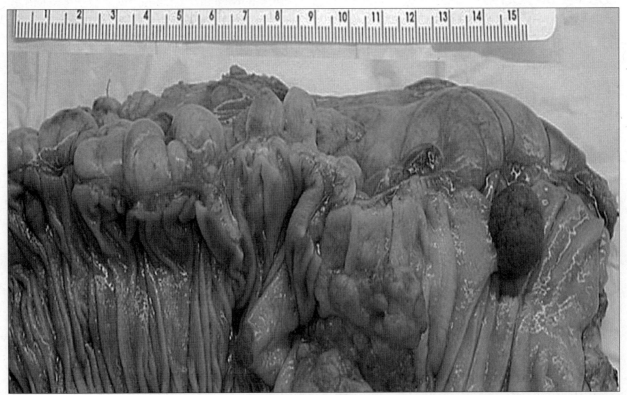

loss of DNA (allelic loss) at the site of a tumor-suppressor gene (the adenomatous polyposis coli *APC* gene) on the long arm of chromosome 5 (5q21); allelic loss at the site of a tumor-suppressor gene located on chromosome 18q (the deleted in colorectal cancer *DCC* gene); and allelic loss at chromosome 17p, associated with mutations in the p53 tumor-suppressor gene.[3] Thus, the altered proliferative pattern of the colonic mucosa, which results in progression to a polyp and then to carcinoma, may involve the mutational activation of an oncogene followed by and coupled with the loss of genes that normally suppress tumorigenesis.[3-5] It remains uncertain whether the genetic aberrations always occur in a defined order. Based on this model, however, cancer is believed to develop only in those polyps in which most (if not all) of these mutational events take place.[3-4]

The likelihood of an adenomatous polyp becoming a cancer depends on the gross appearance of the lesion, its histopathology, and size. Adenomatous polyps may be pedunculated (stalked) or sessile (flat-based) with more cancers developing frequently in sessile polyps.[4-5] Histologically, adenomatous polyps may be tubular, villous (i.e., papillary), or tubulovillous. Villous adenomas, most of which are sessile, become malignant more than three times as often as tubular adenomas. The likelihood that any polypoid lesion in the large bowel contains invasive cancer is related to the size of the polyp, being negligible (<2%) in lesions <1.5 cm, intermediate (2% to10%) in lesions 1.5–2.5 cm in size, and substantial (10%) in lesions >2.5 cm.[3]

Because many colon cancers start in polyps, they should, if possible, be removed when found to prevent colorectal cancer.

ANATOMY OF THE COLON AND RECTUM

The colon (or large intestine) may be divided into the cecum, ascending colon, transverse colon, descending colon, and sigmoid colon.[1-2] The colon serves as a reservoir for the liquids (chyme) emptied into it through the ileocecal valve, from the small intestine. It has a much larger diameter than the small intestine, where the liquid material is made into a solid matter by the reabsorption of water, recycling of materials back into the lymphovascular system, and the rest formed into waste product, the feces.

Epidemiology
PREVALENCE AND INCIDENCE

Cancer of the large intestine is second only to lung cancer as a cause of cancer death in the United States: 153,760 new cases occurred in 2007, and 52,180

deaths were due to colorectal cancer. The incidence rate has remained relatively unchanged during the past 30 years, while the mortality rate has decreased, particularly in females. Colorectal cancer generally occurs in persons older that 50 years.[3-5]

- ❖ Each year about 130,000 people are diagnosed with colorectal cancer. Most of the people who develop colorectal cancer are over 50 years old.
- ❖ Women are more likely to develop cancer of the colon, and men are more likely to develop cancer of the rectum in the USA.
- ❖ Globally, cancer of the colon and rectum is the third leading cause of cancer in males and the fourth leading cause of cancer in females. The frequency of colorectal cancer varies around the world. It is common in the Western world and is rare in Asia and Africa. In countries where the people have adopted western diets, the incidence of colorectal cancer is increasing.
- ❖ In Western countries, cancer of the large intestine and rectum is the second most common type of cancer and the second leading cause of cancer death.
- ❖ The incidence of colorectal cancer begins to rise at age 40 and peaks between the ages of 60 and 75.
- ❖ The rate for the entire American population is about 50 new instances of colorectal cancer for every 100,000 people each year.
- ❖ About 5% of the people with colon or rectal cancer have cancer in two or more sites in the colon and rectum that do not appear to simply be spread from one site to another.

RISK FACTORS

People with a family history of colorectal cancer have a higher risk of developing the cancer themselves. A family history of polyps also increases the risk of colorectal cancer. People with ulcerative colitis or Crohn's disease are at greater risk as well; this risk is related to the person's age when the disease developed and the length of time the person has had the disease. Greater exposure to air and water pollution, particularly to industrial cancer-causing substances (carcinogens), may play a role in the development of the colorectal cancer.[3-5]

Diet

People at highest risk tend to consume a high-fat, low-fiber diet. Diets high in proinflammatory fats are believed to predispose humans to colorectal cancer.[6] In countries with high colorectal cancer rates, the fat intake by the population is much higher than in countries with low cancer rates. It is believed that the breakdown products of fat metabolism can be one of the mechanisms that lead to the formation of cancer-causing chemicals (carcinogens).[7] Diets high in saturated fats and animal fats tend to move the biochemistry of the body toward inflammation by the promotion of arachidonic acid and prostaglandin series 2 formation (PGE2). Diets high in vegetables and high-fiber foods, such as whole-grain breads and cereals, may rid the bowel of these carcinogens and help reduce the risk of cancer.[8-9]

Diets high in factory-farmed animal meats are high in arachidonic acid, a proinflammatory cytokine that promotes PGE2 synthesis and a overall proinflammatory state. Wild animal meats, such as venison, buffalo, and elk) are low in fat and leaner than chicken or turkey meats, and do not promote proinflammatory pathways. Diets high in these processed meats are also associated with the ingestion of animal fecal anaerobes in the gut microflora. These non-endogenous anaerobes are found in large amounts in the feces of patients with colorectal adenomas and cancer.[8-9]

Diet is thus considered an environmental factor associated with socioeconomic class and Western civilization. Colon cancer mortality correlates to the amount of calories, proteins, and bad fats consumed, as well as to an elevation in serum cholesterol concentrations and coronary artery disease.[10] Populations in Western civilization that do not eat the standard American diet (SAD), such as the Mormons and Seventh Day Adventists, have a significantly lower incidence and mortality rate from colorectal cancer.[11] In juxtaposition, those cultures that have adopted a Western diet, such as Japan, have seen an increase in colorectal cancer in their population.[12]

Fiber

Soluble and non soluble plant fibers directly affect the colonic milieu and mucosa, aiding in complete fecal elimination and colonic epithelial health. A diet high in fruits and vegetables not only provides this needed fiber to the diet but also is rich in anti-inflammatory antioxidants needed for health cellular activity.[13]

Obesity and Insulin Resistance

Obesity resulting from high-calorie diets and lack of physical activity leads to insulin resistance that causes an increase in circulating insulin levels. This higher circulatory level of insulin creates a pro-inflammatory state and increases the amount of circulating insulin-like growth factor type I (IGF-I). IGF-I stimulates the proliferation of the intestinal mucosa, depresses the innate immuno-surveillance mechanisms, and disrupts other endocrine functions.[14-16]

Figure 3: Risk Factors for the Development of Colorectal Cancer
- High fat and low fiber diet
- Obesity and insulin resistance
- Smoking
- Streptococcus bovis bacteremia
- Ulcerative colitis
- Hereditary syndromes (autosomal dominant inheritance)

Smoking

Cigarette smoking has been linked to the development of colorectal adenomas. This is statistically significant for those who have smoked for over 35 years or more, although there is no biological explanation directly linked to this development discovered at this time.[17]

Streptococcus bovis

Streptococcus bovis, a fecal bacterium associated with the development of endocarditis and septicemia, exposes people to a higher risk of developing colon cancer. Associated with this infection is the development of occult colorectal tumors and other gastrointestinal cancers.[18]

Ulcerative colitis

Colon cancer is a recognized complication of chronic UC. The risk for cancer begins to rise after 8 to 10 years of colitis. The risk of developing colon cancer in a patient with UC also is related to the location and the extent of the disease.[19]

Current estimates of the cumulative incidence of colon cancer associated with ulcerative colitis are 2.5% at 10 years, 7.6% at 30 years, and 10.8% at 50 years. Patients at higher risk of cancer are those with a family history of colon cancer, a long duration of colitis, extensive colon involvement, and primary sclerosing cholangitis (PSC).[19]

Colorectal cancer that is associated with UC and other IBD syndromes has a favorable outcome when caught at an early stage. Yearly examinations of the colon often are recommended thereafter. During these examinations, biopsies can be taken to search for precancerous changes in the cells of the colon lining. When precancerous changes are found throughout the colon, complete removal of the colon may be necessary to prevent colon cancer.[19]

Hereditary Syndromes

Among first-degree relatives of colon cancer patients, the immediate family members have an 18% risk of developing colon cancer in their lifetime. This is three times greater than the risk among the general population of the United States. Even though family history of colon cancer is an important risk factor, 80% of colon cancers occur sporadically in patients with no family history of colon cancer. Only about 20% of cancers are associated with a family history of colon cancer, and only 5 % of colon cancers are due to hereditary colon cancer syndromes.[20]

In hereditary colon cancer syndromes, the patient has inherited cancer-causing genetic defects from one or both of the chromosomes of the parents. Chromosomal damage causes genetic defects that lead to the formation of colon polyps and later to colon cancer.[20] In sporadic polyp and cancer development absent of any family history, the chromosome damages are acquired and develop in a cell during adult life. The damaged chromosomes can only be found in the polyps and the cancers that develop from that cell. However, in hereditary colon cancer syndromes, the chromosome defects are inherited at birth and are present in every cell in the body[21] Patients who have inherited the hereditary colon cancer syndrome genes are at risk of developing a large number of colon polyps, usually at young ages, and are at very high risk of developing colon cancer early in life. They are at risk of developing cancers in other organs because of these denatured, inherited chromosomal aberrations.[22]

Familial Adenomatous Polyposis

Also known as FAP or polyposis coli, this hereditary colon cancer syndrome results in affected family members developing countless numbers (hundreds and often thousands) of colon polyps starting during the teenage years of development. Unless the condition is detected and treated early (which may involve removal of the colon), a person affected by FAP is almost sure to develop colon cancer from these polyps. Cancers usually develop by the fortieth decade of life and these patients are also at risk of developing other cancers, such as cancers in the thyroid gland, stomach, and the ampulla (the part where the bile ducts drain into the duodenum just beyond the stomach).[23]

It has been shown clinically that NSAIDS and COX-2 inhibitors can decrease the number and size of polyps formed in these patients, although this effect is temporary and related to the continuation of the anti-inflammatory therapy, while not really reducing the risk of cancer development statistically.[24,25] Patients are monitored with a flexible sigmoidoscopy until the age of 35 and then colonoscopy and barium enema are used. Using a test for occult blood is not an adequate screening device because of the lack of sensitivity and specificity for colon cancer. DNA testing from peripheral mononuclear cells for the APC gene mutation is an accurate screening test that also can lead to a definitive diagnosis prior to the development of polyps and cancer.[26]

Attenuated Familial Adenomatous Polyposis

AFAP is a milder version of FAP. Affected family members develop less than 100 colon polyps. Regardless, these people are still at very high risk of developing colon cancers at young ages and they are also at risk of having gastric polyps and duodenal polyps develop.[22-26]

Adenomatous Polyposis Coli

FAP is associated with a mutation/deletion on the long arm of chromosome 5: **APC** gene called adenomatous polyposis coli (APC). The result of this loss of allele functions results in the absence of tumor suppressor genes, which would otherwise inhibit neoplasm growth. This genetic defect leads to abnormal cellular proliferation with the impaired DNA that does not limit this growth.[22-26]

Hereditary Nonpolyposis Colon Cancer

HNPCC, also known as Lynch syndrome, is a hereditary colon cancer syndrome where affected family members develop colon polyps and cancers, usually in the right ascending colon, in their third and fourth decade of life. The average age of onset of cancer development is under 50 years old, which is 10 to 15 years younger than the average age in the general population to develop colon cancer. Certain HNPCC patients are also at a higher risk of developing uterine cancer, stomach cancer, ovarian and endometrial cancers, and cancers of the ureters and the biliary tract. The recommendation is that these patients undergo colonoscopy biennially beginning at 25 years of age. If the patient is female, she should also have intermittent pelvic ultrasonography and endometrial evaluation. HNPCC is associated with germline mutations of several genes, particularly *hMSH2* on chromosome 2 and *hMLH1* on chromosome 3. These mutations lead to errors in DNA replication and are thought to result in DNA instability because of defective repair of DNA mismatches, resulting in abnormal cell growth and tumor development.[27]

MYH Polyposis Syndrome

This recently discovered hereditary colon cancer syndrome typically affects patients with the development

Hereditable (Autosomal Dominant) Gastrointestinal Polyposis Syndromes

Syndrome	Distribution of Polyps	Histologic Type	Malignant Potential	Associated Lesions
Familial adenomatous polyposis	Large intestine	Adenoma	Common	None
Gardner's syndrome	Large and small intestines	Adenoma	Common	Osteomas, fibromas, lipomas, epidermoid cysts, ampullary cancers, congenital hypertrophy of retinal pigment epithelium
Turcot's syndrome	Large intestine	Adenoma	Common	Brain tumors
Lynch syndrome (nonpolyposis syndrome)	Large intestine (often proximal)	Adenoma	Common	Endometrial and ovarian tumors
Peutz-Jeghers syndrome	Small and large intestines, stomach	Hamartoma	Rare	Mucocutaneous pigmentation; tumors of the ovary, breast, pancreas, endometrium
Adenomatous polyposis coli				
MYH Polyposis Syndrome				
Hereditary Nonpolyposis Colon Cancer				
Juvenile polyposis	Large and small intestines, stomach	Hamartoma, rarely progressing to adenoma	Rare	Various congenital abnormalities
Attenuated Familial Adenomatous Polyposis				

(Adapted from McPhee S. CURRENT Medical Diagnosis and Treatment 2009. New York, NY: McGraw Hill, 2009.)[4]

of 10 to 100 polyps occurring around the fortieth decade of life, which represents a high risk of developing colon cancer.[28]

Gardner's Syndrome

This syndrome involves a gene mutation with congenital hypertrophy of the retinal pigmented epithelial tissue and soft tissue with bony tumor formation and additional tumor and cancerous growths in the colon.[23]

Turcot's Syndrome

These malignancies appear in the central nervous system with polyposis coli. Tumors will usually present by the age of 25, and if not treated surgically, will develop into cancer in almost all patients by the age of 40.[23]

Assessment

SIGNS AND SYMPTOMS

Colorectal cancer grows slowly and does not cause symptoms for a long time, making early detection difficult. Symptoms depend on the type, location, and extent of the cancer. Fatigue and weakness resulting from occult bleeding (bleeding not visible to the naked eye) may be the patient's only symptom and can easily be misconstrued for hemorrhoidal bleeds. A tumor in the left (descending) colon is likely to cause obstruction at an earlier stage because the left colon has a smaller diameter and the stool is semi-solid. Cancer tends to encircle this part of the colon, causing alternating constipation and frequent bowel movements before obstruction.

Patients may seek medical treatment because of cramping and abdominal pain or severe abdominal pain and constipation. A tumor in the right (ascending) colon does not cause obstruction until late in the course of the cancer progression because the ascending colon has a large diameter and the contents flowing through it are liquid. By the time the tumor is discovered, it may be so large that it can be palpated through the abdominal wall.

Most colon cancers bleed, usually slowly. The stool may be streaked or mixed with blood, but often the blood cannot be seen; a test of the stool for occult blood is needed to detect it. In order for this Hemacult test to give an accurate detection, 3 different samples are taken 3 days in a row from the patient's stool.

The most common first symptom of rectal cancer is bleeding during a bowel movement. Recurrent hematochezia, tenesmus, and urgency to defecate may all be clinical indicators of rectal cancer. Whenever the rectum bleeds, even if the person is known to have hemorrhoids or diverticular disease, cancer must be considered as part of the differential diagnosis. Painful

bowel movements and a feeling that the rectum has not been completely emptied are other symptoms of rectal cancer. Sitting may be painful, but otherwise the person usually feels no pain from the cancer itself unless it spreads to tissue outside the rectum.

These nonspecific symptoms of colon cancer can be confused with any IBD or diverticular disease.

Colorectal cancer must be ruled out in any patient who is more than 40 years old and who reports a change in bowel habits and hematochezia or who has unexplained iron deficiency anemia or occult blood in the stools.[1-5,29]

SCREENING AND DIAGNOSIS

Early diagnosis depends on routine screening for occult blood. To help ensure accurate test results, the patient should eat a high-fiber diet that is free of red meat for 3 days before providing a stool sample. If blood is detected, further testing and diagnostics are needed. Many experts recommend regular screening for colorectal cancer beginning at age 50, due to the high risk of colorectal cancer developing in the later decades of life. Several screening methods are available.[30]

Digital rectal examination

One approach is to undergo a digital rectal examination (DRE) and a test to detect hidden blood in the stool (fecal occult blood testing/Guiac or Hemacult) every year, although some colorectal cancers can be missed with DRE and Hemacult only.

Sigmoidoscopy

Some experts also suggest that the colon and rectum be examined with sigmoidoscopy or, preferably, with colonoscopy starting at age 50. Sigmoidoscopy allows the doctor to examine the lower portion of the colon; colonoscopy allows examination of the entire colon. Any polyps found are surgically removed, and the examination is repeated in a year. If no polyps are found, testing can be repeated in 5 to 10 years depending on family history (genetic predisposition) and co-morbidities.[31]

CT, MRI, and PET

CT scan is used to obtain abdominal and pelvic images to assist in preoperative staging and to determine metastases, but is much less accurate in determining the level of local extension of the tumor or spread to the lymphatics. To determine if there is hepatic spread, an ultrasonography (US) is more accurate than a CT. For rectal cancer, a pelvic MRI or endorectal US is used to provide accurate information about the depth of the penetration of the cancer

Genes Altered in Colon Cancer

	Gene	%Tumors	Action
Tumor Supp.	APC	>60	
	DCC	>60	Adhesion
	p53	>60	Regulation
Oncogenes	Myc	2	Regulation
	K-ras	50	Signaling
	Cyclins	5	Regulation
	Neu/HER2	5	Growth

(Adapted from Harrison's Textbook of Clinical Oncology. New York, NY: Churchill and Livingston; 1995.)[3]

through the rectal wall and the pararectal lymph nodes. A chest CT is obtained to look for distal metastases and a PET is used to determine the recurrence of colorectal cancer, but is not used for staging.[32]

Colonoscopy

Colonoscopy is the diagnostic procedure of choice in patients with a clinical history suggestive of colon cancer or in patients with an abnormality suspicious for cancer detected on radiographic imaging. Colonoscopy permits biopsy for pathologic confirmation of malignancy. Colonoscopy is been advocated by the American College of Gastroenterology as the preferred screening modality in average-risk patients.[30,31] In patients who are between the ages of 50 and 75 old who underwent a screening colonoscopy there is only a 0.1% risk of serious injury from the procedure.[33] Colonoscopy is regarded as the most sensitive test for detecting adenomas and colorectal cancer. Colonoscopy permits biopsy for pathologic confirmation of malignancy.[32]

In patients in whom colonoscopy is unable to reach the cecum (< 5% of cases) or when a nearly obstructing tumor precludes passage of the colonoscope, barium enema or CT colonography examination can be performed.[32]

Virtual Colonoscopy

Virtual colonoscopy is a term used to describe a colonography. This screening test uses computed tomography (CT) scanning without an actual colonoscope. Many people avoid colonoscopy because the test is cumbersome or because they fear the examination itself. Although a virtual colonoscopy is less intrusive, the colon must still be cleansed the same as for colonoscopy. If abnormalities are detected with virtual colonoscopy, colonoscopy must then be performed so that a biopsy can be done or a polyp removed.[34]

GENETICS AND TUMOR MARKERS

Blood tests are not used to diagnose colorectal cancer, but they can help to monitor the effectiveness of treatment after a tumor has been removed. For example, if levels of carcinoembryonic antigen (CEA) are high before surgery to remove a known cancer and low after surgery, monitoring for another increase in the CEA level may help detect an early recurrence of the cancer. Two other cancer markers, CA 19-9 and CA 125, are similar to CEA and are sometimes elevated in colorectal cancer. Serum levels must be used in conjunction with other findings and may be useful in the decision of active treatment.[35]

Carcinoembryonic Antigen[36]

CEA is primarily used in patients with colon cancer and sometimes breast cancer and other sites. It is used primarily to monitor persistent, metastatic, or recurrent disease. Serum levels predict recurrence independently of staging. CEA should fall back to normal levels postoperatively within 6 to12 weeks. It can predict recurrence earlier than other methods with a rise in serum levels that can be seen 2 to 6 months before clinical evidence of recurrence is found. In approximately half of patients, there may be a latent phase of 4 to 6 weeks from onset of changes in CEA after completion of therapies. CEA screening is not recommended because of low sensitivity and specificity, especially in early stages of disease.

CEA at time of diagnosis is related to prognosis, staging and likelihood of recurrence:

- ❖ >5 ng/ml before treatment suggests localized disease with a favorable prognosis.
- ❖ >10 ng/ml suggests extensive disease and a poor prognosis.

Staging of Colorectal Cancer

Joint Committee Classification	TNM			Duke's Class
Stage 0 Carcinoma in situ		N0	M0	
Stage I Tumor invades submucosa	T1	N0	M0	Duke's A
Tumor invades muscularis propria	T2	N0	M0	Duke's B_1
Stage II Tumor invades into subserosa or into nonperitonealized percolic or perirectal tissues	T3	N0	M0	Duke's B_1 or B_2
Tumor perforates the visceral peritoneum or directly invades other organs or structures	T4	N0	M0	Duke's B_2
Stage III Any degree of bowel wall perforation with lymph node metastasis				
One to three pericolic or perirectal lymph nodes involved	Any T	N1	M0	Duke's C_1
Four or more pericolic or perirectal lymph nodes involved	Any T	N2	M0	Duke's C_2
Metastasis to lymph nodes along a vascular trunk	Any T	N3	M0	
Stage IV Presence of distant metastasis	Any T	Any N	M1	Duke's D

Adapted from American Joint Commission on Cancer, 2009.[37]

❖ >20 ng/ml are usually associated with metastatic disease and can correlate with breast and pancreatic cancer as well as colon cancer.

Note that metastasis can occur with levels < 20 ng/ml and that values < 2.5 ng/ml do not rule out primary, metastatic, or recurrent disease.[36]

Conventional Treatment for Colorectal Cancer

STAGING[37]

Staging the colorectal cancer is an important step in the determination of what the treatment options are for each case. Prognosis of the patient's long-term survival is also gauged by the initial staging of the colorectal cancer. The TNM system is currently used by professionals, replacing Duke's system of staging. Treatment options are dependent on the stage of the cancer.

Survival Rates[37]

STAGE 0: Cancer is limited to the inner layer (lining) of the large intestine (colon) covering the polyp. More than 95% of people with cancer at this stage survive at least 5 years.

STAGE 1: Cancer spreads to the space between the inner layer and muscle layer of the large intestine. (This space contains blood vessels, nerves, and lymph vessels.) More than 90% of people with cancer at this stage survive at least 5 years.

STAGE 2: Cancer invades the muscle layer and outer layer of the colon. About 55% to 85% of people with cancer at this stage survive at least 5 years.

STAGE 3: Cancer extends through the outer layer of the colon into nearby lymph nodes. About 20% to 55% of people with cancer at this stage survive at least 5 years.

STAGE 4: Cancer spreads to other organs, such as the

liver, lungs, or ovaries, or to the lining of the abdominal cavity (peritoneum). Fewer than 1% of people with cancer at this stage survive at least 5 years.[37]

Early detection and periodic monitoring

Colon cancer is most likely to be cured if it is removed early, before it has spread. Cancers that have grown deeply or through the wall of the colon have often spread, even if metastases (spread) cannot be detected. Following the detection of an adenomatous polyp, especially a tubullovillous adenoma, the entire colon should be visualized endoscopically or radiographically, noting that synchronous lesions are found in about one-third of cases. Colonoscopy should then be repeated periodically, even in the absence of a previously documented malignancy, since such patients have a 30% to 50% probability of developing another adenoma and are at a higher-than-average risk for developing a colorectal carcinoma. Adenomatous polyps are thought to require >5 years of growth before becoming clinically significant; colonoscopy need not be carried out more frequently than every 3 years.[30-36]

SURGERY

Surgery, the main treatment for colorectal cancer, is curative in about 70% of cases.[27] In most cases of colon cancer, the cancerous segment of the intestine and any nearby lymph nodes are removed surgically, and the remaining ends of the intestine are joined. When people have colon cancer that has penetrated the wall of the large intestine and spread to a very limited number of nearby lymph nodes, chemotherapy after surgical removal of all visible cancer may lengthen survival time, although the effects of these treatments are often modest.[27]

Surgical resection of the primary colon or rectal cancer is the treatment of choice for any patient who has a resectable lesion. Colectomy with regional lymph node dissection is performed to determine the staging, which then guides the adjuvant therapy strategies.[34] Even patients with extensive disease benefit from resection of the colonic tumor with a reduction in intestinal obstruction and bleeding.

For rectal cancer, the type of operation depends on how far the cancer is located from the anus and how deeply it has grown into the rectal wall.[27] In rectal cancers, the surgery is dependent on the level of the tumor that is above the anal verge as well as the

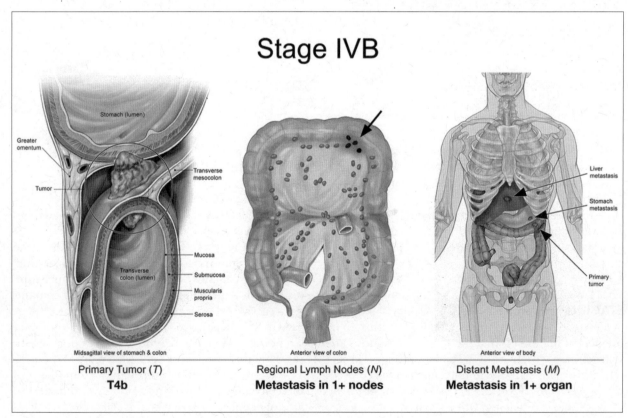

Stage IVB

Primary Tumor (*T*)	Regional Lymph Nodes (*N*)	Distant Metastasis (*M*)
T4b	**Metastasis in 1+ nodes**	**Metastasis in 1+ organ**

Midsagittal view of stomach & colon — Stomach (lumen), Greater omentum, Tumor, Transverse colon (lumen), Transverse mesocolon, Mucosa, Submucosa, Muscularis propria, Serosa

Anterior view of colon

Anterior view of body — Liver metastasis, Stomach metastasis, Primary tumor size and depth of penetration.[27] Transanal excision is performed in patients with small (<4 cm), mobile, well differentiated tumors that are less than 8 cm from the anal verge and appear to be localized. Other patients will require either a low anterior resection with a colorectal anastomosis or an abdominoperineal resection with a colostomy, depending on the distance from the anal verge.[27,36]

Colostomy

In patients who have an unresectable cancer, palliation may be with a diverting colostomy. The complete removal of the rectum and anus leaves the person with a permanent colostomy, which is a surgically created opening between the large intestine and the abdominal wall. The contents of the large intestine empty through the abdominal wall into a colostomy bag. If possible, however, only part of the rectum is removed, leaving a rectal stump and the anus intact. Then the rectal stump is rejoined to the end of the large intestine. In a colostomy, the large intestine is cut. The part that remains connected to the large intestine is brought to the skin surface through an opening that has been formed. The part is then stitched to the skin. Stool passes through the opening and into a disposable bag.[38]

Prognosis after Surgery

The outlook after surgery for colorectal cancer very much depends on the stage of the cancer at diagnosis.[35,36] However, it also depends on how well the person responds to treatment and their general health. More than 90% of people with colorectal cancer that is limited to the inner lining of the colon or rectum or that has grown no further than the layer of tissue just under the inner lining will live at least 5 years after treatment. However, if the cancer extends into nearby lymph nodes or has spread to other organs, the likelihood of living at least 5 years after treatment is greatly decreased.[39,40]

Even after successful treatment, colorectal cancer recurs in about one third of people within 3 to 5 years. Chemotherapy and radiation therapy after surgery have reduced the likelihood of recurrence for many people, but both can cause many side effects. Regular examinations by a doctor are important. Doctors recommend that most people undergo blood tests to look for carcinoembryonic antigen (CEA), an indicator of some kinds of cancer cells, every 2 to 3 months for 2 to 5 years after treatment. Colonoscopy should be performed every 2 to 3 years to look for evidence that the cancer has recurred and for new tumors or polyps.[39,40]

Figure 13: Predictors of Poor Outcome Following Total Surgical Resection of Colorectal Cancer

- Tumor spread to regional lymph nodes
- Number of regional lymph nodes involved
- Tumor penetration through the bowel wall
- Poorly differentiated histology
- Perforation
- Tumor adherence to adjacent organs
- Venous invasion
- Preoperative elevation of CEA titer (>5.0 ng/mL)
- Aneuploidy
- Specific chromosomal deletion (e.g., allelic loss on chromosome 18q)

CHEMOTHERAPY AND RADIOTHERAPY

When rectal cancer has penetrated the rectal wall and spread to a very limited number of nearby lymph nodes, chemotherapy after surgical removal of all visible cancer may lengthen survival time. Radiation therapy after surgical removal of visible rectal cancer may help control the growth of any residual tumors, delay a recurrence, and lengthen survival time. Chemotherapy may be suggested as a form of treatment before or after surgery.

When cancer has spread to lymph nodes far from the colon or rectum, to the lining of the abdominal cavity, or to other organs, the cancer cannot be cured by surgery alone. Survival time is typically only about 7 months. Chemotherapy with fluorouracil and/or irinotecan may be given after surgery as part of the treatment for colorectal cancer that has spread widely, but the chemotherapy usually has little effect on how long the person survives. The doctor usually discusses end-of-life care with the person, the family, and other healthcare practitioners.[42]

DESICCATION

For people who cannot tolerate surgery because of poor health, treatment may involve drying out and shrinking the tumor in a procedure called desiccation. Desiccation is performed with a probe that applies an electrical charge to the surface of the tumor (cautery device) or with a device that dries the tumor with electrified Argon gas (Argon plasma coagulator). Both devices can be passed through a colonoscope. Desiccation may relieve symptoms and lengthen survival time modestly by reducing tumor mass but rarely cures the cancer.[41]

COMBINATION THERAPY

A further important advance has been the FDA approval of oxaliplatin for combination adjuvant therapy. Large, well-designed studies of adjuvant therapy for stage III colon cancer reported a higher rate of disease-free survival at 5 years for patients treated with a combination of oxaliplatin, fluorouracil, and leucovorin (FOLFOX) (66%) than with fluorouracil and leucovorin (FL) alone (59%). The addition of oxaliplatin is associated with an increased incidence of diarrhea and sensory neuropathy, which generally is reversible. Based on these studies, FOLFOX currently is the preferred adjuvant therapy for most patients with Stage III disease. Current studies are evaluating oral capecitabine in combination with oxaliplatin. The role of combination adjuvant therapy of FOLFOX plus a biologic agent (bevacizumab, cetuximab, or panituxumab) also is under investigation.[44]

Even when the cancer has spread widely, surgery is sometimes performed to relieve the intestinal obstruction and ease symptoms. When the cancer has spread only to the liver, chemotherapy drugs can be injected directly into the artery supplying the liver (chemo-artery embolization). A small pump inserted surgically beneath the skin or an external pump worn on a belt allows the patient to be mobile during the treatment. This treatment may provide more benefit than ordinary chemotherapy, but more research is needed. When cancer has spread beyond the liver, this approach has no advantage.[43]

Chemotherapy strategies[36]

- **Neoadjuvant** or **primary systemic chemotherapy:** may be used before surgery to destroy cancer cells. It also allows the physician to determine the effectiveness of a particular regimen on the tumor.
- **Adjuvant chemotherapy:** may be used after surgery or radiation, may further target any possible cancer cells that were not removed during surgery and to prevent the cancer from spreading to other parts of the body.
- **Systemic chemotherapy:** plays an important role in the treatment of patients with locally advanced or metastatic cancer.

Conventional Adjuvant Therapy[36]

Adjuvant chemotherapy and radiotherapy have been demonstrated to improve overall and tumor-free survival in selected patients with colon cancer, selected by staging and clinical presentation.

Stage I

Because of the excellent 5-year survival rate (90% to 100%), no adjuvant therapy is recommended.

Stage II (Node-negative Disease)

The expected 5-year survival rate is 80%. A benefit from adjuvant chemotherapy has not been demonstrated in most controlled trials for stage II colon cancer (see discussion for stage III disease). However, otherwise healthy patients with stage II disease that is at higher risk for recurrence (perforation, T4, poor differentiation on histology) may benefit from adjuvant chemotherapy.[45]

Stage III (Node-Positive Disease)

With surgical resection alone, the expected 5-year survival rate is 30% to 50% if clear margins are obtained. Postoperative adjuvant chemotherapy significantly increases disease-free survival as well as overall survival by up to 30% and is recommended for all patients, especially if the surgical resection margins are not clear. In stage III colorectal cancer, patients treated for 6 months with intravenous 5-FU and leucovorin (folinic acid) who have one to three involved nodes have a 5-year survival of 65%, and those with more than three involved nodes have a 5-year survival of up to 40%.[40] Therefore, until recently, adjuvant therapy with 5-FU and leucovorin was most widely used for stage III disease. An important recent advance was the development of an oral 5-FU analog, capecitabine, which obviates the need for intravenous infusions. This oral monotherapeutic has reduced the rate of side effects and gives the same rate of disease free survival. Hand-foot syndrome, otherwise known as PPE or Palmar-Plantar Erythrodysesthesia, is still a clinical side effect that manifests even with the oral monotherapy. Hand-foot syndrome includes neuropathy, as well as vesicular blistering on the palms of the hands and the soles of the feet coupled with intolerance to temperature changes of hot and cold.

Stage IV (Metastatic Disease)

More than 20% of patients have metastatic disease at the initial diagnosis, with another 30% eventually developing metastatic disease. Some of these patients with metastatic disease to the liver or the lungs that have less than three tumors may benefit from resection with a long-term, more than 5-year survival rate of 35% to 55%.[40] For those who do not have resectable disease, local treatments to ablate the metastatic lesions may provide long-term control and favorable prognosis. Cryosurgery, radiofrequency ablation, embolization, and hepatic intra-arterial chemotherapy (chemo-ablation) have been used successfully in unresectable hepatic metastatic disease. The goal in patients with stage IV metastatic disease is to slow tumor progression while maintaining a reasonable quality of life. The majority of patients with metastatic disease do not have resectable (curable) disease, but due to a number of recent advances in adjuvant chemotherapeutic strategies, the average survival rate of stage IV disease is 2 years.[39-40]

Intravenous 5-FU and folinic acid (leucovorin) or the oral 5-FU analog capecitabine prolong median survival to about 11 months. However, the addition of either oxaliplatin (FOLFOX) or irinotecan (FOLFIRI) to 5-FU and folinic acid provides further improvement in median survival (15 to 20 months).[40] Currently, either FOLFOX or FOLFIRI is the preferred first-line treatment regimens for most patients with metastatic colorectal cancer. For convenience, oral capecitabine (instead of intravenous 5-FU and leucovorin) can be used in combination with oxaliplatin; however, combinations with irinotecan should not be used due to increased toxicity (diarrhea). The role of combination therapy with both oxaliplatin and irinotecan is under investigation.[39,40]

The most recent advance in the treatment of metastatic colon cancer is the development of the biologic agents, cetuximab, panitumumab, and bevacizumab. The role of these agents is rapidly evolving. Cetuximab and panitumumab are monoclonal antibodies to EGFR; bevacizumab is a monoclonal antibody to vascular endothelial growth factor (VEGF). Combination therapy with bevacizumab and FOLFOX or FOLFIRI prolongs mean survival 2 to 5 months compared with either regimen alone. Therefore, many oncologists are now using one of these combinations for initial therapy of metastatic disease. Bevacizumab may cause serious thromboembolic events (including stroke and myocardial infarction) in 5% of patients.[46]

When these combination therapies (FOLFOX or FOLFIRI) do not stay the disease progression, the protocol then is to switch to alternative regimens. Cetuximab and panitumumab are used in protocols for patients whose disease has progressed despite first line interventions. These chemotherapies are also under investigation as combination with first-line therapeutic protocols.[39,40,44,46]

Adjuvant Therapy for Rectal Cancer

When comparing colon cancer to rectal cancer, rectal cancer has a lower long-term survival rate with higher rates of local tumor recurrence at least 25% rate.[40] This is due to the difficulty to achieve clear surgical margins and a combination therapy of fluorouracil as a radiation sensitizing agent is used with radiation therapy. This has been shown to increase disease-free survival rates while decreasing pelvic recurrence and is a standard recommendation for patients with stage II and III disease.[44,45]

It has long been controversial whether chemoradiation should be administered preoperatively ("neoadjuvant") or postoperatively ("adjuvant"). Neoadjuvant therapy may decrease the size of the tumor before surgery (tumor downstaging), allowing more patients to undergo curative resection with sphincter preservation rather than abdominoperineal resection.[47] When initial imaging studies suggest stage I disease, surgery may be performed first, followed by postoperative chemoradiation in patients found at surgery to have more advanced (stage II or III) disease. A recent, large, randomized controlled trial reported that preoperative therapy led to better patient treatment compliance, reduced local recurrence and toxicity, and a higher number of sphincter-preserving resections. Therefore, preoperative chemoradiation increasingly is recommended for patients with distal rectal cancers that are determined to be stage II or III by endorectal ultrasound or MRI.[47]

Follow-Up after Surgery

The standard follow up protocol is that patients should be evaluated every 3-6 months for 3-5 years with blood work, history, physical examination, and a CEA level. For patients who had a preoperative colonoscopy, a repeat should be performed one year after surgery. For patients who did not undergo a full colonoscopy preoperatively, they should have one done within 3 to 6 months after surgery, as well as 1 year afterward. These surveillance colonoscopies are looking for metachronous polyps or signs of recurrent cancer. A rise in CEA of a new onset of symptoms should warrant a chest and abdominal CT to look for recurrent and metastatic disease. If the CT scan is negative but the signs and symptoms persist, a PET scan is more sensitive for the detection of occult metastatic disease. Rectal cancer has a high incidence of local tumor extension and recurrence; a sigmoidoscopy should be performed every 3 to 6 months for 3 years.[35-37,40-41,47]

Naturopathic Approaches to Treating Colorectal Cancer

Naturopathic Therapeutic Protocol
1. Lower risk
2. Support adjuvant radiotherapy and chemotherapy
3. Reduce side effects
4. Prevent metastasis
5. Counsel patients

1. LOWER RISK
Folic Acid
A meta-analysis of 7 cohort and 9 case-control studies examined the association between folate consumption and colorectal cancer risk. The results offer some support for the hypothesis that folate has a small protective effect against colorectal cancer, but confounding by other dietary factors could not be ruled out.[50] A larger study, the Nurse's Health Study, followed nurses taking a multivitamin supplement for 15 years or more, has shown that folic acid decreased colon cancer by up to 75% if folate was among the ingredients.[49]

Camelia sinensis
Green tea is chemopreventive for oral and colon cancers.[50] Oral consumption of green tea reduces PGE2 in a dose-dependent manner in colonic cells. PGE2 is elevated in colon cancer cells and stimulates growth-signaling pathways. It is additionally associated with invasiveness properties.[50] Green tea has inhibitory actions on almost all steps of carcinogenesis. Clinical trials bear this out.[51] A published meta-analysis of all cohort and case-control studies assessing breast cancer incidence and breast cancer recurrence resulted in 7 observational reports that met inclusion criteria. The pooled relative risk for the highest levels of green tea consumption on the risk of developing breast cancer was 0.79 (95% CI, 0.62-1.01; p=0.064). The highest levels of green tea consumption [typically >5 cups daily] showed a pooled relative risk of 0.56 (95% CI, 0.38-0.83; p = 0.0041) for stage I and II disease.[51]

Green tea acts to suppress proliferation and induce p53 activation; EGCG in green tea induces p53 tumor suppressor gene mediatied apoptosis activity.[52] EGCG has been demonstrated in a number of *in-vitro* models to increase DNA repair.[53] This effect is the result of EGCG's influence on the excision-repair system. Rats exposed to heterocyclic amines demonstrated significantly reduced mutagenicity and increased

DNA repair in hepatocytes when fed green tea extract.[54] Green tea acts to suppress proliferation: topoisomerase. *In-vitro* data demonstrates the ability of EGCG to inhibit topoisomerase I. Topoisomerase is critical during DNA transcription and replication by facilitating the unwinding of the DNA helix to allow proper function of large enzymatic machinery. Topoisomerases have been shown to maintain both transcription and replication.[55] Green tea acts to suppress proliferation: p21. EGCG from green tea blocks MCF-7 (ER+ breast cancer cells) in G1 by inducing p21, a cell cycle inhibitor. EGCG from *Camellia sinensis*, baicalein from *Scutellaria baicalensis,* and *Cimicifuga racemosa* extracts each increase apoptosis in CLL cells.[56] All of these herbals interrupt VEGF survival signals, resulting capase activation, and subsequent cell death. Cimicifuga induces capases in MCF-7 cells.[57]

2. SUPPORT ADJUVANT RADIOTHERAPY AND CHEMOTHERAPY
Radiotherapy with Green Tea and Vitamin E
This original research set out to look at vitamin E (natural vitamin E, d-alpha-tocopherol, VE) and EGCG with original hypothesis that these antioxidants may be antagonistic during radiation treatment (XRT). Data suggested that tumor growth was 10% slower in EGCG fed mice and tumor growth was 3% slower in VE fed mice. EGCG and VE protected normal tissues from severe XRT related soft tissue reactions. Intramural apoptosis in the EGCG and VE concentrations were 8.3 fold and 1.3 fold increase as compared to control groups. Tumor cell invasiveness was decreased by 25% with EGCG and VE compared to control groups. VE and EGCG appear to concentrate in tumors; mechanism and significance of this is unknown.[58]

EGCG (*in vivo*) and VE (*in vitro*) significantly slow tumor growth, which is likely due to increased apoptosis and decreased cell proliferation. Anti-angiogenic RNA expression in the EGCG tumors may explain the slower tumor growth. VE and EGCG did not reach statistical significance in increasing radiation resistance in implanted tumors. VE and EGCG significantly decrease radiation reactions in normal tissues. In familial polyposis, ellagic acid and EGCG are chemopreventive.[58]

3. REDUCE SIDE EFFECTS
Glutathione
In one study, glutathione improved survival of patients with advanced colorectal cancer receiving

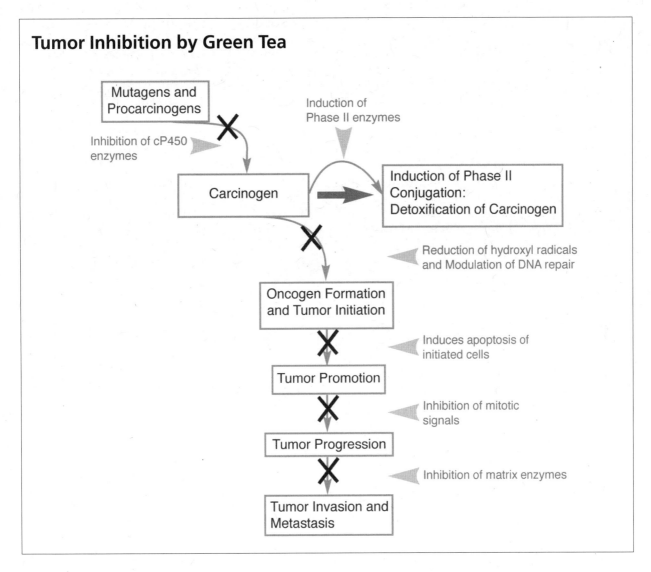

Tumor Inhibition by Green Tea

Mutagens and Procarcinogens

Inhibition of cP450 enzymes

Induction of Phase II enzymes

Carcinogen

Induction of Phase II Conjugation: Detoxification of Carcinogen

Reduction of hydroxyl radicals and Modulation of DNA repair

Oncogen Formation and Tumor Initiation

Induces apoptosis of initiated cells

Tumor Promotion

Inhibition of mitotic signals

Tumor Progression

Inhibition of matrix enzymes

Tumor Invasion and Metastasis

5-FU/oxaliplatin.[59] Glutathione reduces neuropathy in patients treated with ovarian cancer without decreasing the antitumor activity.[60,61] Glutathione reduces neuropathy.[62] Glutathione improved survival of patients with advanced colorectal cancer receiving 5-FU/oxaliplatin.[59]

4. PREVENT METASTASIS
Modified Citrus Pectin

Fractionated citrus pectin powder (modified citrus pectin, or MCP) binds to galectin-3 receptors on cancer cells, preventing micro and distant metastasis. Galectin-3 proteins bind to cancer cell surface lectin receptor sites and interfere with the ability of the cancer cells to aggregate and attach to healthy cells. In one study, MCP was shown to prevent melanoma cells from adhering to laminin and asialofetuin-induced homotypic aggregation, thereby preventing metasta-

tic spread.[63] The metastatic process involves adhesion of tumor cells to target organs through specific cell receptors. MCP significantly inhibited the adhesion of prostate, breast, melanoma and laryngeal carcinoma cells to epithelium, thus suggesting interference with a non-tumor specific common event in the metastatic cascade.[64] MCP added to the media of prostate cancer cells reduced cell growth. Its action may in part be explained by its ability to modulate the expression of protein molecules involved in cell cycling.[65]

Dosage: 1 tbsp t.i.d. (or 6 g b.i.d.) before surgery, stopping the evening before when no longer allowed food or liquids. Mix with a small amount of hot water, swallow quickly, and then follow with strong tasting juice, such as grape juice or apple juice.

Vitamin C

In one study, vitamin C increased sensitivity of colon cancer cells to cisplatin.[66] Vitamin C improves antineoplastic activity of doxorubicin, cisplatin, and Taxol in human beast carcinoma cells *in vitro*.[67] VC increased sensitivity of etoposide and cisplatin by stabilizing p53, which increases Bax, thereby sensitizing HeLa cells to cell-cycle arrest and cell death/apoptosis.[66,67]

Alpha Lipoic Acid (ALA)

Alpha lipoic acid (ALA) reduces cumulative polyneuropathy, but precaution should be used with this endogenous antioxidant and should only be used after standard chemotherapy sequences have been completed or in between during 'chemo breaks'.[68]

Melatonin

MLT blocks mitogenic effects of tumors that promote hormones and growth factors, down regulates 5-lipoxygenase expression and acts a biological response modifier.[71,72] It protects against chemotherapy toxicity and has over 600+ specific publications of MLT and cancer. Greater than 100 of these are specific human studies.

Melatonin (MLT) prevents neuropathy, inhibits cancer cell growth, and potentiates the beneficial effects of chemotherapy and radiation while reducing their side effects.[69,70] MLT can block the mitogenic effects of tumor promoting hormones and growth factors. MLT down-regulates 5-lipoxygenase gene expression. MLT directly slows growth of some prostate cancer cell lines,[73,74] while reversing LHRH resistance in prostate cancer.[75]

In a randomized double blind trial, MLT was studied versus supportive care in 1440 patients with untreatable solid tumors. They were given 20 mg q.h.s. of MLT as the active treatment proband arm. In the active group the frequency of cachexia, asthenia, thrombocytopenia, and lymphocytopenia was significantly lower than in those who received supportive care alone. The percentage of patients with disease stabilization and the % per 1 year survival were both significantly higher in patients concomitantly treated with MLT than in those treated with supportive care alone.[76]

A second study evaluated the influence of MLT on the efficacy of toxicity of chemotherapy in a group of 200 patients with metastatic chemotherapy-resistant cancer. Patients were randomized to receive chemotherapy alone or chemotherapy and MLT at 20 mg q.h.s. Patients in the active group showed an objective tumor response rate significantly higher than in those without MLT. MLT induced a significant decline in the frequency of chemotherapy induced asthenia, thrombocytopenia, stomatits, cardiotoxicity,

and neurotoxicity.[77] Melatonin 20 mg q.h.s. in a European study showed patients who received chemotherapy with MLT had a 1-year survival rate and the objective tumor regression rates were significantly higher in the MLT group (P<0.001).[77] A study *in vitro* comparing Cisplatin vs Cisplatin + MLT for cultured ovarian cancer cell lines showed MLT enhanced Cisplatin sensitivity in two ovarian cell lines.[78]

Summary of melatonin activity as integrative therapeutic
- Physiological antitumor activity
- Antiproliferative action
- Stimulation of anticancer immunity
- Modulation of oncogene expression
- Anti-inflammatory
- Anti-oxidant
- Anti-angiogenic effects
- Inhibits cytokines

Dosage: 10-20 mg q.h.s.

Vitamin D and Calcium

Calcium and vitamin D protect the colonic epithelium against colon cancer by reducing the concentration of bile acids and therefore decreasing a stimulatory effect on cellular proliferation.[79] Colon cancer epidemiology has shown that incidence is higher in areas that get less sunshine. The body needs the UV light exposure to convert chemicals in your skin into vitamin D, which the system uses to metabolize calcium. Calcium supplementation in cancer patients has shown statistically significant survival rates.[80] Taking calcium supplements with vitamin D may be chemopreventative as well as epigenetically preventive. Large population studies have shown a lower risk of colon cancer development associated with higher levels of vitamin D, which may reduce the risk of developing colon cancer by 60%.[81]

Arabinex

Arabinogalactans found in arabinex bind to lectins specific to hepatic parynchema and prevents liver metastasis. They also serve as a good source of fiber that is able to increase short-chain fatty acid production, particularly butyrate, which is an energy source of colon cells and helps colon cells to repair and rejuvenate while protecting colon cells from developing cancer. By decreasing ammonia production in liver, increasing beneficial gut bacteria, stimulating natural killer cell activity, stimulating the immune system, and blocking metastasis of tumor cells to the liver, arabinex can be chemopreventative as well as curative to colon cancer.[82]

Chemotherapeutic and Naturopathic Integrated Therapies

Chemotherapeutic	Naturopathic	Daily Dose	Caution
5-Fu Leucovorin (folinic acid)	*To increase effectiveness:* MCP Actifolate Tri-methylated forms of folic acid	1 scoop bid 800 mcg qd	
	To reduce toxicity: Glutamine Mushrooms Folinic Acid	10 g tid, swish & swallow Stametes 7, Turkey Tails	
Oxalipalatin (FOLFOX) Irinotecan (FOLFIRI)	*To increase effectiveness:* Minimal Essential Multivitamin EPA	1 qd-bid 2-3 g qd	
	To reduce toxicity: Glutamine Mushrooms	10 g tid, swish & swallow Stametes 7, Turkey Tails, 1-2each up to tid	
Flourouracil	*To increase effectiveness:* Vitamin D3	2000-5000 IU qd	
	To reduce toxicity: Topical castor oil for Hand/Foot syndrome (PPE) Glutamine Alpha lipoic acid	PPE prevention and TX 10 g tid, swish & swallow	Use during breaks in therapy, not with therapy
Monoclonal Ab EGFR Cetuximab Panitumumab	*To increase effectiveness:* Green tea *To reduce toxicity:* Glutamine Mushrooms	5-10 cups qd 10 g tid, swish & swallow Stametes 7, Turkey Tails, 1-2each up to tid	
Monoclonal Ab VEGF Bevocizumab	*To increase effectiveness:* Green tea *To reduce toxicity:* Calcium	5-10 cups qd 1200 mg qd (with vitamin C and magnesium)	
Gemcitabine Tarceva	*To increase effectiveness:* Green tea *To reduce toxicity:* Melatonin	5-10 cups qd 20 mg qhs	

References

1. Guyton AC, Hall JE. Textbook of Medical Physiology. 10th ed. New York, NY: WB Saunders Co.;2000.

2. Moore, KL, AF Dalley, and AMR Aqur. 2009. Clinically Oriented Anatomy. 6th ed. Baltimore, MD: Lippincott Williams & Wilkins;2009.

3. Young, RC. Harrison's Internal Medicine, online. Chapter 87, Gastrointestinal Tract Cancer, Robert J. Mayer.

4. McPhee SJ, Papadakis MA. Eds. Gonzales R, Zeiger R. 2009. CURRENT Medical Diagnosis & Treatment. 48th ed.

5. www.medcinenet.com

6. Silviera ML, Smith BP, Powell J, Sapienza C. Epigenetic differences in normal colon mucosa of cancer patients suggest altered dietary metabolic pathways. Cancer Prevention Research 2012;5(3):374-84.

7. Meyerhardt JA, et al. Association of dietary pattern with cancer recurrence and survival in patients with Stage III colon cancer. JAMA. 2007; 298:754-64.

8. Dahm CC, Keogh RH, Spencer EA, Greenwood DC, Key TJ, Fentiman IS, et al. Dietary fiber and colorectal cancer risk: a nested case-control study using food diaries. J Natl Cancer Inst. 2010;102:614-626.

9. Larsson SC, Orsini N, Wolk A. Vitamin B6 and risk of colorectal cancer: a meta-analysis of prospective studies. JAMA. 2010;303:1077-83.

10. Beresford S, Johnson K, Ritenbaugh C, et al. Low-fat dietary pattern and risk of colorectal cancer: the Women's Health Initiative Randomized Controlled Dietary Modification Trial. JAMA. 2006;295:643-54.

11. Reddy BS: Dietary fat and its relationship to large bowel cancer. Cancer Res 41 (9 Pt 2): 3700-705, 1981.

12. Minami Y, Nishino Y, Tsubono Y, et al. Increase of colon and rectal cancer incidence rates in Japan: trends in incidence rates in Miyagi Prefecture, 1959-1997. J or Epid 2006;16(6):240-248.

13. Vargas PA, Alberts DS: Colon cancer: the quest for prevention. Oncology (Huntington); 7(11 suppl): 33-40, 1993.

14. Martínez ME, Giovannucci E, Spiegelman D, et al.: Leisure-time physical activity, body size, and colon cancer in women. Nurses' Health Study Research Group. J Natl Cancer Inst. 1997;89 (13): 948-55.

15. Giovannucci E, Ascherio A, Rimm EB, et al. Physical activity, obesity, and risk for colon cancer and adenoma in men. Ann Intern Med. 122(5):327-34:1995.

16. Calle EE, Rodriguez C, Walker-Thurmond K, et al. Overweight, obesity, and mortality from cancer in a prospectively studied cohort of U.S. adults. N Engl J Med. 348 (17): 1625-38, 2003.

17. Neugut AI, Jacobson JS, DeVivo I. Epidemiology of colorectal adenomatous polyps. Cancer Epidemiol Biomarkers Prev. 1993 Mar-Apr;2(2):159-76.

18. Boleij A, Schaeps RMJ, Tjalsma H. Association between Streptococcus bovis and colon cancer. J of Clin Micro. 2009;47(2):516.

19. Eaden JA, Abrams KR, Mayberry JF. The risk of colorectal cancer in ulcerative colitis: a meta-analysis. Gut 2001;48:526-535.

20. Fearon ER, Vogelstein B: A genetic model for colorectal tumorigenesis. Cell. 1990;61(5): 759-67.

21. Willett W: The search for the causes of breast and colon cancer. Nature. 1989;338 (6214): 389-94.

22. Potter JD: Reconciling the epidemiology, physiology, and molecular biology of colon cancer. JAMA . 1992 Sep 23-30;268 (12): 1573-77.

23. www.cancer.gov/cancertopics/pdg/genetics/colorectalcancer. 2012.

24. Ruder EH, Laiyemo AO, Graubard BI, et al.: Non-steroidal anti-inflammatory drugs and colorectal cancer risk in a large, prospective cohort. Am J Gastroenterol. 2011;106 (7): 1340-50.

25. Hinz B, Brune K. Cyclooxygenase-2–10 years later. J Pharmacol Exp Ther. 300;(2): 367-75.

26. Stryker SJ Wolff BG Culp CE, et al. Natural history of untreated colonic polyps. Gastroenterology. 1997;93 (5):1009-13.

27. www.cancer.org/Cancer/ColonandRectumCancer/ colorectal-cancer . 2012.

28. Cheadle JP, Sampson JR. Exposing the myth about base excision repair and human inherited disease. Oxford Journals. 2003:1-28; hmg.oxfordjournals.org/content/early/2003/hmg.ddg259.full.pdf

29. www.mayoclinic.com/health/colon-cancer/Dsection=symptoms. 2012.

30. Winawer SJ, Zauber AG, Ho MN, et al. Prevention of colorectal cancer by colonoscopic polypectomy. The National Polyp Study Workgroup. N Engl J Med.1993;329 (27):1977-81.

31. Atkin WS, Edwards R, Kralj-Hans I, et al. Once-only flexible sigmoidoscopy screening in prevention of colorectal cancer: a multicentre randomised controlled trial. Lancet. 2010;375 (9726):1624-33.

32. Klessen C, Rogalla P, Taupitz M. Local staging of rectal cancer: the current role of MRI. Eur Radiol 2007;17(2):379-89.

33. Duncan JE, Sweeney WB, Trudel JL et al. Colonoscoy in the elderly: low risk, low yield in asymptomatic patients. Dis Colon Rectum 2006;49(5):646-51.

34. www.mayoclinic.com/health/virtual-colonoscopy/MY00624 2012

35. Duffy MJ, van Dalen A, Haglund C, et al. Tumour markers in colorectal cancer: European Group on Tumour Markers)EGTM guidelines for clinical use. Eur J of Cancer. 2007;43:1348-1360.

36. www.asco.org/CancerPolicyandClinicalAffairs 2006 guidelines for clinical practice.

37. American Joint Committee on Cancer (AJCC). 2002. AJCC Cancer Staging Manual 6th ed. New York, NY: Springer-New York;2002. www.springeronline.com

38. www.nlm.nih.gov/medlineplus/ostomy.html 2012

39. American Cancer Society: Cancer Facts and Figures 2012. Atlanta, GA: American Cancer Society, 2012. Available online. Accessed January 5, 2012.

40. Howlader N, Noone AM, Krapcho M, et al. SEER Cancer Statistics Review, 1975-2008. Bethesda, MD: National Cancer Institute; 2011. Also available online. Accessed December 1, 2011.

41. Van der Voort van Zijp J, Hoekstra HJ, Basson MD. Evolving management of colorectal cancer. World J Gastro. 2008;14(25):3956-67.

42. Moertel CG, Fleming TR, Macdonald JS, et al. Levamisole and fluorouracil for adjuvant therapy of resected colon carcinoma. N Engl J Med. 1990;322 (6): 352-58.

43. Krook JE, Moertel CG, Gunderson LL, et al. Effective surgical adjuvant therapy for high-risk rectal carcinoma. N Engl J Med. 1991;324 (11): 709-15.

44. Bruera G, Santomaggio A, Cannita K, et al. Poker association of weekly alternating 5-fluorouracil, irinotecan, bevacizumab and oxaliplatin (Fir-B/Fox) in first line treatment of metastatic colorectal cancer: a phase II study. BMC Cancer. 2010;10:567.

45. Kopetz S, Freitas D, Calabrich AFC, Hoff PM. Adjuvant chemotherapy for Stage II colon cancer. Onco 2008;22(3):260-70.

46. Veronese ML, O'Dwyer PJ. Monoclonal antibodies in the treatment of colorectal cancer. Euro J Cancer 2004;40(9):1292-1301.

47. www.cancer.gov/cancertopics/pdq/treatment/colon...page9. 2012.

48. Sanjoaquin MA, Allen N, Couto E, Roddam AW, Key TJ. Folate intake and colorectal cancer risk: a meta-analytical approach. Int J Cancer. 2005 Feb 20;113(5):825-28.

49. Giovannucci E, Stampfer MJ, Colditz GA, et al. Multivitamin use, folate and colon cancer in women in the Nurse's Health Study. Ann Intern Med 1998; 129(7):517-24.

50. Li N, Sun Z, Han C, Chen J. The chemopreventive effects of tea on human oral precancerous mucosa lesions.

Proc Soc Exp Biol Med. 1999;220(4):218-24.

51. Seely D, Mills E, Wu P, Guyatt G. Green tea in the prevention of breast cancer and breast cancer recurrence: a systematic review and meta-analysis of observational studies. Int Cancer Ther 2005;4(2):144-55.

52. Sah JF, Balasubramanian S, Eckert RL, Rorke EA. Epigallocatechin-3-gallate inhibits epidermal growth factor receptor signaling pathway: evidence for direct inhibition of ERK1/2 and AKT kinases. J Biol Chem. 2004;279:12755-62.

53. KurodaY. 1999. Antimutagenic and anticarcinogenic activity of tea polyphenols. Mutat Res. 436;69-97.

54. Weisburger JH. Second international scientific symposium on tea and human health: an introduction. Proc Soc Exp Biol Med. 1999;220(4):193-94.

55. Lin JK, Liang YC, Lin-Shiau SY. Cancer chemoprevention by tea polyphenols through mitotic signal transduction blockade. Biochem Pharmacol. 1999;58(6):911-15.

56. Lee YK, ND Bone, AK Stege, TD Shanafelt, DF Jelinek and NE Kay. VEGF receptor phosphorylation status and apoptosis is modulated by a green tea component, epigallocatechin-3-gallate (EGCG), in B-cell chronic lymphocytic leukemia. Blood. August 1; 104(3):788-94.

57. Hostanska K, Nisslein T, et al. Cimicifuga racemosa extract inhibits proliferation of estrogen receptor positive and negative human breast carcinoma cell lines by induction of apoptosis. Breast Cancer Res Treat. 2004 Mar;84(2):151-60.

58. Lawenda BD, et al. Dietary Antioxidant Supplementation During Radiation Therapy: Potential for Radiation Protection of Tumors. Department of Radiation Oncology, Naval Medical Center, San Diego, CA;2004.

59. Stoehlmacher J, Park DJ, Zhang W, Groshen S, Tsao-Wei DD, Yu MC, Lenz HJ. Association between glutathione S-transferase P1, T1, and M1 genetic polymorphism and survival of patients with metastatic colorectal cancer. J Natl Cancer Inst. 2002 Jun 19;94(12):936-42 .

60. Colombo N, Binc, et al. Weekly cisplatin +/- glutathione in relapsed ovarian carcinoma. Int J Gynecol Cancer. 1995;5(2): 81-86.

61. Tiwari RK, Mukhopadhyay B, Telang NT, Osborne MP. Modulation of gene expression by selected fatty acids in human breast cancer cells. Anticancer Res. 1991 Jul-Aug;11(4):1383-88.

62. Cascinu S, Catalano V, Cordella L, Labianca R, Giordani P, Baldelli AM, Beretta GD, Ubiali E, Catalano G. Neuroprotective effect of reduced glutathione on oxaliplatin-based chemotherapy in advanced colorectal cancer: a randomized, double-blind, placebo-controlled trial. J Clin Oncol. 2002 Aug 15;20(16):3478-83.

63. Inohara H, Raz A. Effects of natural complex carbohydrate (citrus pectin) on murine melanoma cell properties related to galectin-3 functions. Glycoconj J. 1994 Dec;11(6):527-32.

64. Naik H, Pilat MJ, Donat T. Inhibition of in vitro tumor cell-endothelial adhesion by modified citrus pectin: a pH modified natural complex carbohydrate. Proc Am Assoc Cancer Res. 1995;36:A377.

65. Hsieh TC, Wu JM. Changes in cell growth, cyclin/kinase, endogenous phosphoproteins and nm23 gene expression in human prostatic JCA-1 cells treated with modified citrus pectin. Biochem Mol Biol Int. 1995;37:833-41.

66. Catani MV, Costanzo A, Savini I, Levrero M, Laurenzi VD, Wang JY, Melino G, Avigliano L. Ascorbate up-regulates MLH1 (Mut L homologue-1) and p73: implications for the cellular response to DNA damage. Biochem J. 2002 Jun 1;364(Pt 2):441-47.

67. Kurbacher CM, Wagner U, Kolster B, et al. Ascorbic acid (vitamin C) improves the antineoplastic activity of doxorubicin, cisplatin, and paclitaxel in human breast carcinoma cells in vitro. Cancer Lett. 1996 Jun 5;103(2):183-89.

68. Muhammad Wasif Saif. Oral calcium ameliorating bexliplatin-induced peripheral neuropathy. J Appl Res. 2004 January 1; 4(4): 576-82; _atiroglu, L. Kabasakal, S. Arbak, S. Öner, F. Ercan, M. Keyer-Uysal. The protective effect of melatonin on cisplatin nephrotoxicity. The Journal of Fundamental Clinical Pharmacology. 2000 Nov-Dec:553-60. Published Online: Aug 26, 2009.

69. Hara M, et al. Melatonin, a pineal secretory product with antioxidant properties, protects against cisplatin-induced nephrotoxicity in rats. Journal of Pineal Research. 2001 Apr;30(3):129-38.

70. Wilson AL, Melatonin blocks the stimulatory effects of prolactin on human breast cell growth culture. Brit J Cancer. 1995;72:1435-40.

71. Steinhilber D, Brungs M, et al. The nuclear receptor for melatonin represses 5-lipoxygenase gene expression in human B lymphocytes. J Biol Chem. 1995;270:7037-40.

72. Toma JG, Amerongen HM, Hennes SC, et al. Effects of olfactory bulbectomy, melatonin, and/or pinealectomy on three sublines of the Dunning R3327 rat prostatic adenocarcinoma. J Pineal Res. 1987;4:321-38.

73. Marelli MM, Limonta P, Maggi R, Motta M, Moretti RM. Growth-inhibitory activity of melatonin on human androgen-independent du 145 prostate cancer cells. Prostate. 2000;45:238-244.

74. Lissoni P, Cazzaniga M, et al. LHRH analogue in metastatic prostate cancer by the pineal hormone melatonin: efficacy of LHRH analogue plus melatonin in patients progressing on LHRH analogue alone. Eur Urol. 1997;31(2):178-81.

75. Lissoni P. Is there a role for melatonin in supportive care? Supp. Care Cancer. 2000 Mar;10(2):110-16.

76. Lissoni P, Barni S, Mandalà M, et al. Decreased toxicity and increased efficacy of cancer chemotherapy using the pineal hormone melatonin in metastatic solid tumour patients with poor clinical status. Eur J Cancer. 1999 Nov;35(12):1688-92.

77. Futagami M, Sato S, Sakamoto T, et al. Effects of melatonin on the proliferation and cis-diamminedichloroplatinum (CDDP) sensitivity of cultured human ovarian cancer cells. Gynecol Oncol. 2001 Sep;82(3):544-49.

78. Murray M, et al. How to Prevent and Treat Cancer with Natural Medicine. New York, NY: Riverhead Books/Penguin Putnam Inc; Chapter 4:103-104.

79. Baron JA, Beach M, Mande JS, et al. Calcium supplements for the prevention of colorectal adenomas. Calcium polyp prevention study group. New Engl J Med. 1999;340:101-07.

80. Garland CF, Garland FC, Gorham ED. Calcium and vitamin D. Their potential roles in colon and breast cancer prevention. Ann NY Aca Sci. 1999;889:107-19.

81. Alschuler LN, Gazella KA. Alternative Medicine Magazine's Definitive Guide to Cancer: An Integrated Approach to Prevention, Treatment, and Healing (Alternative Medicine Guides). Berkley, CA: Ten Speed Press;2007.

82. Ahsan H, et al: Family history of colorectal adenomatous polyps and increased risk for colorectal cancer. Ann Intern Med. 1998;128:900.

83. Bernstein CN, et al: Cancer risk in patients with inflammatory bowel disease: a population-based study. Cancer. 2001;91:854.

84. Bruce WR, et al: Possible mechanisms relating diet and risk of colon cancer. Cancer Epidemiol, Biomarkers Prev. 2000;9:1271.

85. Forman D: Meat and cancer: A relation in search of a mechanism. Lancet. 1999;353:686.

86. Giovannucci E: An updated review of the epidemiologic evidence that cigarette smoking increases risk of colorectal cancer. Cancer Epidemiol, Biomarkers, Prev. 2001; 10:725.

87. Greenberg ER, et al: A clinical trial of antioxidant vitamins to prevent colorectal adenoma. N Engl J Med. 1994;333:141.

88. Fuchs CS, et al: A prospective study of family history and the risk of colorectal cancer. N Engl J Med. 1994;331:1669.

89. Fuchs CS, et al. Dietary fiber and the risk of colorectal cancer and adenoma in women. N Engl J Med. 199;340:169.

90. Jänne PA, Mayer RJ: Chemoprevention of colorectal cancer. N Engl J Med. 2000;342:1960.

91. Schatzkin A, et al: Lack of effect of a low-fat, high-fiber diet on the recurrence of colorectal adenomas. N Engl J Med. 2000;342:1149.

92. Syngal S, et al: Benefits of colonoscopic surveillance and prophylactic colectomy in patients with hereditary nonpolyposis colorectal cancer mutations. Ann Intern Med. 1998;129:787.

93. Vogelstein B, et al: Genetic alterations during colorectal-tumor development. N Engl J Med. 1988;319:595.

94. Byers T, et al: American Cancer Society guidelines for screening and surveillance for early detection of colorectal polyps and cancer. CA Cancer J Clin. 1997;47:154.

95. Cotton PB, et al: Computed tomographic colonography (virtual colonoscopy): a multicenter comparison with standard colonoscopy for detection of colorectal neoplasia. JAMA. 2004;291:1713.

96. Desch CE, et al: Colorectal cancer surveillance: 2005 update of an American Society of Clinical Oncology practice guidelines. J Clin Oncol. 2005; 23:8512.

97. Fenlon HM, et al: A comparison of virtual and conventional colonoscopy for the detection of colorectal polyps. N Engl J Med. 1999;341:1496.

98. Ransohoff DF, Sandler RS. Screening for colorectal cancer. N Engl J Med. 2002;346:40.

99. Andre T, et al: Oxaliplatin, fluorouracil, and leucovorin as adjuvant treatment for colorectal cancer. N Eng J Med.2004;350:2343.

100. Chan I, Cunningham D: Adjuvant therapy in colon cancer-what, when and how? Ann Oncol. 2006;17:1377.

101. Compton C, et al: American Joint Committee on Cancer Prognostic Factors Consensus Conference. Colorectal working group. Cancer. 2000;88:1739.

102. Cunningham D, et al: Cetuximab monotherapy and cetuximab plus irinotecan in irinotecan-refractory metastatic colorectal cancer. N Engl J Med. 2004;351:337.

103. DeGramont A, et al: Leucovorin and fluorouracil with or without oxaliplatin as first-line treatment in advanced colorectal cancer. J Clin Oncol. 2000;18:2938.

104. Douillard JY, et al: Irinotecan combined with fluorouracil compared with fluorouracil alone as first-line treatment for metastatic colorectal cancer: A multi center randomised trial. Lancet. 2000;355:1041.

105. Hurwitz H, et al: Bevacizumab plus irinotecan, fluorouracil and leucovorin for metastatic colorectal cancer. N Engl J Med. 2004;350:2335.

106. International multi center pooled analysis of B2c colon cancer trials (IMPACT B2) Investigators. Efficacy of adjuvant fluorouracil and folinic acid in B2 colon cancer. J Clin Oncol. 1999;17:1356.

107. Kapiteijn E et al: Preoperative radiotherapy combined with total mesorectal excision for resectable rectal cancer. N Engl J Med. 2001;345:638.

108. Minsky BD: Adjuvant therapy of resectable rectal cancer. Cancer Treat Rev. 2002;28:181.

109. O'Connell JB, et al: Colon cancer survival rates with the new American Joint Committee on Cancer. 6th ed. staging. J Natl Cancer Inst. 2004;96:1420.

110. Saltz LB et al: Irinotecan plus fluorouracil and leucovorin for metastatic colorectal cancer. N Engl J Med. 2000;343:905.

Pathophysiology

Leukemia is the term used for cancer that affects the blood cells. Leukemia literally means "many white cells in the blood." White blood cells are produced by the bone marrow, the soft spongy center of bones. They then pass from the bone marrow into the blood stream and lymph system, where they differentiate to the different cell lines. Normal, healthy blood is made up of plasma and three types of blood cells: white blood cells, red blood cells, and platelets.

White blood cells fight infection and disease, differentiating to fight bacterial, viral, or allergic responses. Red blood cells carry oxygen, iron, and carbon dioxide to and from the cells of the body. Platelets (also called thrombocytes) help form blood clots to control bleeding. Blood cells are made in the bone marrow, the soft, spongy middle part of the bones. In adults, most bone marrow can be found in the hips, ribs, spine, and skull. The immature blood cells in the marrow are called blasts.

LYMPHOCYTIC AND MYELOGENOUS LEUKEMIA

There are two kinds of abnormal white blood cells that cause leukemia. If the cancer cells are lymphoid, the disease is called lymphocytic leukemia. If they are myeloid cells, the disease is myelogenous leukemia. Leukemia can also be acute or chronic. Acute leukemia cancer cells are immature blasts and grow quickly, which makes them more virulent, while chronic leukemia cells are a combination of immature and mature cells, which grow more slowly and are usually less deadly. The myeloid leukemias are a group with heterogenous characterization of infiltrates found in the blood, bone marrow, and other tissues of the hematopoietic system. These leukemias form a spectrum of malignancies that range from rapidly fatal to slow growing and have traditionally been designated as either acute of chronic.[1]

ACUTE LEUKEMIA

In acute myelogenous leukemia (AML) and acute lymphocytic leukemia (ALL), the original acute leukemia cell goes on to form about a trillion more leukemia cells. These cells are described as "nonfunctional"

because they do not work like normal cells. They also crowd out the normal cells in the marrow, which, in turn, causes a decrease in the number of new normal cells made in the marrow. This results in low red cell counts, which creates anemia. The lack of normal white cells impairs the body's ability to fight infections. A shortage of platelets results in bruising and easy bleeding.[2]

CHRONIC LEUKEMIA

In chronic myelogenous leukemia (CML), the leukemia cell that starts the disease makes blood cells in all three cell lines (red cells, white cells, and platelets) that function almost like normal cells. The number of red cells is usually less than normal, resulting in anemia. But many white cells and sometimes many platelets are still made. Even though the white cells are nearly normal in how they work, their counts are high and continue to rise.[3] This can cause serious problems if the patient does not get treatment.

Types of leukemia[6]

There are six types of leukemia, which are usually identified according to their growth speed (acute or chronic) and the cancer cell type (lymphocytic or myelogenous).[2-9]

- Acute lymphocytic leukemia (ALL): This type of leukemia is the most commonly found in children and in adults over the age of 65. Very few cases of ALL are adults age 20 to 65.
- Acute myelogenous leukemia (AML): This type of leukemia almost always affects adults and is rarely seen in children. It is also called acute non-lymphocytic leukemia (ANLL).
- Chronic lymphocytic leukemia (CLL): This leukemia usually affects adults over age 55, and sometimes is found in younger adults, but it almost never affects children.
- Chronic myelogenous leukemia (CML): This leukemia almost always affects adults and is extremely rare in children.
- Hairy cell and acute promyelocytic peukemia (APL): These two forms of leukemia are extremely rare in both adults and children.

If untreated, the white cell count can rise so high that blood flow slows down and anemia becomes severe.[4]

In chronic lymphocytic leukemia (CLL), the leukemia cell that starts the disease makes too many lymphocytes that do not function. These cells replace normal cells in the bone marrow and lymph nodes. They interfere with the work of normal lymphocytes, which weakens the patient's innate immune response. The high number of leukemia cells in the marrow may crowd out normal blood-forming cells and lead to a low red cell count or anemia. A very high number of leukemia cells building up in the marrow also can lead to low neutrophil and platelet counts.[4]

Epidemiology

PREVALENCE AND INCIDENCE
CLL and ALL
CLL is the most prevalent leukemia in Western countries, most often found in older adults but rarely in children, while being more common in males than in females, and in whites more than in blacks. In the United States, more than 8000 new cases are diagnosed annually. This type of leukemia is uncommon in Asia.[5]

ALL is chiefly found in children and young adults. Childhood ALL has also been found to be correlated to higher socioeconomic groups. Children with Down syndrome (Trisomy 21) have an increased risk for ALL and AML. Exposure to high energy radiation in early childhood development has shown to increase the risk of developing T cell ALL.[7] A form of ALL, Burkitt's leukemia also occurs in children, usually in developing countries, and is associated with an EBV infection that has persisted since infancy.[7]

The etiology of ALL in adults is unknown, but it is a common leukemia among middle-aged and geriatric adults. AML is still the most common leukemia in older patients. As an adult, the risk for developing ALL is increased by environmental exposures to industrial and agricultural chemicals, cigarette smoke, and radiation.[8]

AML and CML
The annual incidence of AML in the United States is on average 4 per 100,000 people, with a higher propensity in males than in females (4.4 vs. 3.0).[8] AML incidence increases with age, with only 1.7 people <65 years old and 16.2 in those >65 years old. Notable is a significant increase in occurrence rates during the past 10 years. Heredity can play a part in the etiology of AML as well as exposures to chemicals

(benzenes especially indicated), radiation, and other occupational hazards. Drugs used to treat other cancers have also shown to increase the risk of these patients for developing AML.[9]

People with Down syndrome (trisomy 21), Klinefelter syndromes (XXY and variants), and Patau syndrome (trisomy 13) show an increased incidence of AML. Diseases that are inherited with associated excessive chromatin fragility also have an increased chance of AML occurrence (Fanconi anemia, Bloom syndrome, ataxia telangiectasia, Kostmann syndrome). Interestingly, it was found that those who survived the atomic bombing of Japan during WWII had an increased incidence of myeloid leukemias that peaked 5 to 7 years after the exposure. Chemical exposures linked to benzene (a solvent used in chemical, plastic, rubber, pharmaceuticals) have a direct correlation with an increased incidence of AML. Cigarette smoking and exposure to petroleum products, paint, embalming fluids, ethylene oxide, herbicides, and pesticides have also shown a direct correlation to an increased incidence of AML.[10]

Anticancer Chemotherapeutics
Anticancer chemotherapeutics are the leading cause of treatment associated with AML. Alkylating agents are the largest offending group, and the associated leukemias occur on average 4 to 6 years after exposure, especially in those people with aberrations in chromosome 5 and 7. Topoisomerase II inhibitors have associated leukemias developing from 1 to 3 years after exposure, especially in those people with aberrations on chromosome 11q23. Taking chloramphenicol, phenylbutazone, methoxypsoralen, and chloroquine can result in bone marrow failure and AML.[11]

IMMUNOLOGY AND GENETICS
Burkitt's is the most aggressive lymphoid leukemia, with a phenotype of mature follicle center IgM bearing B cells. Leukemias that bear the immunologic cell surface phenotype of a more primitive cell line (like pre-B ALL, CD10+) are usually less aggressive and more susceptible to a curative therapy than the more mature appearing cells in Burkitt's leukemia.[12]

The stage of differentiation of the malignant cell line does not necessarily reflect the stage at which the genetic mutation gave rise to that malignant cell line. Follicular lymphoma is a case in point. It has the cell surface phenotype of a follicle center cell, but also has the characteristic chromosomal translocation t(14;18), which involves the antiapoptotic bcl-2 gene

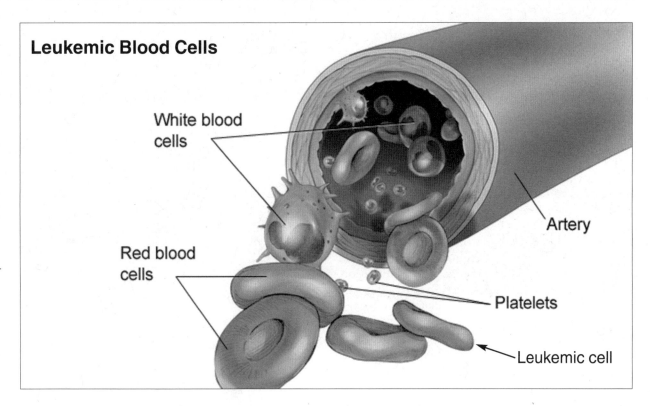

Leukemic Blood Cells

White blood cells

Red blood cells

Artery

Platelets

Leukemic cell

next to the immunoglobulin heavy chain gene. In typical B cell CLL, trisomy 21 mutation conveys a poor prognosis. In ALL (for both adults and children), genetic abnormalities give important prognostic data: Patients with the t(9;22) have a poorer prognostic outlook than patients who do not have this translocation. Other genetic abnormalities that occur frequently in adult ALL are the t(4;11) and the t(8;14).[13]

Statistics have shown that the first mutation is associated with females, younger age groups, and high white cell counts, while the second is associated with males of an older age group with frequent CNS involvement. Both have an associated poor prognosis. In childhood ALL, an associated hyperdiploidy has been shown to give a more favorable prognosis.[14]

Assessment
SIGNS AND SYMPTOMS

Signs and symptoms vary based on the type of leukemia. Each type of leukemia may have other symptoms or signs that prompt a medical examination, but the best advice is to get a complete evaluation if the person has a lasting low grade fever, unexplained weight loss, tiredness, or shortness of breath as persistent symptoms.

AML

AML patients often present with nonspecific symptoms that can begin gradually or abruptly but are usually a consequence of anemia, leukocytosis, leucopenia, thrombocytopenia, frank neutroperia, or another leukocyte dysfunction. Over half of these patients typically have symptoms for more than 3 months before the leukemia is diagnosed. Over half of these presenting complaints are fatigue as the first symptom, with weakness being the most common complaint at the time of diagnosis. Weight loss with associated anorexia is also a common complaint. Fever without a known infection is presented by 10% of patients, and 5% of patients present with abnormal hemostasis, such as easy bruising or bleeding.[15]

Other symptoms that are less frequent are bone pain, lymphadenopathy, nonspecific cough, headache, and diaphoresis (sweating). Very rarely there is a tumor mass located in the soft tissues of the breast, ovary, cranial or spinal dura, bone, lung, gastrointestinal tract, or prostate. This tumor is a mass of leukemic cells called a granulocytic sarcoma or chloroma. This is a rare presentation and is more common in people with the t(8;21) translocations. Fever, hepatosplenomegaly, lymphadenopathy, sternal tenderness, hemorrhage, and systemic infection are often found upon initial diagnosis. GI bleed, intrapulmonary hemorrhage, and intracranial hemorrhage are more often associated with acute promyelocytic leukemia (APL).[16]

Monocytic AML may have associated coagulopathy with extremes degrees of leukocytosis and thrombocytopenia. In AML, retinal hemorrhages are found in 15% of patients, as well as infiltration of the gingivae, skin, sort tissues, or meninges with leukemic blasts at the time of diagnosis (FAB M4 and M5).[17]

Anemia is usually present and can be severe with varying degrees of other hematologic findings, such as splenomegaly. The anemia is usually normochromic normocytic with a decreased erythropoiesis, resulting in a reduced reticulocyte count and a decreased erthrocyte survival due to the accelerated destruction and active blood loss.[18] Between 24% and 40% of patients have counts <5000/L and 20% have counts >100,000/L. Fewer than 5% have no detectable leukemic cells in the blood at all. There may be poor neutrophil function, and the function is usually an impaired phagocytosis with a migration and morphologically abnormal lobulation of the cells with a noted deficient granulation. Platelet counts are <100,000/L and are common in 75% of patients at the time of diagnosis; approximately 25% have counts <25,000/L. Functional and morphological platelet abnormalities can be observed, which include large and bizarre shapes with abnormal granulation and inability of platelets to aggregate or adhere to each other normally.[19]

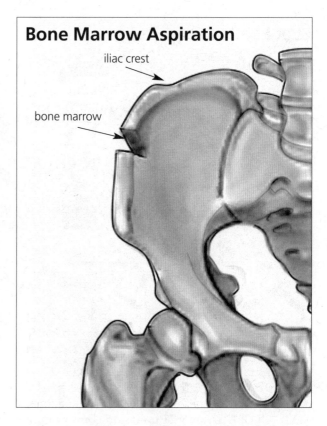

Bone Marrow Aspiration

iliac crest

bone marrow

Acute Leukemia Symptoms[15]

- Tiredness or no energy
- Shortness of breath during physical activity
- Pale skin
- Mild fever or night sweats
- Slow healing of cuts and excess bleeding
- Black-and-blue marks (bruises) for no clear reason
- Pinhead-size red spots under the skin
- Aches in bones or joints (for example, knees, hips or shoulders)
- Low white cell counts, especially monocytes or neutrophils

CLL and CML

People with CLL or CML may not have any symptoms. Some patients learn they have CLL or CML after a blood test as part of a regular checkup. Sometimes a person with CLL may notice enlarged lymph nodes in the neck, armpit, or groin and go to the doctor. The person may feel tired or short of breath (from anemia) or have frequent infections if the CLL is more severe. In these cases, a blood test may show an increase in the lymphocyte count.

CML signs and symptoms tend to develop slowly. People with CML may feel tired and short of breath while doing everyday activities; an enlarged spleen (leading to a "dragging" feeling on the upper left side of the belly), night sweats, weight loss, pallor to the skin, and afternoon fatigue are classic symptoms.[10]

Acute promyelocytic leukemia (APL)

Characteristic of this subtype of acute myeloid leukemia is the presence of multiple cells with Auer rods in their cytoplasm. Auer rods are not present in all patients with acute myelogenous leukemia, but their presence is pathognomonic of leukemia that is myeloid rather than lymphoid. This particular subtype of acute myeloid leukemia is associated with acute disseminated intravascular coagulation.[20]

DIAGNOSIS

CML

CML patients are initially evaluated by a CBC and complete chemistry study, which enables a snapshot of organ functions. This should be followed by a bone marrow biopsy with genetic and immunologic studies, as well as a lumbar puncture. The lumbar puncture is necessary to rule out any CNS involvement. CML prognosis is dependent upon the genetic characteristics of the cancer, the patient's age, white cell counts, major organ function, and overall clinical status.[21]

CLL

CLL patients are also evaluated by a CBC and complete chemistry, as well as a serum protein electrophoresis and bone marrow biopsy. These patients often have imaging studies of the chest and abdomen looking for pathologic lymph nodes (> 2 cm).[22]

PROGNOSIS

Patients with typical B cell CLL can be divided into three major prognostic groups:

1. Those with only blood and bone marrow involvement by leukemia but no lymph node involvement, organomegaly, or signs of bone marrow failure have the best outcomes.
2. Those patients that have lymphadenopathy and organomegaly have intermediate prognosis.
3. Those patients with bone marrow failure (hemoglobin <100g/L or 10g/dl) or with a platelet count of <100k/L have the worst outcome.

It is important to distinguish between the pathogenesis of anemia or thrombocytopenia as the prognosis is adversely affected when either or both are due to a progressive marrow infiltration or loss of productive marrow. If, however, either or both of these conditions are due to an autoimmune disturbance or from hypersplenism (which can develop during the course of the disease), the prognosis is improved as the condition can usually be reversed with treatment of glucocorticoids for the autoimmune disease or splenectomy for the hypersplenism.[23]

Bone Marrow Findings

Bone marrow aspirate smears are now the gold standard for diagnosing leukemias. For a diagnosis of acute or chronic leukemia to be confirmed, it must be classified by an examination of the bone marrow. Replacement of the cellular component of the marrow by immature or undifferentiated cells must exceed 30% of the cellularity for a positive diagnosis (the World Health Organization recommends 20% for a diagnosis of AML).[24]

Anemia and thrombocytopenia

Bone marrow infiltrates are created by clonal proliferation of precursor cells that lead to infiltration of bone marrow by replacing normal hematopoesis, which creates anemia and thrombocytopenia.

- Anemia: normochromic, normocytic: hemoglobin <11.0 g/dL
- Thrombocytopenia: platelets <100,000/uL, prolonged partial thromboplastin and prothrombin times
- Reduced fibrinogen (DIC) is possible, especially

with acute promyleocytic leukemia (APL).
- Thrombocytosis with platelet anisocytosis may be found in CML.[25]

Blood Chemistry Abnormalities

- Possible blood chemistry abnormalities include elevated lactate dehydrogenase (LDH), uric acid, hepatic enzymes, calcium (rare).[26]

Acute Leukemias

- Hallmark: anemia and thrombocytopenia with circulating blasts
- 10% of patients will present without circulating blasts
- Extreme shift to the left of WBCs: metamyelocyts, myelocytes, promyelocytes and blasts[26]

Tumor Lysis Syndrome (Oncological Emergency)

- Elevated LDH, uric acid, phosphorus, potassium, and calcium due to rapid release of intracellular products from malignant cells after cytotoxic therapy
- Important in all rapidly proliferating tumors
- Leukemias, lymphomas, small cell cancers[27]

Chronic Myeloid Leukemia

- Hallmark: greater percent of myelocytes than metamyelocytes
- WBC count at diagnosis usually > 50 x 109/L (range 20-800)
- WBC differential shows virtually all cells of the neutrophilic series (mature neutrophils to myeloblasts)
- Usually find absolute basophilia and eosinophilia[28]

Chronic Lymphocytic Leukemia

- Hallmark: isolated lymphocytosis
- WBC >20,000/uL; 75% to 98% lymphocytes
- CLL lymphocytes: clonal B-cells arrested in B-cell differentiation pathway
- Although mature appearing, these cells are functionally immature
- Prolymphocytes up to 55%
- Decreased percentages of T-cells and NK cells
- Hypogammaglobulinemia is common, especially in advanced stage, and may find polyclonal or less commonly monoclonal increases in gamma globulin
- Cytogenics: useful prognostic indicators[22]

Acute Myeloid Leukemia (SWOG and MRC Studies)[29]

Favorable:

- Inv (16), t(16;16), t(8;21), t(15;17)

- CR 84-91%, 5-year survival 55-65%

Intermediate:

- Normal, +8, +6, -y
- CR 76-86%, 5-year survival 38-41%

Unfavorable:

- Monosomy 5, Monosomy 7
- CR 55-63%, 5-year survival 11% to14%

Chronic Myeloid Leukemia

- Ph chromosome present in almost all CML cells
- Unfavorable: trisomy 8, trisomy 19, isochromosome 17q[30]

Acute Lymphogotic Leukemia

- Favorable: t(12;21), hyperdiploid state
- Unfavorable: t(1;19), t(8;14), t(2;8), t(8;22), t(9;22)[30]

Chronic Lymphoid Leukemia

- Favorable: del13q, 13q14
- Unfavorable: Trisomy 12 associated with advanced stage disease and higher proliferation rate
- del 17p13 associated with disruption of p53, increased incidence Richters transformation, more prolymphocytes, advanced stage, chemoresistance, poor prognosis[30]

Chronic Lymphocytic leukemia

- B cell: CD19, CD20, CD21, CD24; CD11c (variably expressed)
- T cell: CD2, CD5, CD7
- Rituximab: monoclonal antibody directed toward CD20[30]

Histopathology

Note infiltration with small, mature-appearing lymphocytes typical of chronic lymphocytic leukemia. A persistent unexplained lymphocyte count in the peripheral blood of > 5000/mcL establishes the diagnosis of chronic lymphocytic leukemia.[30]

Acute Lymphocytic Leukemia (ALL)

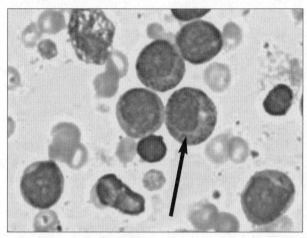

The cells are heterogeneous in size, have round or convoluted nuclei, high nuclear/cytoplasmic ratio, and absence of cytoplasmic granules.

Chronic Lymphocytic Leukemia (CLL)

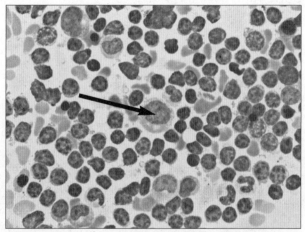

Peripheral white blood cell count is high due to increased numbers of small, well-differentiated, normal-appearing lymphocytes. Leukemia lymphocytes are fragile, and substantial numbers of broken, smudged cells are usually also present on the blood smear.

Acute Myeloid Leukemia (AML)

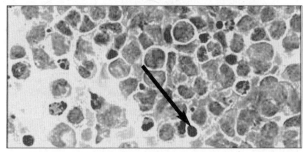

Among the many different types of acute myeloid leukemia, promonocytes have a very characteristic appearance with nuclei that show a delicate folding pattern, almost like a piece of tissue paper that has been crumpled a bit. If you had a case of acute leukemia and most of the cells looked like this, you would think about acute monocytic leukemia – and you would request an NSE to prove it.

Chronic Myclogenous Leukemia (CML)

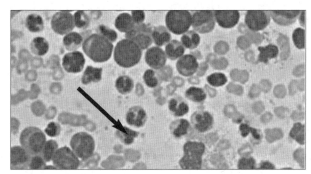

In CML there are few blasts; certainly not 20% or more seen AML. In CML, the tyrosine kinase is permanently in the "on" position, so the cells are dividing and proliferating even when they shouldn't be.

Hairy Cell Leukemia

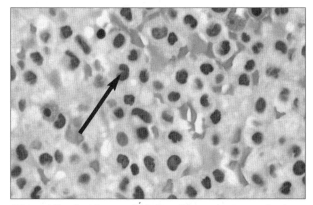

These cells often have a "fried egg" appearance and a loose infiltrating look in the marrow compartment.

CML Diagnosis

The defining diagnostic characteristic for CML is the clonal expansion of a hematopoietic stem cell that possess a reciprocal translocation between chromosomes 9 and 22. This translocation causes a head to tail fusion of the breaking point cluster region gene on chromosome 22q11 and an ABL (the Abelson murine leukemia virus) gene on chromosome 9q34.[21] If left untreated, this disease will rapidly transition from a chronic phase to an accelerated phase and into a blast crisis. The etiology of this disease remains unknown, although there has been recent study and speculation of a viral etiology, due to incidences of CML found higher in spouses of patients with CML. Cigarette smoking has been shown to accelerate a progression of the disease to a blast crisis.[31] Radiation exposure by studying the atomic bomb survivors of WWII shows a delay in the development of CML up to 6 years.[32] There was no increase found in the survivors of the Chernobyl accident, which suggests that only a large dose of radiation induces CML.[34]

Auer Rods

Auer rods are elongated structures seen in malignant cells of the neutrophil lineage. Mostly, they are seen in myeloblasts – but you can see them in any stage of maturation (even in mature neutrophils). They are really just linear groupings of primary granules (therefore, you only see Auer rods in neutrophilic cells – not monocytes, or red cells, or any other type of cell). When you see an Auer rod, you know two things:
1. The population of cells you're looking at is malignant
2. The malignancy is one that involves the neutrophil series.

Staging and Grading

There are several staging systems used in charting the progress of cancer cells depending on the type and subtypes of the leukemia. Some are more specific and precise than others.

Staging Systems for Assessing Leukemia[6]
- FAB (French-American-British)
- Morphologic and Cytochemical
- WHO (World Health Organization)
- Preceptor Cell

FAB Classification[34]

Leukemias are first divided into acute and chronic subtypes with chronic leukemias subdivided into lymphoid or myeloid origins. Acute leukemias of lymphoid cells are further subdivided based on morphologic characteristics by the French-American-British (FAB) group, which has become the standard classification system. This morphology is based on bone marrow aspirate cell smears.

Acute Myeloid Leukemia (AML)
- Hallmark: presence of Auer rods is pathognomonic
- FAB M0: minimally differentiated
- FAB M2: differentiated
- FAB M3 (Acute promyelocytic leukemia): usually associated with t(15;17)
- FAB M4 (Acute myelomonocytic leukemia): includes variant with abnormal eosinophils
- FAB M5 (Acute monoblastic leukemia): associated with poor prognosis features, including extramedullary disease, hyperleukocytosis, 11q23 abnormalities, flt3 mutations, coagulopathy, CNS involvement
- FAB M6 (Acute erythroleukemia)
- FAB M7 (Acute megakaryoblastic leukemia): rare with poor overall survival; may be seen with trisomy 21

Acute Lymphoblastic Leukemia (ALL)
Classified from FAB L1 to L3 as in AML.

Morphologic and Cytochemical Classification
AML can be further categorized into biologically distinct groups based on morphology, cytochemistry, and immunophenotyping of the cells. Cytogenetics and molecular mapping may also aid in distinguishing these groups.[35]

AML is diagnosed by the presence of 20% or more myeloblasts in the blood or bone marrow (WHO classification). Myeloblasts have nuclear chromatin that is uniformly lacelike in appearance and large nucleoli (2 to 5 per cell). Specific cytoplasmic granules called Auer rods are pathoneumonic. Nuclear folding and clefting are usual characteristics of monocytoid cells. A positive myeloperoxidase reaction is found in >3% if the blasts may be the only diagnostic feature that distinguishes AML from ALL.[35]

- M0: Minimally differentiated leukemia
- M1: Myeloblastic leukemia without maturation
- M2: Myeloblastic leukemia with maturation
- M3: Hypergranular promyelocytic leukemia
- M4: Myelomonocytic leukemia
- M4Eo: Variant: Increase in abnormal marrow eosinophils
- M5: Monocytic leukemia

- M6: Erythroleukemia (DiGuglielmo's disease)
- M7: Megakaryoblastic leukemia

World Health Organization Classification
Whereas the FAB classification system looks for the presence of 30% myeloblasts in the marrow, the WHO modified this classification schema by reducing the number of blasts required for diagnosis and incorporating the molecular (including cytogenetic), morphologic (multilineage dysplasia), and clinical features (like a prior hematologic disorder) in defining this disease.[36]

I. AML with recurrent genetic abnormalities
- AML with t(8;21)(q22;q22);AML1(CBF)/ETO
- AML with abnormal bone marrow eosinophils [inv(16)(p13q22) or t(16;16)(p13;q22);CBF/MYH11]
- Acute promyelocytic leukemia [AML with t(15;17)(q22;q12) (PML/RAR and variants]
- AML with 11q23 (MLL) abnormalities

II. AML with multilineage dysplasia
- Following a myelodysplastic syndrome or myelodysplastic syndrome/myeloproliferative disorder
- Without antecedent myelodysplastic syndrome

III. AML and myelodysplastic syndromes, therapy-related
- Alkylating agent–related
- Topoisomerase type II inhibitor–related
- Other types

IV. AML not otherwise categorized
- AML minimally differentiated
- AML without maturation
- AML with maturation
- Acute myelomonocytic leukemia
- Acute monoblastic and monocytic leukemia
- Acute erythroid leukemia
- Acute megakaryoblastic leukemia
- Acute basophilic leukemia
- Acute panmyelosis with myelofibrosis
- Myeloid sarcoma

PRECURSOR B CELL CLASSIFICATIONS
Further classification can be made based on precursor cell characteristics.[37]

Precursor B Cell Neoplasms and Precursor B Cell Lymphoblastic Leukemia/Lymphoma
The most common cancer in childhood is B cell ALL.

Although this can present as a lymphoma, this presentation is rare in both adults and children. The malignant cell in these patients is the precursor B cell. Most patients present with signs of bone marrow failure, infection due to peripheral blood cytopenias, and the physical/clinical symptoms of pallor, fatigue, bleeding, and fever.[38] Peripheral blood smears show counts that reflect anemia and thrombocytopenia, but also may show leucopenia, a normal leukocyte count or leukocytosis, all based on the number of circulating malignant cells. Extranodal sites of the disease are frequently involved and usually manifest as lymphadenopathy, hepatosplenomegaly, CNS disease, testicular enlargement, or cutaneous infiltration.[38]

Diagnosis is made by bone marrow biopsy, which will show infiltration of malignant lymphoblasts. Immunophenotyping shows a pre-B cell malignancy that is characterized by cytogenetic abnormalities, which confirms the diagnosis. Poor prognosis is associated with B cell ALL that has very high white blood cell counts, the presence of CNS involvements, and unfavorable cytogenetic abnormalities. In adults with B cell lymphoblastic leukemia and the $t(9;22)$ translocation, the outlook is poor.[39]

Treatment of precursor B cell leukemias usually involves a remission induction with combination chemotherapy. This includes a high-dose systemic therapy and even intrathecal chemotherapy to eliminate CNS disease, then a period of continual therapy to prevent relapse and possibly effect a cure. The cure rate in children is 85%, while in adults it is only about 50%.[40] This is due to the high proportion of adverse cytogenetic abnormalities seen in adults with this type of leukemia. In a few patients who present with a disease that is confined to the lymph nodes, there has been a statistically high cure rate reported.

Precursor T Cell Malignancies and Precursor T Cell Lymphoblastic Leukemia/Lymphoma

These T cell malignancies can present as either ALL or as an aggressive lymphoma. These leukemias are more common in children and young adults, with an increased frequency in males as compared to females. Precursor T cell ALL will present with bone marrow failure, neutropenia, and thrombocytopenia less often than B cell ALL. Usually these patients have an extremely high WBC, mediastinal mass, lymphadenopathy, and hepatosplenomegaly. Precursor T cell lymphoblastic lymphoma is usually found in young males who present with a large mediastinal mass and pleural effusions. Whether presenting as leukemia or lymphoma, this cancer tends to metasta-

size to the CNS, and CNS involvement is often present at initial evaluation and diagnosis.[41]

Children with precursor T cell ALL seem to benefit the most from intensive remission inductive therapies, and the majority with these consolidation regimens can be cured of their disease. Older children and young adults with precursor T cell lymphoblastic lymphoma are usually treated with leukemia regimens, and if their disease is localized, have an excellent prognosis. The older the patient, the worse the prognosis. Adults with precursor T cell lymphoblastic lymphoma who have high levels of LDH or bone marrow infiltrates or CNS involvement usually are treated with bone marrow transplantation due to their poorer prognosis.[42]

Mature (Peripheral) B Cell Neoplasms and B Cell Chronic Lymphoid Leukemia/Small Lymphocytic Lymphoma

This is the most common type of lymphoid leukemia, and accounts for 7% of non Hodgkin's lymphomas (NHL). This type of cancer can present as either a leukemia or lymphoma. Diagnosis of typical B cell CLL is made when there is an increased number of circulating lymphocytes (>4x 109/L and usually >10x 109/L) with an associated monoclonal B cell displaying the CD5 antigen. Finding bone marrow infiltrate with these cells confirms the diagnosis. The peripheral blood smear will typically show 'smudge' or 'basket' cells, which are nuclear remnants of cell damaged by the physical stress of making the blood smear.[43]

Cytogenetic studies reveal trisomy 12 found in 25% to 30% of patients, as well as some abnormalities found on chromosome 13. If the physical/clinical presentation includes lymphadenopathy and a lymph node biopsy is done, a hemopathology can make a definitive diagnosis of this leukemia based on morphology and immunophenotyping. From 70% to 75% of these patients will also have bone marrow involvement and positive monoclonal B lymphocytes found in the circulating cells. For this reason, typical B cell CLL is often found incidentally with CBC, but physical complaints often accompany this, including fatigue, frequent infections, and new lymphadenopathy. If a patient presents with autoimmune hemolytic anemia or autoimmune thrombocytopenia, this diagnosis should be considered. B cell CLL has also been associated with red cell aplasia.[44]

B Cell Lymphoid Malignancies and B Cell Prolymphocytic Leukemia

This leukemia shows blood and bone marrow infiltrations by large lymphocytes with prominent nucleoli.

These patients have high white blood cell counts, splenomegaly with minimal lymphadenopathy. Prognosis is poor for these patients with chances of complete response to treatment rare.[43]

B Cell Lymphoid Malignancies and Hairy Cell Leukemia

This is also a rare disease usually found in older males with a typical presentation of pancytopenia and splenomegaly. These malignant cells have a 'hairy' appearance due to projections on light and electron microscopy, while showing a characteristic staining pattern with tartrate-resistant acid phosphatase. Usually bone marrow cannot be aspirated and a biopsy will show a pattern of fibrosis with diffuse infiltration by the malignant cells. These patients are prone to immunodeficiency types of infective events, like *Mycobacterium avium intracellulare* (MAC) and vasculitis. This leukemia is responsive to chemotherapy with interferon, pentostatin, or cladribine, which is the preferred treatment. Complete clinical remissions have occurred with this chemotherapy, and the majority of these patients can have long-term disease-free survival.[45]

Conventional Treatments for Leukemias

Treatment for patients without any manifestations of the disease other than bone marrow involvement and lymphocytosis can take a watchful waiting approach. These patients have an average survival rate of >10 years without any therapy ever required. If the patient has an adequate number of normal circulating cells, is asymptomatic but considered to be in an intermediate stage due to lymphadenopathy or hepatosplenomegaly, the watchful waiting approach may still be taken. The average survival rate is approximately 7 years and most usually will require some treatment in the first few years of follow up.[47]

GLUCOCORTICOID THERAPY

Patients who present with bone marrow failure will require immediate therapy. The average survival rate is only 1.5 years. Immuno-specific presentations of B cell CLL should be managed without antileukemia drugs to start. Glucocorticoid therapy for autoimmune cytopenias or globulin replacement therapy for hypogammaglobulinemia anemia should be administered first regardless of an antileukemia therapy. Patients who present primarily as a lymphoma with a low IPI score have an average 5-year survival rate of 75%, but those with a high IPI score have an average 5-year survival rate of <40% and usually are more likely to need early interventional therapy.[47]

CHEMOTHERAPY
Chlorambucil, Fludarabine, and Alemtuzimab

The most common treatment is single agent chemotherapy, such as chlorambucil or fludarabine, which may be administered in combination. Chlorambucil can be administered orally and has fewer side effects than fludarabine, which is administered through IV and causes immunosuppression.[48] However, fludarabine has more biological activity against this cancer and is the only drug associated with a significant incidence of complete remission. For this reason in younger aged patients, this is the treatment of choice. It can also be used as a second line interventional chemotherapeutic for those patients whose cancer was unresponsive to chlorambucil. Chlorambucil is usually the chemotherapy of choice in the elder population with this cancer. Many of the patients who present with lymphoma will receive the combination chemotherapy used in lymphoma (CVP and CHOP).[50]

Alemtuzimab (anti-CD52) is another therapeutic strategy, but it kills both B and T cells and therefore has more immunocompromise than rituximab. In younger patients with this cancer, bone marrow transplantation may be used. Allogeneic bone marrow transplantation can be curative, but it is also associated with more treatment related mortality, and therefore is discouraged.[51]

TREATING AML

Once a diagnosis of AML is confirmed, progression toward rapid treatment with a complete evaluation should ensue. Beyond clarifying the subtype of leukemia, an initial evaluation of the major organ systems function should include the cardiovascular, pulmonary, renal, and hepatic systems. All prognostic factors should be assessed before initiating treatment, and leukemic cells should be obtained pretreatment and cryopreserved for future use as new tests and ther-

Hyperuricemia

About 50% of AML patients present with mild to moderate elevation of uric acid, with only 10 % showing marked elevations. Chemotherapy may worsen hyperuricemia, especially with the side effects of nausea and vomiting leading to increased dehydration. Patients are usually started on corrective and kidney sparing drug therapies like allopurinol or recombinant uric oxidase (rasburicase) but hydration alone can be key. If there are high concentrations of lysozyme (a marker for monocytic differentiation) may indicate renal tubular dysfunction which again can be aggravated by chemotherapy.[52]

New Chemotherapies
SELECTED NEW AGENTS UNDER STUDY FOR TREATMENT OF ADULTS WITH AML[54]

Class of Drugs	Example Agent(s)
MDR1 modulator	Cyclosporine analogues, PSC-833
Demethylating agent	Decitabine, 5-azacytidine
Histone deacetylase inhibitor	Depsipeptide, suberoylanilide hydroxamic acid (SAHA), MS275, Valproic Acid
Heavy metals	Arsenic trioxide, antimony
Farnesyl transferase inhibitors	R115777, SCH66336
FLT3 inhibitors	SU11248, PKC412, MLN518
HSP-90 antagonists	17-Allylaminogeldanamycin (17-AAG)
BCR/ABL PDGFR/c-kit inhibitor	Imatinib (ST1571, Gleevec)
Protein kinase C inhibitor	Bryostatin, UCN-01, CGP41251
Cell cycle inhibitor	Flavopiridol
Humanized antibodies	-chain, HLA-DR)
Toxin-conjugated antibodies	Gemtuzumab ozogamicin (Mylotarg)
Radiolabeled antibodies	Yttrium-90-labeled human M195
Cytokines	Recombinant human interleukin (IL) 2 and IL-12
Anticytokines	Antivascular endothelial growth factor (Avastin)

apeutics are made available. Patients with AML should also be initially evaluated for infections.[46]

Possible Transfusion
Most AML patients present with anemia and/or thrombocytopenia, and if replacement of blood components is required, it should begin immediately. Platelet transfusion is justifiable and necessary if the qualitative platelet dysfunction (or the presence of an infection) can increase the chances of hemorrhage, even if the platelet count is only moderately decreased.[53]

Induction and Remission
The treatment of a newly diagnosed patient with AML is divided into two phases, the induction and postremission phases. The goal is to induce complete remission, and once that is obtained, to use therapies to prolong survival and possibly achieve cure. The first phase of

intensified therapy will use traditional chemotherapies, such as cytarabine and anthracyclines, in patients under the age of 60. This second phase is considered a consolidation period and the therapies chosen are often based on the patient's age. In older patients intensive therapy may be deferred and consolidation therapies are more actively pursued.[55]

Induction chemotherapy for patients other than those with APL usually consists of combination chemotherapy with cytarabine (cytosine arabinoside) and an anthracycline. Cytarabine is a cell cycle S-phase specific antimetabolite that becomes phosphorylated intracellularly to an active triphosphate form that interferes with DNA synthesis. Anthracyclines are DNA intercalators with their primary action as an inhibitor of topoisomerase II, which leads to DNA breaks. Anthracycline therapy usually is daunorubicin IV on days 1 to 3; and idarubicin for 3 days in conjunction with cytarabine giving a continuous 7- day infusion cycle. The addition of etoposide may improve the duration of a remission.[56]

After induction therapy, the bone marrow is examined to see if the leukemia has been eradicated. If >5% blasts exist with 20% cellularity, the treatment regimen proceeds to a retreatment with cytarabine and an anthracycline similar to induction therapy, but for 5 and 2 days. After two inductions if a patient fails to achieve remission, the procedure is to undergo an allogeneic stem cell transplant, if a donor that matches exists. This is usually only used for patients under the age of 70.[56]

About 65% to 75% of adults with AML will achieve complete remission with induction therapy. Two thirds of these achieve remission after a single course of the therapy, while the remaining one third requires two courses. About 50% of AML patients who do not achieve remission after two courses have a drug resistant form of leukemia, and 50% do not achieve remission because of fatalities from complications with bone marrow aplasia or impaired recovery of normal stem cells. As the age of the patients increase, a higher induction treatment related mortality rate is seen, as well as an increase in resistant leukemia disease.[56]

Postremission
Once remission has been achieved, a postremission therapy is given to achieve cure. These options include standard chemotherapy, and autologous and allogeneic bone marrow transplants. Once again, based on the patient's age and clinical status, the optimal treatment strategy is chosen. APL is usually treated with chemotherapy plus retinoic acid with 70% to 80% of patients remaining in long-term remission. Arsenic trioxide has been used in relapse diseases and is currently under investigation for primary therapy.[57]

Cure rates for patients with an average risk associated with their AML disease are 35% to 40% for chemotherapy, 50% for autologous transplantation, and 50% to 60% for allogeneic transplantation. Some types of AML with better cytogenetic factors have an improved prognosis, with 40% to 60% cure rate with chemotherapy and 70% with autologous transplantation (2-9). The prognosis is favorable for adults with AML under the age of 60 with 70% to 80% achieving complete remission. In those patients who undergo postremission chemotherapy in high doses, there is a cure rate of 35-40% with high dose cytarabine shown to be the best therapeutic choice.[57]

In younger adults, allogenic bone marrow transplantation is curative in 50-60% of the cases. In older

adults who can withstand the treatment, autologous bone marrow transplantation may be superior to chemotherapy with 50% cure rates. The cure rates for older patients are generally very low (10% to 15%) even when they are able to achieve remission and receive postremission chemotherapy.[57]

TREATING CML
Once a patient is diagnosed with CML, treatment is usually initiated immediately using Gleevac (imatinib mesylate), and while this does not cure CML, it does keep it under control for many patients as long as they continue its use. In other patients, Sprycel (dasatinib) and Tasigna (nilotinib) block the *BCR-ABL* cancer gene and are used for CML patients who are resistant or intolerant to prior therapies, including Gleevac. These drugs are taken orally.[58]

Stem Cell Transplantation
The only treatment that is considered curative is allogeneic stem cell transplantation. This treatment is most successful in patients of a younger age, and those with a matched donor may have success up to the age of 60.[59]

Naturopathic Approaches to Treating Leukemias
Naturopathic protocols for treating leukemias are similar to therapeutic strategies for managing lymphomas. The chronic anemia associated with leukemias may be improved with integrative naturopathic strategies to support the red blood cell formation and capacity to carry oxygen and iron. Melatonin should not to be used in any of the lymphomas, leukemias or myelogenous cancers because it could affect the cellular differentiation and make matters worse, immunological speaking.

Naturopathic Therapeutic Protocol
1. Manage anemia
2. Avoid immune modulating therapies, specifically melatonin
3. Stop metastasis: Herbs, nutraceuticals
4. Counsel patients
5. Manage conventional therapy side effects

---

1. MANAGE ANEMIA
Amino Acid Chelate
Using an amino acid chelate form of iron (glycinate, succinate, gluconate) with added vitamin B-6 and B-12 will allow some relief from the anemia by increasing

absorption of the iron and therefore decreasing the amount needed to be taken. This can be recommended in doses of 100-150 mg in divided daily doses with food.

2. AVOID IMMUNE MODULATING THERAPIES, SPECIFICALLY MELATONIN
Melatonin

As a standard of naturopathic care, immune modulating therapies, such as melatonin, should be considered contraindicated for hematological malignancies. In one study, there was a significant increase in growth of myeloma cells when melatonin was administered.[60,61] The investigators were looking for the effect of melatonin on the proliferation of normal lymphocytes and certain T-lymphomas and myelomas under *in-vitro* conditions. In human and mouse lymphocytes and T-lymphoblastoid cell lines, melatonin significantly inhibited the incorporation of [3H] thymidine, but the influence of melatonin on myeloma cells provoked an increase in cell proliferation. The data demonstrates a chief pineal indole affect selectively in the processes of lymphoblastoid cell growth.[60]

In the second study, there was a significant elevation in melatonin upon serum analysis. It was postulated by the research team that "the patients with multiple myeloma showed significantly higher mean melatonin serum levels than healthy subjects (21.6 +/- 13.5 versus 12.1 +/- 4.8 pg/ml; $p < 0.001$). This behavior could actually represent a phenomenon secondary to an altered endocrine-metabolic balance caused by an increased demand of the developing tumor. On the other hand, the increased melatonin secretion might be considered as a compensatory mechanism due to its antimitotic action and therefore as an effort to secrete substances capable of regulating neoplastic growth."[61]

However, several studies have indicated that melatonin may help some leukemias, and their side effects of lymphocytopenia and thrombocytopenia. In a study looking at conventional chemotherapy side effects on normal blood cell production caused by toxicity, FDA approved drugs such as Nuepogen, a granulocyte colony stimulating factor (G-CSF), and Leukine, a granulocyte macrophage colony stimulating factor (GM-CSF), affected these conventional side effects. A combination of low dose interleukin 2 (IL2) decreased chemotherapy-induced lymphocytopenia with a decreased number of lymphocytes in the peripheral circulation noted in the cancer patients.[62]

For patients with bloodborne cancers, an IL-2/melatonin combination is also promising. Twelve patients (nonresponsive to standard therapies) evaluated the efficacy and tolerability of a combination of low-dose IL-2 plus melatonin in advanced malignancies of the blood, including non-Hodgkin's lymphoma, Hodgkin's disease, acute myelogenous leukemia, multiple myeloma, and chronic myelomonocytic leukemia. IL-2 was given 6 days a week for 4 weeks, along with oral melatonin (20 mg a day). Cancer was stabilized and the melatonin/IL-2 therapy was well-tolerated.[62]

Several *in-vivo* and *in-vitro* studies have shown how T-helper-2 lymphocytes are a peripheral target of melatonin,[63] and how hematopoietic rescue via T-cell-dependent, endogenous granulocyte-macrophage colony-stimulating factor was induced by melatonin.[64]

Mycomedicinals have shown promise in the treatment of blood borne cancers and their side effects. However, Reishi has been found to stimulate B lymphocytes, so therefore should be contraindicated for long-term supplementation.[65]

3. STOP METASTASIS
Curcumin

This flavonoid, found in tumeric, shows promise in stopping the spread of bone marrow cancer. A study published by researchers at the University of Texas Anderson Cancer Center discovered that curcumin can stop the activation process that leads to the spread of myeloma cell lines by the down-regulation of the activation of nuclear factor-kappa B and IKappa Balpha kinase.[66] Curcumin also turns on apoptosis in cancer cells. These two functions make curcumin a

Chemotherapeutic and Naturopathic Integrated Therapies

Chemotherapeutic	Naturopathic	Daily Dose	Caution
AML combination induction therapy in preparation for allogeneic stem cell transplant: Cytosine arabinoside (cytarabine)	*To increase effectiveness:* Amino acid chelate forms of iron (glycinate, succinate, gluconate) with added vitamin B-6 and methylated B-12 and added glandular liver fractions[104]	100-200 mg in divided daily doses with food	
Anthracyclines (danorubicin, idarubicin) Etoposide	*To reduce toxicity:* Mycomedicinals, esp. Trametes (turkey tails) specifically indicated for leukemias[105]		
AML post remission therapy: Retinoic acid Arsenic trioxide and antimony are under investigation for relapse disease	*To increase effectiveness:* Curcumin also specifically indicated for leukemias[106] Meriva (see page 68 for protocol)[107] Green tea specifically indicated for leukemias[108] *To reduce toxicity and side effects* See page 68 (Integrated Premedications) for protocols for managing: Mucositis Nausea Vomiting Diarrhea[109] Glutamine	500-1000 mg qd-tid 5-10 cups qd 10 gm tid, swish & swallow	
CML: Imatnib mesylate (gleevac) Dasatinib (sprycel) Nilotinb (tasigna) Allogeneic stem cell transplant[110]			

Note: Chemotherapies used in induction therapy are also used in post remission therapy as well as allogenic and autologous bone marrow transplants promising long-term supplement for fighting these blood/bone marrow cancers.

Herbal Extracts

Tumeric and 32 other medicinal herbals were investigated for their cancer inhibition by researchers at the School of Pharmacy of Howard University. These studies spanned several years and 36 extracts of the 32 herbs were evaluated as anticancer agents. The herbs included *Ginkgo biloba, Cimicifuga racemosa, Echinacea spp., Piper methysticum, Serenoa repens, Glycyrrhiza glabra, Dioscorea spp., Passiflora incarnate, Tanecetum, Vaccinium spp., Vitex agnus-castus, Urtica spp., Valeriana* and *Humulus.* The researchers then took cells infected with Epstein-Barr virus early antigen (EBV-EA) and exposed these cells to a tumor promoter. Tumeric was found to be the most potent anti-EBV-EA agent, 10x more so than passionflower, which was the next highest in activity. Several of the medicinal herbals inhibited the EBV-EA in cells exposed to the tumor promoter by more than 90%." We report for the first time the activities of 16 new medicinal plants as potential cancer chemopreventive agents," the researchers wrote. "Our results indicate new and potential applications of these herbal remedies as cancer chemopreventive agents since they are already in clinical use in the human population."[67]

References

1. Guyton AC, Hall JC. Textbook of Medical Physiology. 10th ed. St Louis, MO: WB Saunders Co.;2000.

2. Moore, KL, AF Dalley, and AMR Aqur. Clinically Oriented Anatomy. 6th ed. Baltimore, MD: Lippincott Williams & Wilkins;2009.

3. Young, RC. Harrison's Internal Medicine, online. Chapter 89, Pancreatic Cancer, Yu Jo Chua, David Cunnignham.

4. McPhee SJ, Papadakis M. Eds. Gonzales R, Zeiger R. Online Eds. 2009. CURRENT Medical Diagnosis & Treatment. 8th ed.

5. www.medcinenet.com

6. American Joint Committee on Cancer (AJCC). AJCC Cancer Staging Manual. 6th ed. New York, NY: Springer-New York, www.springeronline.com

7. http://www.cancer.org

8. http://www.cdc.gov

9. www.ricancercouncil.org

10. http://www.cancer.net/patient/Cancer+Types/Leukemia +-+Acute+Myeloid+-+AML/ci.Leukemia+-+Acute+Myeloid+-+AML.printer Oncologist-approved cancer information from the American Society of Clinical Oncology; 2012.

11. Praga C, Bergh J, Bliss J, et al. Risk of acute myeloid leukemia and myelodysplastic syndrome in trial of adjuvant epirubicin for early breast cancer: correlation with doses of Epirubicin and Cyclophosphamide. Am Soc Clin Onoc. 2005;23(18):4179-91.

12. www.cancer.gov/dictionary?cdrid=256548

13. Doubek M, et al. Acute myeloid leukemias with recurrent genetic abnormalities: frequent assessment of minimal residual disease and treatment of molecular relapse with chemotherapy. Leukemia. 2005;19:885-88.

14. http://www.cancer.gov/newscenter/pressreleases/2009/ alltarget Gene Abnormality Found To Predict Childhood Leukemia Relapse. 2009.

15. http://www.cancer.org/Cancer/Leukemia-Acute-MyeloidAML/DetailedGuide/leukemia-acute-myeloid-myelogenous-diagnosed. 2012

16. Biswas S, Chakrabarti S, Chakraborty J, et al.Childhood acute leukemia in West Bengal, India with an emphasis on uncommon clinical features. Asian Pacific J Cancer Prev. 2009;10:903-06.

17. Tallman MS, Haesook TK, Paietta E, et al. Acute monocytic leukemia (French-American-British classification M5) does not have a worse prognosis than other subtypes of acute myeloid leukemia: a report from the Eastern Cooperative Oncology Group. JCO. 2004;22(7):1276-86.

18. Brody JI, Finch SC. Serum factors of acquired hemolytic anemia in leukemia and lymphoma. J Clin Invest. 1961;40(2):181-87.

19. http://www.harrisonspractice.com/practice/ub/view/ Harrisons%20Practice/141173/all/Acute_Myeloid_Leukemia

20. http://www.cancer.gov/cancertopics/pdq/treatment/ childAML/HealthProfessional/page7. 2012.

21. http://www.cancer.org/Cancer/Leukemia-Chronic MyeloidCML/DetailedGuide/leukemia-chronic-myeloid-myelogenous-diagnosis. 2011.

22. http://www.cancer.org/Cancer/Leukemia-Chronic LymphocyticCLL/DetailedGuide/leukemia-chronic-lymphocytic-diagnosis. 2011.

23. Kalil N, Cheson BD. Chronic lymphocytic leukemia. The Oncologist 1999;4(5):352-69.

24. http://www.nlm.nih.gov/medlineplus/ency/article/ 003934.htm 2012

25. Troup SB, Swisher SN, Young LE. The anemia of leukemia. The Am J Med 1960;28(5):751-63.

26. Seiter K, Besa EC, et al. Acute myelogenous leukemia workup. Drugs, disease & procedures. 2012. Emedicine.medscape.com/article/197802-workup

27. Howard SC, Jones DP, Pui CH. The tumor lysis syndrome. N Engl J Med. 2011;364:1844-54.

28. Faderl S, Talpaz M, Estrov Z, et al. The biology of chronic myeloid leukemia. N Engl J Med. 1999;341:164.

29. Slovac ML, Kopecky KJ, Cassileth PA, et al. Karyothypic analysis predicts outcome of preremission and postremission therapy in adult acute myeloid leukemia: a Southwest Oncology Group/Eastern Cooperative Oncology Group study. Blood. 2000;96(13):4075-83.

30. Slovak ML, Kopecky KJ, Wolman SR, et al. Cytogenetic correlation with disease status and treatment outcome in advanced stage leukemia post bone marrow transplantation: a Southwest Oncology Group study (SWOG-8612). Leuk Res. 1995;19(6):381-88.

31. Herr R, Ferguson J, Myers N, Rovira D, Robinson WA. Cigarette smoking, blast crisis, and survival in chronic myeloid leukemia. Am J Hematol 1990;34(1):1-4.

32. Ichimaru M, Ichimaru T, Mikami M, et al. Incidence of leukemia in a fixed cohort of A-bomb survivors and controls. Hiroshima and Nagasaki Oct. 1950-Dec. 1978 RERF tech report 1981:13-81.

33. Hatch M, Ron E, Bouville A, et al. The Chernobyl disaster: Cancer following the accident at the Chernobyl nuclear power plant. Epid Rev. 2005;27(1):56-66.

34. Aul C, Giagounidis A, Germing U. Bone marrow morphology and classification systems in a myelodysplatic syndromes. Cancer Treat Rev. 2007;33(1):S2-S5.

35. Liso V, Bennett J. Morphological and cytochemical characteristics of leukaemic promyelocytes. Best Practic & Res Clin Haematology. 2003;16(3):349-55.

36. http://www.who.int/classifications/atcddd/en/ . 2012.

37. http://www.uptodate.com/contents/clinical-manifestations-pathologic-features-and-diagnosis-of-precursor-b-cell-acute-lymphoblastic-leukemia-lymphoma. 2012.

38. http://www.cancer.net/patient/Cancer+Types/Leukemia+-+B-Cell?sectionTitle=Symptoms%20and%20Signs .2012.

39. Lazarus HM, Richards SM, Chopra R, et al. Central nervous system involvement in adult acute lymphoblastic leukemia at diagnosis: results from the international ALL trial MRC UKALL XII/ECOG E2993. Blood 2006;108(2):465-72.

40. Stock, W. Adolescents and young adults with acute lymphoblastic leukemia. Hematology. 2012;1:21-29.

41. t cell malignancies and t cell lyphoblastic leukemia/lymphoma. T cell acute lymphoblastic leukemia(T-ALL), FISH clinical information. Mayo Clinic Interpretive Handbook. 2012.

42. http://emedicine.medscape.com/article/203556-overview Tuscano M, Besa EC. Lymphoblastic Lymphoma. Drugs, Diseases &Procedures. 2011.

43. Nelson BP, Variakojis D, Peterson LC. Leukemic Phas of B-Cell Lymphomas mimicking chronic lymphocytic leukemia and variants at presentation. Mol Path. 2002;15(11):1111-20.

44. Juliusson G, Gahrton G. 5 Cytogenetics in CLL and related disorders. Baillierre's Clin Haematology. 1993;6(4):821-48.

45. http://www.ncbi.nlm.nih.gov/pubmedhealth/PMH0001618/ Hairy cell leukemia. ADAM Medical Encyclopedia PubMed Health. 2010.

46. Stalfelt AM, Brodin H. Costs over time in conventional treatment of acute myeloid leukaemia. A study exploring changes in treatment strategies over two decades. J Intern Med. 1994;236(4):401-09.

47. Hodgson K, Ferrer G, Montserrat E, Moreno C. Chronic lymphocytic leukemia and autoimmunity: a systemic review. Haematologica. 2011;96(5):752-61.

48. http://www.webmd.com/cancer/tc/leukemia-treatment-overview Leukemia treatment overview. 2011.

49. Jackson GH. Use of fludarabine in the treatment of acute myeloid leukemia. Hematol J. 2004;5 suppl 1:S62-7.

50. Rai KR, Peterson BL, Appelbaum FR, et al. Fludarabine compared with chlorambucil as primary therapy for chronic lymphocytic leukemia. New Eng J Med. 2000;343(24):1750-57.

51. Lundin J, Kimby E, Bjorkholm M, et al. Phase II trial of subcutaneous anti-CD52 monoclonal antibody alemtuzumab (Campath-1H)as first line treatment for patients with B-cell chronic lymphocytic leukemia (B-CLL). Blood 2002;100(3):768-73.

52. Krakoff IH. Use of allopurinol in preventing hyperuricemia in leukemia and lymhoma. Cancer 1966 (online 2006);19(11):1496-98.

53. Dawson MA, Avery S, McQuilten ZK, et al. Blood transfusion requirements for patients undergoing chemotherapy for acute myeloid leukemia how much is enough? Haematol. 2007;92(7):996-97.

54. http://www.cancer.gov/cancertopics/pdq/treatment/adultAML/Patient/page3 National Cancer Institute: Adult Acute Myeloid Leukemia treatment overview. 2012.

55. Rowe JM. Optimal induction and post remission therapy for AML in first remission. Hematol Am Soc Hematol Educ Program. 2009:396-405.

56. http://emedicine.medscape.com/article/2005126-overview Kotiah SD. Acute Promyelocytic Leukemia Treatment Protocols. Drugs, Diseases & Procedures. 2012.

57. Ghavamzadeh A, Alimoghaddam K, Ghaffari SH. Treatment of acute promyelocytic leukemia with aresenic trioxide without ATRA and/or chemotherapy. Ann Onco. 2005;17(1):131-34.

58. Kantarjian HM, Hochhaus A, Saqlio G, et al. Nilotinib versus imatinib for the treatment of patients with newly diagnosed chronic phase, Philadelphia chromosom-positive chronic myeloid leukaemia: 24 month minimum follow up of the phase 3 randomised ENESTnd trail. Lancet Onco. 2011;12(9):841-51.

59. Stamatovic D, Balint B, Tukic L, et al. Allogenic stem cell transplant for chronic myeloid leukemia as a still promising option in the era of the new target therapy. Vojnosanit Preql. 2012;69(1):37-42

60. Persengiev SP, Kyurkchiev S. Selective effect of melatonin on the proliferation of lymphoid cells. Int J Biochem. 1993 Mar;25(3):441-44.

61. Tarquini R, Perfetto F, Zoccolante A, Salti F, Piluso A, De Leonardis V, Lombardi V, Guidi G, Tarquini B. Serum melatonin in multiple myeloma: natural brake or epiphenomenon? Anticancer Res. 1995 Nov-Dec;15(6B):2633-37.

62. http://www.worldhealth.net/news/melatonin/Melatonin Posted on 2008-03-19 09:14:53 in Hormones & Pharmacological Agents

63. http://www.ncbi.nlm.nih.gov/entrez/query.fcgi?cmd= Retrieve&db=pubmed&dopt=Abstract&list_uids=7629695 T-helper-2 lymphocytes as a peripheral target of melatonin. JPinealRes.1995Mar;18(2):84-89.

64. http://www.ncbi.nlm.nih.gov/entrez/query.fcgi?cmd= Retrieve&db=pubmed&dopt=Abstract&list_uids=8162592 Hematopoietic rescue via T-cell-dependent, endogenous granulocyte-macrophage colony-stimulating factor induced by the pineal neurohormone melatonin in tumor-bearing mice. Cancer Res. 1994 May 1;54(9):2429-32.

65.Zhang J, Tang Q, Zimmerman-Kordmann M, Reutter W, Fan H. Activation of B lymphocytes by GLIS, a bioactive proteoglycan from Ganoderma lucidum Life Sci. 2002 Jun 28;71(6):623-38.

66. Bharti AC, Donato N, Singh S, Aggarwal BB. Curcumin (diferuloylmethane) down-regulates the constitutive activation of nuclear factor-kappa B and Ikappa Balpha kinase in human multiple myeloma cells, leading to suppression of proliferation and induction of apoptosis. Blood. 2003 Feb 1;101(3):1053-62.

67. Kapadia GJ, Azuine MA, Tokuda H, Hang E, Mukainaka T, Nishino H, Sridhar R. Inhibitory effect of herbal remedies on 12-o-tetradecanoylphorbol-13-acetate-promoted Epstein–Barr virus early antigen activation. Pharmacol Res. 2002 Mar;45(3):213-220.

Pathophysiology

Lung cancer is a disease of uncontrolled cell growth in tissues of the lung. This growth may lead to metastasis, which is the invasion of adjacent tissue and infiltration beyond the lungs. The majority of primary lung cancers are carcinomas of the lung, derived from epithelial cells.

The human body is capable of living without food for several weeks, without water for a few days, but only a few minutes without oxygen. Every cell in the body is dependent on oxygen to be in constant supply in order to produce energy, grow, repair, and replicate itself while maintaining its own vital functions for life. That oxygen provided to the cell must be brought into the body, cleaned, cooled, heated, and humidified and then delivered in the right amounts dependent on the type of cell. This is the normal function of the pulmonary system.

The physiology of the system includes the diaphragm and chest muscles, nose and mouth, pharynx and trachea, and the bronchial tree that leads to the lungs, each with several lobes. The lungs give the bloodstream oxygen that is then taken throughout the rest of the body. Each cell exchanges oxygen with carbon dioxide as metabolic waste, which is returned to the lungs and expelled.

The bloodstream, the heart, and the brain are all involved in making this mechanism work. The heart creates the pumping force that moves the blood at a precise speed and pressure throughout the entire body including the brain. The brain directs all of the systems synchronistic smooth muscles function via the autonomic nervous system.

This system is susceptible to damage caused by inhaling toxic materials or irritants that can affect the large pulmonary surface area and thus affect the body's oxygen supply, while also denaturing cells and turning on inflammation. This system is so intricately laced with the cardiovascular system that pulmonary disease can also cause heart disease; in fact, disease in any one of its linked parts can lead to disease or damage to other vital organ systems.[1-2]

A person at rest breathes about 6 liters of air a minute. Heavy exercise can increase the amount to over 75 liters per minute. During an 8-hour work day of moderate activity, the amount of air breathed may be as much as 8.5 m^3 (300 cubic feet). The skin, with its surface area of approximately 1.9 m^2 (20 sq. ft.) is commonly thought to have the greatest exposure to air of any body part. However, in reality the lungs have the greatest exposure, with a surface area exposed to air of 28 m^2 (300 sq. ft.) at rest and up to 93 m^2 (1,000 sq. ft.) during a deep breath.[1-2]

NON-SMALL AND SMALL LUNG CANCER

We tend to categorize lung cancer by the size of the cell: Non-small cell lung cancer (NSCLC) and small cell lung cancer (SCLC). In turn, NSCLC is broken down into four different categories by type of cell growth: squamous or epidermoid, adenocarcinoma, large cell, and undifferentiated. SCLC is also known as oat cell carcinoma by the microscopic resemblance of the small cell to a grain of oats.[3]

Non-Small Cell Lung Cancer

Non-small cell carcinomas are the most common lung cancers. NSCLC is the most common type of lung cancer, with approximately 150,000 new cases reported in the USA in 2004.[3,4] The majority of NSCLC develops in former or current cigarette smokers with an overall 5-year survival rate at 15%, which is unchanged in the last two decades.[4]

NSCLC: Squamous Cell Carcinoma

Squamous cell carcinoma commonly starts in the bronchi and may not spread as rapidly as other lung cancers.[5]

NSCLC: Adenocarcinoma

Adenocarcinoma usually develops on the outer boundaries of the lungs and is more commonly found in women than in men.[6]

Histopathology

There are three main sub-types of lung cancer: adenocarcinoma, squamous cell lung carcinoma, and large cell lung carcinoma. Nearly 40% of lung cancers are adenocarcinoma. This type of cancer usually originates in peripheral lung tissue. Most cases of adenocarcinoma are associated with smoking; however, among people who have smoked fewer than 100 cigarettes in their lifetimes ("never-smokers"), adenocarcinoma is the most common form of lung cancer. A subtype of adenocarcinoma, the bronchioloalveolar carcinoma, is more common in female never-smokers, and may have different responses to treatment.

Squamous Cell Carcinoma

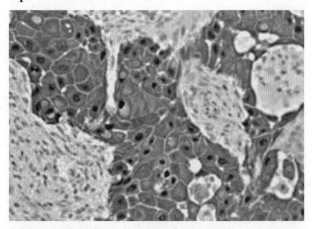

Adenocarcinoma

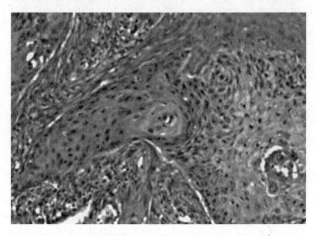

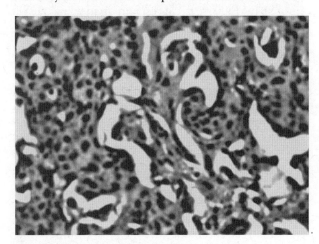

Non-small Cell Carcinoma

Anatomy of the Lungs

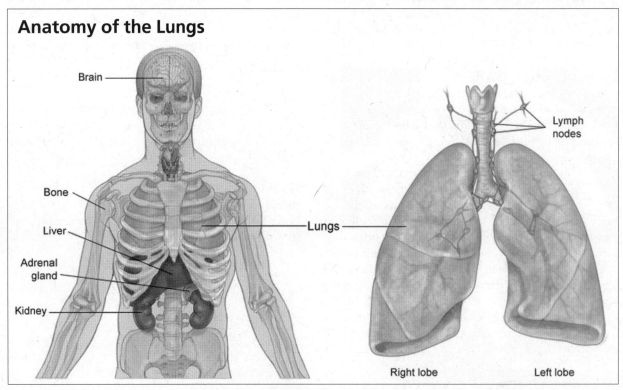

Brain

Bone

Liver

Adrenal gland

Kidney

Lungs

Lymph nodes

Right lobe   Left lobe

Epidemiology
PREVALENCE AND INCIDENCE

Lung cancer, the most common cause of cancer-related death in men and women, is responsible for 1.3 million deaths worldwide annually.[7-8] Lung cancer is the leading cause of cancer deaths, with more than 203,536 new cases diagnosed in 2007 in the United States and more than 158,683 deaths (more than 25% of all cancer deaths). Incidence in males is decreasing: in 1984, 86.5/100,000; in 1995, 73.4/100,000. During 1991-1995, mortality from lung cancer declined 1.6% per year in men, while rates for women were increasing. Since 1987, lung cancer has been in the leading cause of cancer mortality in women. Cigarette smoking causes over 90% of lung cancer in males and over 80% in females.[8]

RISK FACTORS[6]

- Risk of lung cancer is 20x higher for smokers (30 packs per year)
- Risk of lung cancer for a non smoker married to a smoker increases 30%
- Exposure to asbestos or radon are both additive risk factors and independent risk factors
- Chemical exposure (arsenic, asbestos, chromates, nickel, chloromethyl ethers)
- Tuberculosis
- Radiation exposure

Occupational Hazards

A small proportion of lung cancers (about 10% in men and about 5% in women) are caused by substance exposures from an occupational hazard.[8] Working with asbestos, radiation, arsenic, chromates, nickel, chloromethyl ethers, mustard gas, and coke-oven emissions has been linked with lung cancer. The risk of contracting lung cancer is greater in people who are exposed to these substances and who also smoke cigarettes. Air pollution causes about 1% of lung cancer cases.[9] Exposure to radon gas in the home causes lung cancer in less than 1% of cases.[10] Occasionally, lung cancers, especially adenocarcinoma and alveolar cell carcinoma, develop in people whose lungs have been scarred by other lung diseases, such as tuberculosis and fibrosis.[11]

Smoking

Smoking contributes to lung disease in several ways. It impairs the lungs' natural defense mechanisms by irritating the airways and inhibiting the work of macrophages and the mucociliary escalator that expels mucous. Smoking itself it is a leading cause of serious lung and heart disease and certain types of cancers are directly correlated to the activity.[12] It also has a synergistic effect with other pulmonary carcinogens, such as asbestos, chromium and uranium compounds, and arsenic. Synergistic means that the combined effect of two or more substances is greater than the effects of each added together. Smoking increases the risk of lung cancer by 15%, chronic asbestos exposure by 4%, but together they produce a 60% increase in risk, not a 19% increase. As a result, smokers who receive prolonged occupational exposures to other airborne contaminants develop heart and lung disease and cancers more readily than do nonsmokers with comparable exposures, and these diseases progress more rapidly because of the extra burden on the lungs created by smoking with the added deficiency of oxygen readily supplied to the cells for restoration and repair.[13]

Tobacco and Cancer Statistics[14]

- 25% of the adult U.S.A. population smokes
- 25% of those are heavy smokers (>1 pack per day)
- Smoking is the direct cause of 20% of all deaths in the United States and 25% of deaths between ages 35 and 64
- The greater the quantity and duration of smoking, the greater the risk of developing lung cancer.
- About 10% to 12% of all smokers eventually develop lung cancer

Assessment NSCLC

In the diagnosis of NSCLC, several strategies can be used to take for a precise cellular sample of the lesion. Often in early stages of the cancer growth, the lesion may be found incidentally on chest x-ray. This positive finding should be followed with a CT of the chest and a sputum cytology or a fiberoptic bronchoscopy with an aspiration cytology of suspicious nodes. Pleural effusions may be even more diagnostically precise. A mediastinoscopy may often be used in extensive disease with a biopsy of suspected metastatic lesions taken at that time.[15]

NSCLC SYMPTOMS AND COMPLICATIONS

The symptoms of lung cancer depend on its type, its location, and the way it spreads.[16]

Cough: Usually, the first and most common symptom is a persistent cough. Patients with chronic bronchitis who develop lung cancer often notice that their coughing becomes worse. If sputum can be coughed up, it may be streaked with blood (called hemoptysis).

Hemoptysis: If a lung cancer grows into underlying blood vessels, it may cause severe bleeding, thus causing the hemoptysis.[16]

Atelectasis: Lung cancer may cause wheezing by narrowing the bronchus in or around which it is growing, literally obstructing the airway. Blockage of a bronchus may lead to the collapse of the part of the lung that the bronchus supplies, a condition called atelectasis. Other consequences of a blocked bronchus are shortness of breath, and pneumonia, with coughing, fever, and chest pain.[16]

Chest pain: If the tumor grows into the chest wall, it may produce persistent chest pain.[16]

Horner's syndrome: Lung cancer may grow into certain nerves in the neck, causing a droopy eyelid, small pupil, sunken eye, and reduced perspiration on one side of the face – together these symptoms are called Horner's syndrome.[16]

Pancoast syndrome: Cancers at the top of the lung may grow into the nerves that supply the arm, making the arm painful, numb, and weak. This condition is called Pancoast syndrome.[16]

Voice box damage: Nerves to the voice box may also be damaged, making the voice quality sound hoarse. This damage happens mainly in people whose cancers involve the left lung.[16]

Dysphagia: Lung cancer may grow directly into the esophagus, or it may grow near it and put pressure on it, leading to difficulty in swallowing (dysphagia).[16]

Aspiration: Occasionally, an abnormal channel (fistula) between the esophagus and bronchi develops because of invasion by the cancer, causing severe coughing during swallowing because food and fluid enter the lungs (aspiration).[16]

Superior vena cava syndrome: A lung cancer may grow into the heart, causing abnormal heart rhythms, blockage of blood flow through the heart, or fluid in the pericardial sac surrounding the heart. The cancer may grow into or compress the superior vena cava (one of the large veins in the chest); this condition is called superior vena cava syndrome. Obstruction of this vein causes blood to back up in other veins of the upper body. The veins in the chest wall enlarge. The face, neck, and upper chest wall – including the breasts – swell and become tinged with purple. The condition also produces shortness of breath, headache, distorted vision, dizziness, and drowsiness. These symptoms usually worsen when the person bends forward or lies down.[16]

Pleural effusions: Fluid accumulations around the lung (pleural effusions) occur when the cancer has spread into the pleural space. They can lead to shortness of breath. Severe shortness of breath, low levels of oxygen in the blood, and cor pulmonale may develop if cancer spreads within the lungs.[16]

Paraneoplastic syndromes: Lung cancer may also spread through the bloodstream to the liver, brain, adrenal glands, spinal cord, and bone; less commonly, lung cancer may spread to other parts of the body. The spread of lung cancer may occur early in the disease, especially with small cell carcinoma. Symptoms – such as headache, confusion, seizures, and bone pain – may develop before any lung problems become evident, making an early diagnosis difficult.[16]

These syndromes are not related to the size or location of the lung cancer and do not necessarily indicate that the cancer has spread outside the chest; rather, they are caused by substances secreted by the cancer (hormones, cytokines, and a variety of other proteins).[16]

NSCLC DIAGNOSIS

When a person, especially a smoker, presents with a persistent or worsening cough or other lung symptoms (such as shortness of breath or coughed-up sputum tinged with blood), further testing is needed. Sometimes a shadow on a chest x-ray of someone with no symptoms provides the first clue, although a shadow on an x-ray is not proof of cancer and all suspect x-rays should be followed up with further diagnostics. A chest x-ray can detect most lung tumors, although it may miss small ones. Computed tomography (CT) may show small nodules that do not appear on chest x-rays. CT can also reveal whether the lymph nodes are enlarged. A biopsy of enlarged lymph nodes is often needed to determine if inflammation or cancer is responsible for the lymphadenopathy and to obtain a pathology of the cells in the lymph tissue. A microscopic examination of lung tissue is usually needed to confirm the diagnosis. Sometimes a sample of coughed-up sputum can provide enough material for an examination (called sputum cytology). Bronchoscopy is usually performed to obtain the tissue sample of a lung cancer lesion and suspect metastatic growth.[17]

BRONCHOSCOPY

Bronchoscopy is a direct visual examination of the voice box (larynx) and airways through a flexible viewing tube (a bronchoscope). A bronchoscope has a light at the end that allows a doctor to look down through the larger airways (bronchi) into the lungs. For at least 4 hours before bronchoscopy, the person should not eat or drink. A sedative is often given to ease anxiety, and atropine may be given to reduce the risks of spasm of the voice box and slowing of the heart rate, which sometimes occur during the procedure. The throat and nasal passage are sprayed with an anesthetic, and the flexible bronchoscope is passed through a nostril and into the airways of the lungs.

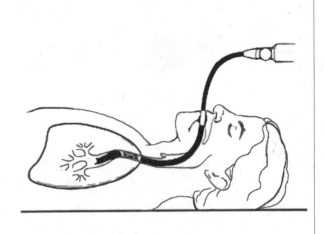

Diagnostic Imaging

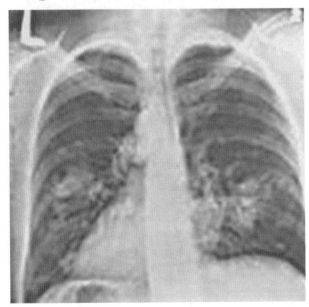

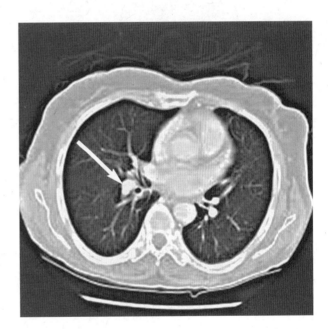

X-ray of adenocarcinoma

The lungs are the two dark areas. The heart and other structures are white areas visible in the middle of the chest. The light areas that appear as subtle branches extending from the center into the lungs are cancerous.

CT scan of adenocarcinoma

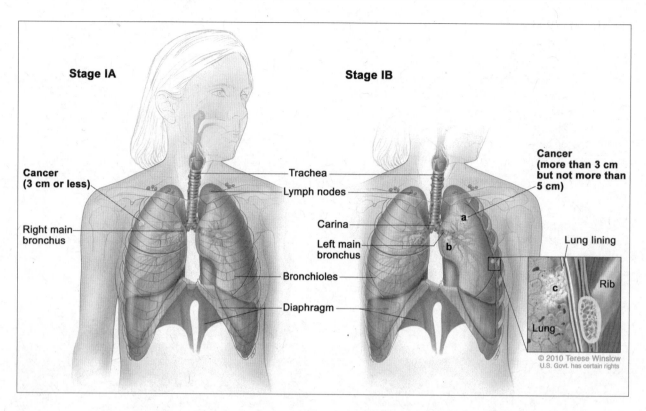

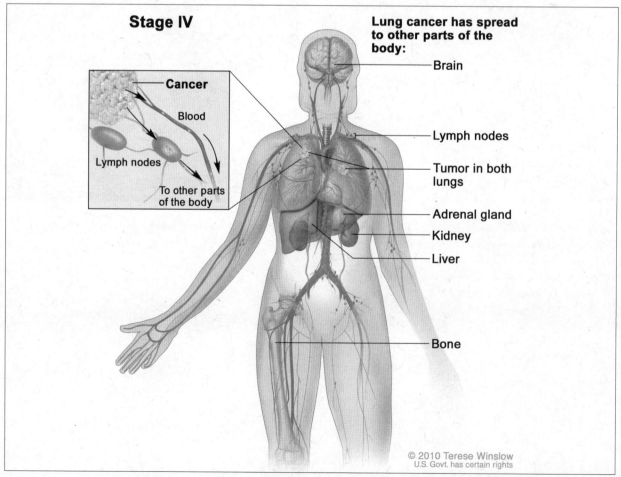

Staging NSCLC

Occult		TX	N0	M0	
Stage 0		Tis	N0	M0	
Stage I		T1-2 N0	M0	45%	
Stage II	T1-2 N1	M0	20-30%		
Stage IIIA	T3	N0-1 M0	15-30%	T1-3 N2 M0	
Stage IIIB	T4	N0-2 M0	<5%	T1-4 N3 M0	
Stage IV	Any T Any N M1		<3%		

(Adapted from AJCC.)[6]

NSCLC Staging and Grading

TNM System
T = Tumor Size
N = Nodal Involvement
M = Distant Metastases

Primary Tumor (T)
- TX Positive sputum or washings, no tumor
- Tis Carcinoma in situ
- T1 Tumor < 3 cm
- T2 Tumor ≥ 3 cm; or involving main stem
- T3 Tumor invading chest wall, diaphragm, mediastinal pleura;   atelectasis or obstructive pneumonitis of entire lung
- T4 Tumor invading mediastinum, heart, great vessels, esophagus, vertebral body; ipsilateral malignant pleural effusion

Regional Nodes (N)
- N0 No regional nodes
- N1 Ipsilateral peribronchial or hilar nodes
- N2 Ipsilateral mediastinal or subcarinal nodes
- N3 Contralateral mediastinal or hilar nodes; any scalene or supraclavicular nodes

Distant Metastases (M)
M0 No distant metastases
M1 Distant metastases

Conventional Treatment for NSCLC

NSCLC SURGERY

Stages 0, I, II, should be initially considered for surgery. Stage I 5-year survival rate is about 45%, Stage II about 20% to 30%. Stage IIIA can be treated surgically and in selected patients 5-year survival rates can be as high as 20% to 35%.[18]

For stage I-II patients unable to undergo surgery, radiation therapy results in 15% to 20% survival. Stages IIIB and IV are not curable surgically. Treatment options include local radiation, chemotherapy, chemopotentiated radiation, or supportive measures only.[19]

Chemotherapy for NSCLC[19]
- Cisplatin, Carboplatin
- Paclitaxel (Taxol)
- Ifosfamide
- Gemcitabine (Gemzar)
- Etoposide (VP-16)
- Cisplatin, Carboplatin, and Taxol are the standards of care in treatment protocols.

Assessment SCLC

Small cell carcinoma, also called oat cell carcinoma, can create its own hormones, which alter body chemistry. SCLC accounts for 25% of lung cancers. The clinical course without treatment is rapid, much more aggressive than NSCLC:[20]
- Limited stage disease with 4 to 5 month survival rate
- Extensive disease with 1 to 2 month survival rate

SCLC DIAGNOSIS

Diagnosis is usually made on a small amount of tissue via histopathology. It is critical that the diagnosis be confirmed by a pathologist experienced in the examination of lung when suspecting a SCLC. A CT of chest and abdomen may aid in staging and grading of the disease, and often a brain scan, bone scan, or PET/CT can be useful in defining the extent of the disease, but rarely influences therapeutic choices.[20]

SCLC STAGING

Staging of a SCLC is the same as for NSCLC with the following exceptions:[21]
- Limited Stage: Tumor is confined to one hemithorax and regional lymph nodes that can be encompassed in a tolerable radiation therapy port. Ipsilateral pleural effusion and supraclavicular adenopathy are often included within the definition of limited stage disease.
- Extensive Stage: Tumor beyond limited stage disease

Conventional Treatment for SCLC

Chemotherapy for SCLC[22]
- Cisplatin, Carboplatin + Etoposide
- Cyclophosphamide, Doxorubicin, Etoposide
- Paclitaxel
- 80% to 90% response, 12-18 month survival in Limited Stage SCLC
- 60% to 80% response, 7-10 month survival in Extensive Stage SCLC

CHEMOTHERAPY FOR NSCLC AND SCLC

These drugs can be used alone or in combination with other traditional chemotherapy agents. Platinum-based chemotherapy may be used as the initial chemotherapy. Common examples of platinum-based agents are Carboplatin and Cisplatin. To help boost the effectiveness of chemotherapy, oncologists may add a taxane drug to the platinum-based chemotherapy. Common examples of taxanes are Paclitaxel and Docetaxel.[23]

Targeted treatments

If the tumor has not responded to at least one previous chemotherapy regimen, oncologists may try a targeted treatment. Targeted treatments work differently from traditional chemotherapy. Some targeted treatments are tablets taken by mouth once a day.[24]

Rash and diarrhea are the most common side effects associated with targeted treatments. They are generally mild to moderate. The rash that may occur with targeted treatments is not an allergic reaction to the drug. Tarceva is the targeted treatment of choice in late stage NSCLC in combination with other chemotherapy regimens. Tarceva affects certain cell activities, blocking tumor cell growth by targeting the protein HER1/EGFR. This protein is important for cell growth in NSCLC. HER1/EGFR is present on the surface of some cancer cells and normal cells.[25]

GENETIC AND SERUM MARKERS

NSCLC and SCLC have some common genetic markers as well as individual markers. By finding positive markers, treatment regimens may be enhanced. These markers can also serve as therapeutic response markers.[26]

Conventional Lung Cancer Treatments[27]

Treatments	Action	Application
Surgery	Removes the tumor. This can be done if the tumor is small and has not spread to other areas of the system.	The patient should be in good overall health to have surgery. Surgery can be the first step in the treatment plan. It is usually done in Stage I-II. Neoadjuvant chemotherapy may be used to make the tumor more resectable.
Radiation	Uses high-energy x-ray beams to shrink the tumor. Radiation treatment destroys any leftover cancer cells not removed by surgery, therefore is a usual follow up to chemotherapeutic interventions.	This may be done before surgery to make it easier to remove the tumor. Radiation can also be done after surgery. This treatment may be used in Stage II-III. However, it can also be used to shrink tumors in advanced NSCLC (Stage IV) to ease pain. If the overall health of the patient is not good enough for surgery or the cancer may have spread to other areas in the body. If so, radiation treatment may be used instead of surgery.
Chemotherapy	Drugs used to destroy cancer cells. Some kinds of chemotherapy may help slow the growth of cancer cells and destroy them.	Chemotherapy may be used with radiation to help shrink the tumor before surgery (neoadjuvant therapies) It may be used after surgery or radiation to destroy any cancer cells that may have been left behind (adjuvant therapies).
Tertiary or Targeted Therapy	Designed to affect only certain cancer cell activities. Helps slow the tumor growth and destroys cancer cells.	Used when at least one previous chemotherapy regimen has not worked to control advanced NSCLC.

Epithelial Growth Factor Receptor (EGFR)
- Also known as HER-1 or c-erbB-1
- Over expressed in a variety of solid tumors, including lung cancers
- Expression of EGFR has been correlated with advanced disease stage and poor prognosis in NSCLC
- Up-regulates matrix metalloproteinase (MMP)-9, a molecule that regulates tumor invasiveness
- EGFR monoclonal antibodies (Iressa, Tarceva, Erbitux)[28]

HER-2/neu
- Most commonly associated with breast cancer, though over expression has also been associated with non-small cell lung cancer (NSCLC)
- Associated with shorter survival times in NSCLC
- Possible use of Herceptin[29]

K-ras
- Ras genes regulate signal transduction pathways that control cell growth
- 40% of NSCLC exhibit mutated ras oncogenes, most commonly K-ras
- In a study of 106 patients with adenocarcinoma of the lung, K-ras mutations were noted exclusively in smokers (43% versus zero), suggesting a causal relationship between smoking, K-ras mutation, and the development of lung cancer.
- Ras monoclonal antibodies in early stages of study
- Zarnestra, Sarsar[30]

Carcinoembryonic Antigen (CEA)
- Only FDA-approved tumor marker for lung cancer
- Elevated preoperative serum concentrations of carcinoembryonic antigen predicted a poor prognosis
- Used for monitoring and prognosis[31]

CEA in smokers vs. non smokers[32]
- Normal for non smokers <3.07 ng/ml
- Normal for smokers <6.17 ng/ml

Small Cell Lung Cancer (SCLC)[33]
- Because of their epithelial cellular origin, virtually all SCLCs are immunoreactive for keratin and epithelial membrane antigen
- May also have neuroendocrine and neural differentiation
- May result in expression of dopa decarboxylase, calcitonin, neuron-specific enolase, chromogranin A, CD56 (neural cell adhesion molecule [NCAM]), gastrin releasing peptide (GRP), and insulin-like growth factor-I (IGF-I)
- One or more of these markers can be found in approximately 75% of SCLC
- SCLC cells can also produce a number of polypeptide hormones, including ACTH and vasopressin
- May cause hormonal syndromes, such as Cushing's syndrome or syndrome of inappropriate antidiuretic hormone secretion (SIADH)

Naturopathic Approaches to Treating LungCancer

Naturopathic therapies are directed by the staging and grading of tumor growth and cell type. The goals are to prevent surgical complications and speed tissue healing post-operatively; prevent recurrence and reduce the risk of metastasis; enhance the innate tumor kill potential of the immune system before and after treatment; and to reduce the side effects from treatment. Counseling patients in a recovery or palliative state remians central to the natuoropathic approach to cancer management. These protocols are not unlike the strategies applied to the other cancers discussed in this textbook, but they are specific to the type of lung cancer cell.

Naturopathic Therapeutic Protocols
1. Prevent recurence and reduce the risk of metastasis
2. Speed tissue healing post-operatively
3. Enhance innate tumor kill potential
4. Reduce side effects
5. Counsel patients

---

1. PREVENT RECURRENCE AND REDUCE RISK OF METSTASIS
Retinoids
The retinoids are chemo-radiosensitization antioxidants that help to control the growth of cancer and repair precancerous lesions, such as lichen planus. These retinoids can also induce cell differentiation, prevent metastasis and secondary cancer growth, and control angiogenesis while stimulating the innate immune system. The carotenoids, such as beta-carotene and vitamin A, belong to this larger family of retinoids.

Anticancer action of retinoids and carotenoids
Retinoids
- Inhibit growth of protein kinase-C [34]
- Reduce oncogene expression [35]
- Reduce transplanted tumor growth [36]
- Reduce tumor size [37]
- Best activity in squamous cell, cervical, and renal cell cancers [38]
- Organ development not affected

Carotenoids [39]
- Induce differentiation
- Inhibit growth of human melanoma cells
- Stimulate the level of cAMP induced differentiation
- Beta carotene increases expression of connexin gene, which functions to hold normal cells together and codes for gap junction in genetic code [40]

Carotenoids and Smoking
Smoking and exposure to occupational chemicals increase the relative risk of developing lung cancer. Some studies have shown that caretinoids can prevent and treat this exposure.[41] Beta-carotene and vitamin A each showed diminished toxicity to local radiation in tumor-bearing mice without diminishing the antitumor effect of the radiation. The tumor-bearing mice that received both the 3,000 rad local tumor radiation supplemented with vitamin A or beta-carotene showed that the antitumor effect or the local radiation was enhanced.[42] Beta-carotene supplementation has shown significant results in TGF-beta-1 immunoreactivity in three cervical epitheal cancer cell lines with regression in 4/10 patients.[43]

Lycopene strongly inhibits proliferation of endometrial, mammary, and lung carcinoma cells. Alpha and beta-carotene were less effective than lycopene as inhibitors.[44] Trans retinoic acid (ATRA) causes apoptosis in certain cancer cell lines, and ATRA combined with Cisplatin induced apoptosis significantly more that with either agent alone. ATRA enhances the cytoxicity of Cisplatin by facilitating apoptosis.[45]

Further investigations into the use of carotenoids as cancer treatment have given mixed results. Even though it seems like a rational choice for the naturopathic physician to prescribe an antioxidant as a chemoradio therapy, there are some cautions that may discourage this practice.

Carotenoid Meta-analysis[46]

Alpha-tocopherol, Beta Carotene Prevention Study (ATBCPS)

- 29,000 Finish smokers studied
- 20 mg synthetic carotene, 50 mg tocopherol, both or placebo
- 18% higher incidence, 8% higher mortality with carotene[72]

Physicians Health Study[47]

- 22,071 male physicians studied
- 50 mg q.d. synthetic carotene or placebo
- No significant differences in lung cancer incidence or deaths from cancer
- No risk associated with non-smoking population
- No significant differences in current or former smokers

Beta-Carotene and Retinol Efficacy Trial (CARET)[48]

- 18,314 smokers, former smokers and workers with asbestos exposure
- Synthetic carotene (30 mg) and retinol (25,000 IU) daily or placebo
- Carotene/retinol group had a 28% increase in lung cancer incidence (218 vs 170), and a 46% increase in lung cancer mortality

---

Based on these findings, most integrative practioners do not recommend beta-carotene as a therapy in lung cancer management, specifically synthetic beta-carotene. Synthetic beta-carotene used in these large numbered studies shows deleterious effects, even in low doses.[49]

However, dietary beta-carotene from raw fruits and vegetable does not have a deleterious effect and shows a 30% reduction in lung cancer incidence in non smokers.[50] In breast cancer cases, high comsumption of carotenes prior to the diagnosis of breat cancer was correlated with an increased survival and a improved favorable outcome,[51] while a significant inverse relationship was shown between dietary intake of beta-carotene and the risk of breast cancer.[52] Beta-carotene induces apoptosis by down-regulation of EGF receptor proteins,[53] and has shown to be active in the prevention of cancer cell initiation but not promotion.[54] Dietary natural carotenoids found in fruits and vegetables are the best delivery of these antioxidants in smokers, with a risk of cancer mortality at 0.3 in those in the lowest quintile.[55]

In summary, natural mixed carotenoids from dietary sources (but not synthetic beta-carotenes) are beneficial in prevention of initiation of a wide variety of cancers, but less effective at reversing the cancer at later stages.

Vitamin A

Vitamin A can promote normal cell differentiation preventively, and toxicity is less frequent than is normally assumed. A safe dose of up to 300,000 IU of vitamin A can be administered safely for up to 2 years.[56] Beta-carotene and vitamin A should not be used with the chemotherapeutic regimen of 5-FU due to a significant reduction in the chemotherapeutic effect.[57]

---

2. SPEED TISSUE HEALING POST-OPERATIVELY
N-acetyl-cysteine (NAC) and reduce glutathione (GSH)

L-cysteine, in its bioavailable form (NAC), is utlized by the CYP450 system in the human physiology functioning as reduced glutathione (r-GSH). Often with smokers, naturopathic physicians recommend the use of NAC to help reduce the destruction of smoking to the lung tissues and to aid in restoration of optimal function pre- and post-smoking cessation. Reduced glutathione protects DNA and p53 suppressor gene, and gives some relief to mucositis diarrhea (28% vs 52% controls).[58] NAC and glutathione stimulates p53, thereby stimulating apoptosis, supports the liver in phase 2 conjugation of the CYP450 system, and can be orally tolerated. NAC elevates p53 activity and apoptosis in cancer cells but not in healthy cells.[58]

While biochemistry shows that NAC changes into r-GSH in the human physiology, NAC may have adverse reactions as an antioxidant, especially with the chemotherapeutic cisplatin. However, GSH helps cisplatin work better and reduces the nephro- and neuro-toxicity associated with it. Oral glutathione is not absorbed as well as the reduced form, and even then caution should be used. Oral doses of GSH range from 1200-2400 mg daily; IV doses are 1500-2000 mg daily.[61,62] Glutathione reduces neurotoxicity of cisplatin without reducing antitumor effects,[59] and appears to increase the effectiveness of cisplatin.[60] In one study, GSH reduced neuropathy of cisplatin, reduced the need for transfusions and treatment delays, and increased response rate to chemotherapeutic.[60]

Dosage: To avoid interfering with conventional treatment, do not use during chemotherapeutic administration: Follow the '3 day rule' (not the day before, day of, or day after chemotherpy). Do not use NAC until the chemotherpy regimen schedule has been completed, unless warranted.[61-62]

3. ENHANCE INNATE TUMOR KILL POTENTIAL
Melatonin

Melatonin acts as a biological response modifier in cancer patients.[63] A pineal secretory product with antioxidant properties, melatonin protects against cisplatin-induced nephrotoxicity.[64] Studies looking at lung cancer specific interactions in integrative therapeutics found that melatonin helps first-line chemotherapeutics while reducing toxicities in NSCLC and SCLC.

4. REDUCE SIDE EFFECTS
CoQ10

CoQ10 is a synonym for ubiquinone, a naturally forming plant chlorophyll that is fat soluble and present in all human cells. It is an essential cofactor in cellular metabolism, specifically in oxidative respiration. As the human body ages, CoQ10 levels diminish. Some prescriptive medications also significantly reduce natural CoQ10. In ischemic tissues, CoQ10 functions as a free radical scavenger and membrane stabilizer, while being the mobile component of the mitochondrial membrane.[69]

When using CoQ10 as a supplemental intervention, caution should be applied to the type and form of CoQ10 that is used. Most of the "cheap" CoQ10 supplements in the market place are synthetic. The synthetic form is not bioidentical to the CoQ10 the human cell uses for restoration and repair. It must be bioavailable in a fat soluble form to cross the phospholipid bilayer of the cell and then cross the mitochondrial membrane to effect the redux oxidation chain that produces the ATP by splitting a molecule of water. CoQ10 is used with vitamin E to protect patients from chemotherapy-induced cardiomyopathies.[69]

CoQ10 is nontoxic even at high dosages and has been shown to prevent liver damage from the drugs Mitomycin C and 5-FU. Adriamycin (Docorubincin)

Melatonin Meta-analysis[65]

NSCLC Studies

- 63 patients with histologically proven metastatic NSCLC who did not respond to first-line cisplatin chemotherapy
- Randomzed to either supportive care alone or melatonin (MLT) at 10 mg q.d. at bedtime
- No therapy related toxicity in the MLT group
- Stabilization of disease was higher in the MLT group (10/31 vs 3/32, p<0.05)
- Mean survival greater for those in the MLT group (7.9 vs 4.1, p<0.025)
- Disease stabilization most frequest in those without liver mets.

Metastatic Lung Cancer Studies[66]

- 50 patients with brain mets from various solid tumors who progressed following radiation and chemotherapy
- Randomized to either supportive care alone (steroids + anticonvulsants) or MLT (20 mg q.h.s)
- Time till progression significantly longer in MLT group (5.9 ± 0.8 mo. Vs 2.7 ± 1.06 mo., p<0.05)
- One year survival significantly higher in the MLT group (9/24 vs 3/26, p<0.05)
- When analyzed by site of primary cancer, only those with a single brain met from lung cancer maintained a significant difference (6/10 vs 2/12).

Inoperable NSCLC and SCLC Studies[67]

- 20 previously untreated patients with inoperable lung cancer (16 NSCLC, 4 SCLC)
- Randomized to receive either carboplatin (5 AUC on day 1) and etoposide (150 mg/m?/day on days 1-3) or carboplatin-etoposide+MLT (40 mg QHS) in cross over fashion
- No effect observed on depth and duration of toxicity for hemoglobin, ANC, or ANC nadir[103]

Integrative Chemotherapy/MLT in Lung Cancer Patients Studies[68]

- 250 metastatic solid tumor patients (104 lung) with poor clinical status
- Randomized to receive chemotherapy or chemotherapy + MLT (20 mg QHS)
- Lung Cancer
  - Cisplatin + etoposide
  - gemcitabine
- The 1-year survival rate and the objective tumor regression rate were significantly higher in patients concomittantly treated with MLT than chemotherapy (CT) alone
- Tumor response rate 42/124 CT + MLT versus 19/126 CT alone (p<0.001)
- 1 year survival rate 63/124 CT + MLT versus 29/126 CT alone (p<0.001)

Chemotherapeutic and Naturopathic Integrated Therapies

Chemotherapeutic	Naturopathic	Daily Dose	Caution
NSLC: In combinations of one another: Cisplatin Carboplatin, Paclitaxel (Taxol) Ifosfamide Gemcitabine (Gemzar) Etopiside (VP-16) all	*To complement effectiveness:* NAC, CoQ10, beta carotene and vitamin A are used specifically for lung cancers	Minimal and essential multivitamin 1-2 qd	Do not use NAC, GSH, CoQ10 (endogenous during chemotherapy antioxidants)
	Melatonin Apoptosin Green Tea	20 mg qhs 5-10 cups qd	
SCLC: Cisplatin Carboplatin Etoposide Cyclophosphamide, Doxorubicin, etoposide, paclitaxel	*To reduce toxicity and side effects:* See page xx for protocols for managing: Mucositis Nausea Vomiting Diarrhea Glutamine	10 tid, swish & swallow	

induced cardiomyopathies have been prevented by concomitant supplementation with CoQ10. CoQ10 reduces free radical formation induced by doxorubicin.[69-71] Research studies in both animals and humans have found that pretreating with coenzyme Q10, at levels of 100 mg per day, reduces cardiac toxicity caused by doxorubicin.[72-74]

Dosage: Recommendations vary upon polypharmacy and comorbidity: general recommendations vary from 100 mg-3000 mg q.d. in divided doses in the literature. Generally, 100-200 mg t.i.d. in a fat-soluble form is optimal.

CoQ10 Anticancer Actions[69-75]

- Affects the function of all cells in the body, making it essential for the health of all human tissues and organs, especially the most metabolically active: heart, immune, gingiva, and gastric mucosa due to the oxidation/reduction electron transport chain in the mitochondria that eventually splits water and makes cellular ATP
- Enhances immune function
- Prevents metastasis and enhances remission in breast cancer
- Acts as an intracellular antioxidant
- Protects gastric mucosa
- Prevents of Adriamycin toxicity in the cardiac muscle
- In study of 32 node positive BRCA patients treated with conventional therapy and 90 mg q.d. of CoQ10 showed better survival time

References

1. Guyton AC, Hall JE. Textbook of Medical Physiology. 10th ed. St Louis, MO: WB Saunders Co.;2000.

2. Moore KL, AF Dalley, AMR Aqur. Clinically Oriented Anatomy. 6th ed. Baltimore, MD: Lippincott Williams & Wilkins;2009.

3. Young, RC. Harrison's Internal Medicine, online. Chapter 89, Pancreatic Cancer, Yu Jo Chua, David Cunningham.

4. McPhee SJ, Papadakis MA. Eds. Gonzales R, Zeiger R. Online Eds. 2009. CURRENT Medical Diagnosis & Treatment. 48th Ed.

5. www.medcinenet.com

6. American Joint Committee on Cancer (AJCC). AJCC Cancer Staging Manual, 6th Ed.New York, NY:Springer-New York, www.springeronline.com.2002.

7. http://www.cancer.org

8. http://www.cdc.gov/cancer/lung/statistics/.2007.

9. Jockel KH, Ahrens W, Wichmann HE, et al. Occupational and environmental hazards associated with lung cancer. In J Epidem.1992;21(2):202-13.

10. http://www.cancer.gov/cancertopics/factsheet/Risk/r adon 2012

11. Cowen, J. Pulmonary TB linked to EGFR mutations in lung cancer. J Thorac Oncol. 2012;7:299-305.

12. Ahrendt, SA, Decker, PA, Alawi, EA, et al. Cigarette smoking is strongly associated with mutation of the k-ras gene in patients with primary adenocarcinoma of the lung. Cancer. 2000;92:1525.

13. Saracci, R, Boffetta, P Interactions of tobacco smoking and other causes of lung cancer. In: Samet, JM eds. Epidemiology of lung cancer;1994:465-93.

14. http://www.cancer.gov/cancertopics/tobacco/statisticssnapshot. 2010.

15. www.cancer.gov/cancertopics/pdq/treatment/nonsmall-cell.../page4.2012.

16. http://www.mayoclinic.com/health/lung-cancer/DS00038/DSECTION=complications. 2012.

17. Van Meerbeck JP, Tournoy KG. Screening and diagnosis of NSCLC. Annals of Onco 2004;15(suppl 4):65-70.

18. www.cancer.gov/cancertopics/pdq/treatment/nonsmall-cell.../page9.2012.

19. http://www.cancer.net/patient/Cancer+Types/Lung+Cancer?sectionTitle=Treatment Oncologist approved cancer information from the American Society of Clinical Oncologist. 2012.

20. www.cancer.gov/cancertopics/pdq/treatment/small-cell-lung/.../page1.National Cancer Institute Home: NCI Home. Cancer Topics. Clinical Trials. Cancer Statistics. 2012.

21. http://emedicine.medscape.com/article/2006716-overview Stevenson M. Small cell lung cancer staging. Drugs, Diseases & Procedures. 2011.

22. Sandler AB. Chemotherapy for small cell lung cancer. Semin Onco 2003;30(1):9-25.

23. Patel N, Adatia R, Mellemgaard A, et al. Variation in the use of chemotherapy in lung cancer. Br J Ca. 2007;96(6):886-90.

24. Sun S, Schiller JH, Spinola M, Minna JD. New molecularly targeted therapies for lung cancer. Sci in Med. 2007;117(10):2740-50.

25. www.tarceva.com/patient/learning/treatment.jsp

26. Rubins JB, Dunitz J, Rubins HB. Serum carcinoembryonic antigen as an adjunct to preoperative staging of lung cancer. J Thorac Cardiovasc Surg. 1998;116(3):412-16.

27. http://www.merckmanuals.com/professional/hematology_and_oncology/principles_of_cancer_therapy/modalities_of_cancer_therapy.html. 2011.

28. Rosell R, Moran T, Queralt BS, et al. Screening for epidermal growth factor receptor mutations in lung cancer. NEJM. 2009;361:958-67.

29. Bunn PA, Helfrich B, Soriano AF, et al. Expression of Her-2/neu in human lung cancer cell lines by immunohistochemistry and fluorescence in situ hybridization and its relationship to in vitro cytotoxicity by trastuzumab and chemotherapeutic agents. Clin Ca Res. 2001;7(10):3239-50.

30. Riely GJ, Marks J, Pao W. KRAS Mutations in non-small cell lung cancer. Proc Am Thorac Soc. 2009;6(2):201-05.

31. Salqia R, Harpole D, et al. Role of serum tumor markers CA 125 and CEA in non small cell lung cancer. Anticancer Res. 2001;21(2B):1241-46.

32. www.labtestsonline.org.au/understanding/analytes/ce a/tab/test

33. Taneja TK, Sharma SK. Markers of small cell lung cancer. World J Surg Onco. 2004;2:10.

34. Prasad KN, Kumar A, Kochupillai V, Cole WC. High doses of multiple antioxidant vitamins: essential ingredients in improving the efficacy of standard cancer therapy. J Am Col Nutr. 1999;18(1):13-25.

35. Prasad KN, Edwards-Prasad J, Kumar S, Meyers A. Vitamins regulate gene expression and induce differentiation oand growth inhibition in cancer cells. Arch Otolaryngol Head Neck Surg. 1993;119(10):1133-40.

36. Cole, W.C., Prasad, K.N. Contrasting effects of vitamins as modulators of apoptosis in cancer cells and normal cells: A review. Nutr. Cancer. 1997;29:97-103.

37. Dahl AR, Grossi IM, Houchens DP, et al. Inhaled isotretinoin (13-cis retinoic acid) is an effective lung cancer chemopreventive agent in A/J mices at low doses: a pilot study. Clin Ca Res. 2000;6(8):3015-24.

38. Motzer RJ, Schwartz L, Law TM, et al. Interferon alfa-2a and 13-cis retinoic acid in renal cell carcinoma: antitumor activity in a phase II trial and interactions in vitro. JCO. 1995;13(8):1950-57.

39. Chew BP, Park JS. Carotenoid action on the immune response. J Nutr. 2004;134(1):2575-615.

40. Zhang LX, Acevedo P, Guo H, Bertram JS. Upregulation of gap junctional communication and connexin43 gene expression by carotenoids in human dermal fibroblasts but not in human keratinocytes. Mol Carcino.1995;12(1):50-58.

41. Shekelle RB, Liu S, Raynor WJ Jr, Lepper M, Maliza C, Rossof AH, Oglesby P, Macmillan-Shryock A, Stamler J. Dietary vitamin A and risk of cancer in the western electric study. The Lancet. 1981 28 Nov;318(8257):1185-1242.

42. Selfter E. Morbidity and mortality reduction et al by supplemental vitamin A or beta - carotene in CBA mice given total body radiation. JNCI. 1984 ;73:1167.

43. Comerci J T Jr, Runowicz CD, Fields AL, Romney SL, Palan PR, Kadish AS, Goldberg GL. Induction of transforming growth factor beta-1 in cervical intraepithelial neoplasia in vivo after treatment with beta-carotene. Clin Can Res. 997(3):157-60.

44. Levy J, Bosin E, Feldman B, Giat Y, Miinster A, Danilenko M, et al. Lycopene is a more potent inhibitor of human cancer cell proliferation than either a-carotene or b-carotene. Nutr Cancer. 1995;24:257-66.

45. Aebi S, Kröning R, Cenni B, Sharma A, Fink D, Los G, Weisman R, Howell SB, Christen RD. all-trans retinoic acid enhances cisplatin-induced apoptosis in human ovarian adenocarcinoma and in squamous head and neck cancer cells. Clin Cancer Res. 1997 Nov;3:2033-38.

46. The effect of vitamin E and beta carotene on the incidence of lung cancer and other cancers in male smokers. The Alpha-Tocohperol, Beta Carotene Cancer Prevention Study Group (No authors listed). N Engl J Med. 1994 Apr 14;330(15):1029-35.

47. Hennekens CH, Buring JE, Manson JE, Stampfer M, Rosner B, Cook NR, Belanger C, LaMotte F, Gaziano JM, Ridker PM, Willett W, Peto R. Lack of effect of long term supplementation with beta carotene on the incidence of malignant neoplasms and cardiovascular disease. N Engl J Med. 1996 May 2;334(18):1145-49.

48. Omenn GS, Goodman GE, Thornquist MD, Balmes J, Cullen MR, Glass A, Keogh JP, Meyskens FL, Valanis B, Williams JH, Barnhart S, Hammar S. Effects of a combination of beta carotene and vitamin A on lung cancer and cardiovascular disease. N Engl J Med. 1996 May 2;334(18):1150-55.

49. Taylor-Mayne S, Janerich DT, Greenwald P, Chorost S, Tucci C, Zaman MB, Melamed MR, Kiely M, McKneally MF. Dietary beta carotene and lung cancer risk in U.S. nonsmokers. J. Natl. Cancer Inst. 1994;86:33-38.

50. Rock CL, et al. Carotenoids, vitamin A and estrogen receptor status in breast cancer. Nutrition and Cancer 1996;25:281-96.

51. Negri E, La Vecchia C, Franceschi S, et al. Intake of selected micronutrients and the risk of breast cancer. Int J Cancer. 1996;65:140-44.

52. Y Muto, J Fujii, Y Shidoji, H Moriwaki, T Kawaguchi, and T Noda. Growth retardation in human cervical dysplasia-derived cell lines by beta-carotene through down-regulation of epidermal growth factor receptor Am J Clin Nutr. 1995;62:1535S-1540S.

53. Grubbs CJ, Eto I, Juliana MM, Whitaker LM. Effect of canthaxanthin on chemically induced mammary carcinogenesis. Oncology.1991;48:239-245.

54. Colditz GA, Branch LB, et. Increased green and yellow vegetable intake and lowered cancer deaths in an elderly population. Am J Clin Nutr.1985;41:32-36.

55. Goodman GE, Christofferson E, Kaplan HG, et al: Phase II trial of retinol in patients with advanced cancer. Cancer Treat Rep. 1986;70:1023-24.

56. Lamson DS, Brignall MS. Antioxidants in cancer therapy; their actions and interactions with oncologic therapies. Altern Med Rev. 1999;4(5):304-29.

57. Teicher BA, Schwartz JL, Holden SA, et al. In vivo modulation of several anticancer agents by beta-carotene. Cancer Chemother Pharmacol 1994;34:235-241.

58. Donnerstag B, et al. Reduced glutathione and S-acetyl-gluathione as slective apoptosis inducing agents in cancer therapy. Cancer Letters 1996;110:63-70.

59. Colombo N, Bini S, Miceli D, et al. Weekly cisplatin +/- glutathione in relapsed ovarian carcinoma. Int J Gynecol Cancer. 1995;5:81-86.

60. Cascinu S, Cordella L, Del Ferro E, et al. Neuroprotective effect of reduced glutathione on cisplatin-based chemotherapy in advanced gastric cancer: a randomized double-blind placebo-controlled trial. J Clin Oncol 1995;13:26-32.

61. Smyth JF, Bowman A, et al. Glutathione reduces the toxicity and improves quality of life of women diagnosed with ovarian cancer treated with cisplatin: results of a double-blind, randomised trial. Ann Oncol. 1997 Jun;8(6):569-73.

62. Cascinu S, Ferro ED, Catalano G. Different doses of granulocyte colony stimulating factor to support a weekly chemotherapeutic regimen in advanced gastric cancer: a randomized study. J Clin Onco 1995. Jan;13(1):26-32.

63. Neri B, De Leonardis V, Gemelli MT, et al. Melatonin as biological response modifier in cancer patients. Anticancer Res, 1998;18:1329-32.

64. Hara M, Yoshida M, Nishijima H, Yokosuko M, Iigo M, Ohtani-Kaneka R, et al. Melatonin, a pineal secretory product with antioxidant properties, protects against cisplatinin-duced nephrotoxicity in rats. J Pineal Res. 2001;30:129-38.

65. Lissoni P, Barni S, et al. Randomized study with the pineal hormone melatonin versus supportive care alone in advanced nonsmall cell lung cancer resistant to a first-line chemotherapy containing cisplatin. Oncology. 1992;49:336-39.

66. Lissoni P, Barni S, et al. A randomized study with the pineal hormone melatonin versus supportive care alone in patients with brain metastases due to solid neoplasms. Cancer. 1994 Feb 1;73(3):699-701.

67. Ghielmini M, Pagani O, de Jong J, Pampallona S, Conti A, Maestroni G, Sessa C Cavalli F. Double-blind randomized study on the myeloprotective effect of melatonin in combination with carboplatin and etoposide in advanced lung cancer. Br J Cancer 1999;80:1058-61.

68. Lissoni P, Barni S, et al. Decreased toxicity and increased efficacy of cancer chemotherapy using the pineal hormone melatonin in metastatic solid tumour patients with poor clinical status. Eur J Cancer.1999 Nov;35(12):1688-92.

69. Folkers K, Vadhanavikit S, Mortensen SA. Biochemical rationale and myocardial tissue data on the effective therapy of cardiomyopathy with coenzyme Q10. In: Proc. Natl. Acad. Sci., U.S.A.2012;82(3):901-04.

70. Gaby AR. The Doctor's Guide to Vitamin B6. Emmaus, PA: Rodale Press;1984; Rev.ed. B6: The Natural Healer. New Canaan, CT: Keats Publishing;1987.

71. Anonymous.Vitamin E and cell injury. Nutr Rev. 1988;46:1367.

72. Judy WV, Hall JH, Toth PD, Folkers K. Double blind-double crossover study of coenzyme Q10 in heart failure. In: Folkers K., Yamamura Y. (eds.) Biomedical and clinical aspects of coenzyme Q, vol. 5. Amsterdam: Elsevier O15-33.

73. Ogura R, Toyama H, Shimada T, Murakami M. The role of ubiquinone (Coenzyme Q10) in preventing Adriamycin-induced mitochondrial disorders in rat heart. J Appl Biochem.1979,1:325.

74. Sugiyama S, Yamada K, Hayakawa M, Ozawa T. Approaches that mitigate doxorubincin induced delayed adverse effects on mitochondrial function. Biochem Mol Biol Int. 1995;36:10010-07.

75. Lenaz G, Fato R, Degli Esposti M, Rugolo M, Parenti Castelli G. The essentiality of coenzyme Q for bioenergetics and clinical medicine. Drugs Exp Clin Res. 1985;11(8):547-56.

Pathophysiology

Lymphoma is a cancer that begins in the lymphatic cells of the immune system and presents as a solid tumor of lymphoid cells. It is treatable with chemotherapy, radiotherapy, and bone marrow transplantation. Lymphoma can be cured depending on the histology, type, and stage of the disease.

LYMPHOID CELL MALIGNANCIES

The malignancies that affect the lymphoid tissues can range from the most indolent to the most aggressive of human malignancies. These cancers arise in the cells that function in the immune system, at different stages of differentiation, which results in a wide range of morphologic and immunologic dysfunction, resulting in a variety of clinical findings.

Malignancies of lymphoid cells that primarily involve the bone marrow and blood present as leukemia. Malignancies that are lymphomas usually present as solid tumors in the lymph or immune system. However, some malignancies of the lymphoid cells can present as either lymphoma or leukemia. Confusingly, the clinical pattern of the disease process can change over the course of the illness; this is usually seen in patients who have lymphoma and then develop manifestation of leukemia over the course of the illness and treatments.[1-2]

LYMPHOMA AND LEUKEMIA CLASSIFICATIONS

The WHO has established a system to classify and distinguish lymphomas from leukemias. The WHO classification takes into account the morphological, clinical, immunologic, and genetic differences among lymphomas.

L1 lymphoid malignancies: small uniform blasts that are typical in childhood acute lymphoblastic leukemia [ALL]

L2 lymphoid malignancies: larger and more variable sized cells

L3 lymphoid malignancies: uniform cells with basophilic and sometimes vacuolated cytoplasm, which is typical in Burkitt's lymphoma cells. Non-Hodgkin's lymphomas are separated from Hodgkin's disease by recognition of the Sterberg-Reed cells.[3]

Hodgkin Disease and Non-Hodgkin Lymphoma
Both Hodgkin lymphoma (formerly known as Hodgkin's disease) and non-Hodgkin lymphoma (also known as non-Hodgkin's lymphoma) are cancers that originate in the lymphocytes. The main difference between Hodgkin and non-Hodgkin lymphoma is in the specific lymphocyte each involves. Non-Hodgkin lymphomas are distinguished from Hodgkin disease by the presence of Reed-Sternberg cells, visible under a microscope.[4]

IMMUNOLOGY AND LYMPHOMAS

All of the lymphoid cells come from a common mother or hematopoietic progenitor cell. This gives rise to the lymphoid, myeloid, erythroid, monocyte, and megakaryocyte lines. Through the activation of an orderly transcription, the cell becomes committed to the lymphoid line and then gives rise to B and T cells.[5] Approximately 90% of all lymphomas are of B cell origin. A cell becomes committed to become a B cell when it rearranges it immunoglobulin genes and causes a sequence of cellular changes, including changing its cell surface phenotype to be characterized as a normal B cell. A cell becomes committed to T cell differentiation after it has migrated to the thymus and rearranged its antigen receptor genes to sequence the events to become a T cell.[5]

By looking at immunoglobulin heavy chain gene rearrangement (HCR) and light chain gene rearrangement or deletion occurrence in early B cell development, the normal stage of differentiation is associated with particular lymphomas, such as ALL (acute lymphoid leukemia), CLL (chronic lymphoid leukemia), and SL (small lymphocytic lymphoma). T cell antigen receptors rearrange in the thymus and mature T cell migrate to nodes and peripheral blood creating specific disease states: ALL, CLL, T cell ALL, TLL (T cell lymphoblastic lymphoma), T-CLL (T cell chronic lymphoid leukemia), CTCL (cutaneous T cell lymphoma), and NHL (non- Hodgkin's lymphoma).[6]

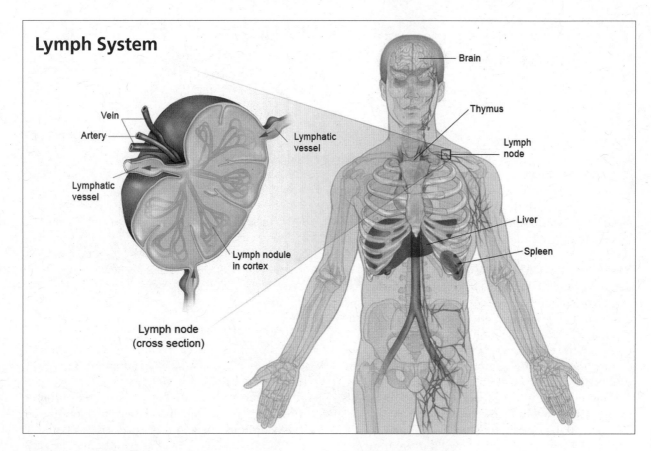

Lymph System

Vein

Artery

Lymphatic vessel

Lymphatic vessel

Lymph nodule in cortex

Lymph node (cross section)

Brain

Thymus

Lymph node

Liver

Spleen

GENETICS AND EPIGENETICS

Lymphoid cancers are associated with recurrent genetic abnormalities, and although not all specific abnormalities have been identified, it is presumed that they exist for all subtypes of lymphoid malignancies. These genetic abnormalities can be identified at a variety of levels, ranging from the gross chromosomal changes found in translocations to additions or deletions. Genes can become rearranged and over expressed or under expressed or bear mutations of specific oncogenes. The altered expression or mutation of specific proteins becomes important in this expression.[7]

Immunoglobulin genes on chromosomes 2, 14 and 22 in B cells are associated with the development of lymphoma. Other non-immunoglobulin genes, like *bcl-6*, may become mutated and in the case of diffuse large B cell lymphoma, this occurs in 30% of patients with this overexpression on chromosome 18. The *bcl-2* protein, which is involved in suppressing apoptosis, has been found to be overexpressed in lymphoma development. There is an associated higher relapse rate in patients whose tumors over-express this protein.[8]

Epidemiology

PREVALENCE AND INCIDENCE
Hodgkin Lymphoma

There is overwhelming evidence that suggests Hodgkin lymphoma is of B cell origin. New incidences of Hodgkin lymphoma appear stable, with approximately 8000 new cases diagnosed annually in the United States.[9] It is more common in whites than in blacks as well as more common in males than in females. There is a bimodal distribution of age at the time of diagnosis, with one peak incidence occurring in patients in their 20s and the other in those in their 80s.[10] In the late age group, other similar appearing anaplastic large cell lymphoma and T cell rich B cell lymphoma also occur and may confuse the diagnosis of Hodgkin lymphoma. Patients in the younger age group diagnosed in the United States most commonly have the nodular sclerosing subtype of Hodgkin lymphoma.[8]

Patients with both primary and secondary immunodeficiency states are more predisposed to developing Non-Hodgkin lymphoma, except with HIV and EBV infections. HIV (human immunodeficiency virus) infection and EBV (Epstein-Barr virus) infection are known risk factors for the development of

Hodgkin lymphoma. HIV infected patients may have a mixed cellularity Hodgkin or a lymphocyte-depleted Hodgkin. EBV infected patients have shown a monoclonal or oligoclonal proliferation of EBV infected cells in 20% to 40% of the patients with Hodgkin lymphoma.[11]

Non-Hodgkin Lymphoma

For reason unknown, non-Hodgkin lymphomas (NHL) increased in frequency in the United States at a rate of approximately 4% per year between the 1950s and the late 1990s. For those same unknown reasons, the rate of this increase in the past few years has been decreasing. Non-Hodgkin lymphomas are more frequent in males and the elderly, as well as patients with immunodeficiency states. This includes patients who have undergone organ transplant and are on immunosuppressing drugs to tolerate the donor organ; patients with inherited immunodeficiency syndromes; patients with sicca syndrome; and patients with rheumatoid arthritis.[11]

There is a geographic pattern to the incidence of non-Hodgkin lymphomas with the expression of patterns of various subtypes that differ geographically. T cell lymphomas are more common in Asia than in Western countries. Certain subtypes of B cell lymphomas, such as follicular lymphoma, are more common in the Western countries. In Latin America and Southern Asia, a specific subtype of non-Hodgkin's lymphoma, known as the angiocentric nasal T/natural killer (NK) cell lymphoma, strikes geographically. In the Caribbean and southern Japan, another subtype of non-Hodgkin lymphoma associated with infection by human T cell lymphotropic virus (HTLV) occurs geographically.[12]

Environmental exposures have been implicated in the occurrence of non-Hodgkin lymphoma, including infectious agents, chemical exposures, medical treatments, agricultural chemicals, and viral infections. There is an association between non-Hodgkin's development and exposure to agricultural chemicals. Patients treated for Hodgkin's disease can develop non-Hodgkin lymphoma. HTLV-1 infects T cells and leads directly to the development of adult T cell lymphoma (ALT) in a small percentage of patients infected with the virus. There is a 2.5% lifetime risk.[13]

Infectious Agents

EBV is associated with the development of Burkitt's lymphoma and the occurrence of aggressive non-Hodgkin lymphomas in immunosuppressed patients in Western countries. The majority of these present as primary central nervous system (CNS) lymphomas.

EBV is also associated with the occurrence of extranodal nasal T/NK cell lymphomas in Asia and South America. Infection with HIV also has the predisposition to the development of an aggressive B cell non-Hodgkin's lymphoma. It is postulated that this is due to the overexpression of interleukin 6 (IL6) by HIV infected macrophages. Patients with the bacteria *Helicobacter pylori (H.pylori)* are predisposed to the development of MALT (mucosa associated lymphoid tissue) lymphomas. The bacterium dose not transform the lymphocytes to produce the lymphoma like HIV; instead, a strong immune response is made to the infective bacterium and the chronic antigenic stimulation leads to the development of the neoplasia.[14]

Chronic hepatitis C viral infection (HCV) is associated with the development of lymphoplasmacytic lymphoma. Human herpes virus 8 (HHV8) is associated with the development of lymphoma in HIV infected patients that leads to a primary effusion lymphoma with diffuse lymphadenopathy associated with systemic symptoms of fever, malaise and cachexia called Multicentric Castleman's disease.[15]

Staging

In Hodgkin lymphoma and non-Hodgkin lymphoma staging is similar. Determining an accurate anatomic stage is an important part of the evaluation. The Ann Arbor staging system is commonly used and was originally developed for Hodgkin's disease.[10]

Lymphoid Disorder Confusion[9]

These disorders can present as chronic leukemia and be confused with typical B cell chronic lymphoid leukemia (CLL).

- Follicular lymphoma
- Splenic marginal zone lymphoma
- Nodal marginal zone lymphoma
- Mantle cell lymphoma
- Hairy cell leukemia
- Prolymphocytic leukemia (B cell or T cell)
- Lymphoplasmacytic lymphoma
- Sézary syndrome
- Smoldering adult T cell leukemia/lymphoma

WHO Classification of Lymphoid Malignancies[9]

B Cell	T Cell	Hodgkin Disease
Precursor B cell neoplasm Precursor B lymphoblastic leukemia/lymphoma (precursor B cell acute lymphoblastic leukemia)	Precursor T cell neoplasm Precursor T lymphoblastic lymphoma/leukemia (precursor T cell acute lymphoblastic leukemia)	Nodular lymphocyte-predominant Hodgkin's disease
Mature (peripheral) B cell neoplasms	Mature (peripheral) T cell neoplasms	Classic Hodgkin disease
B cell chronic lymphocytic leukemia/small lymphocytic lymphoma	T cell prolymphocytic leukemia	Nodular sclerosis Hodgkin disease
B cell prolymphocytic leukemia	T cell granular lymphocytic leukemia	Lymphocyte-rich classic Hodgkin's disease
Lymphoplasmacytic lymphoma	Aggressive NK cell leukemia	Mixed-cellularity Hodgkin disease
Splenic marginal zone B cell lymphoma (± villous lymphocytes)	Adult T cell lymphoma/leukemia (HTLV-I+)	Lymphocyte-depletion Hodgkin disease
Hairy cell leukemia	Extranodal NK/T cell lymphoma, nasal type	
Plasma cell myeloma/plasmacytoma	Enteropathy-type T cell lymphoma	
Extranodal marginal zone B cell lymphoma of MALT type	T cell lymphoma	
Mantle cell lymphoma	Subcutaneous panniculitis-like T cell lymphoma	
Follicular lymphoma	Mycosis fungoides/Sézary syndrome	
Nodal marginal zone B cell lymphoma (± monocytoid B cells)	Anaplastic large cell lymphoma, primary cutaneous type	
Diffuse large B cell lymphoma	Peripheral T cell lymphoma, not otherwise specified (NOS)	
Burkitt's lymphoma/ Burkitt's cell leukemia	Angioimmunoblastic T cell lymphoma	
	Anaplastic large cell lymphoma, primary systemic type	

Infectious Agents Associated with Developing Lymphoid Cancers [14]

Infectious Agent	Lymphoid Malignancy
Epstein-Barr virus	Burkitt's lymphoma Post–organ transplant lymphoma Primary CNS diffuse large B cell lymphoma Hodgkin's disease Extranodal NK/T cell lymphoma, nasal type
HTLV-I	Adult T cell leukemia/lymphoma
HIV	Diffuse large B cell lymphoma Burkitt's lymphoma
Hepatitis C virus	Lymphoplasmacytic lymphoma
Helicobacter pylori	Gastric MALT lymphoma
Human herpes virus 8	Primary effusion lymphoma Multicentric Castleman's disease

Ann Arbor Staging System [10]

Stage	Definition
I	Involvement of a single lymph node region or lymphoid structure (e.g., spleen, thymus, Waldeyer's ring)
II	Involvement of two or more lymph node regions on the same side of the diaphragm (the mediastinum is a single site; hilar lymph nodes should be considered "lateralized" and, when involved on both sides, constitute stage II disease)
III	Involvement of lymph node regions or lymphoid structures on both sides of the diaphragm
III 1	Subdiaphragmatic involvement limited to spleen, splenic hilar nodes, celiac nodes, or portal nodes
III 2	Subdiaphragmatic involvement includes paraaortic, iliac, or mesenteric nodes plus structures in III1
IV	Involvement of extranodal sites beyond that designated as "E" More than one extranodal deposit at any location Any involvement of liver or bone marrow
IV A	No symptoms
IV B	Unexplained weight loss of >10% of the body weight during the 6 months before staging investigation Unexplained, persistent, or recurrent fever with temperatures >38°C during the previous month Recurrent drenching night sweats during the previous month
IV E	Localized, solitary involvement of extralymphatic tissue, excluding liver and bone marrow

Assessment
BONE MARROW INFILTRATION[15]

The gold standard for diagnosis is bone marrow infiltration, which may show the following signs in late stage disease:

- Anemia: low RBC, low Hgb, Hrc
- Thrombocytopenia: platelets <100,000/uL signifies high tumor burden
- Leukopenia: absolute neutrophil count <1,000/uL signifies high burden; hyperleukocytosis in B/T-cell lymphoblastic lymphoma
- Sedimentation rate: over normal limits
- LDH : elevated LDH is considered a tumor marker for lymphoma[30]
- Viral infections: increased incidence with:
  - Epstein-Barr Virus (EBV) specifically Burkitt's
  - EpsteiHuman Immunodeficiency Virus (HIV)
  - EpsteiHepatitis B, Hepatitis C
- Hypercalcemia: present in 15% of NHL; more common in HTLV-1 associated adult T-cell lymphoma
- Hyperuricemia: typically seen during initial treatment of rapidly proliferating non Hodgkin lymphoma (NHL)

NHL prognosis
Prognosis for patients with NHL is assigned by using the International Prognostic Index (IPI). This predicts for all subtypes of NHL.[16]

DIAGNOSTIC SEQUENCING
Non Hodgkin Lymphoma

In patients with suspected NHL, evaluation typically starts with a CBC, ESR, and organ function studies; CT scans of the chest, abdomen and pelvis; and a bone marrow biopsy. Although CT (computed tomography) is routinely used to evaluate NHL patients, PET or gallium scans are used for aggressive subtypes like diffuse large B cell lymphoma. Additionally, serum levels of LDH (lactate dehydrogenase), 2-microgloblulin, and serum protein electrophoresis should be included. If NHL is suspected, a series of other tests should be arranged.

1. Lymph node biopsy:[17]
- Used for diagnoses and prognosis
- Immunophenotypic and cytogenetic studies helpful when conventional histology is ambiguous
- Improved detection of minimal disease
- Flow cytometry standardly used to verify
2. Fine-needle aspiration used only when biopsy impossible[17]

3. Bone marrow aspiration:[17]
- If it exhibits positive cells, patient is automatically placed in most advanced stage
- May see atypical cells in peripheral smear with bone marrow involvement
4. Tumor markers[17]
- Beta-2 microglobulin (serum):
  - Useful in indolent lymphomas
  - Prognostic marker
  - Surrogate measure of disease volume
  - Monitors response to therapy
- Lactate dehydrogenase (LDH):
  - Isoenzymes 2 & 3 for pretreatment prognostic variable for survival
  - Isoenzymes 4 & 5 for reflect post-chemotherapy myeloid regeneration
5. Prognostic markers (newer)[17]
- nm23-H1 (serum):
  - Nucleoside dephosphate kinase enzyme activity involved in tumor metastasis regulation
  - Increased levels in aggressive variants
  - 5-year overall survival in patients with diffuse large B-cell NHL
    - <80 ng/mL vs. >80 ng/mL is 78% vs. 6% respectively
- Basic fibroblast growth factor (bFGF) and vascular endothelial growth factor (VEGF)
  - Both potent stimulators of angiogenesis
  - Higher serum levels associated with increased relative risk of death
- BCL-6 gene: improved survival in diffuse large B-cell lymphoma

6. Immunoglobulin studies[17]
- Used to detect hypogammaglobulinemia or monoclonal paraprotein in small lymphocytic lymphoma
- IgM paraprotein may contribute to hyperviscosity symptoms in Waldenstrom's macroglobulinemia (lymphoplasmacytoid lymphoma)

Hodgkin Lymphoma

Like NHL, evaluation of patients with suspected Hodgkin disease typically starts with a CBC, ESR and organ function studies, as well as CT scans of the chest, abdomen and pelvis, and a bone marrow biopsy.[17] Neither a PET scan nor a gallium scan are necessary to stage Hodgkin lymphoma, but in most cases these scans help to assign the anatomic stage and the development of a treatment plan. One of these tests should be performed at the completion of the treatment regimen to evaluate any persistent radiographic abnormalities, with particular interest to the mediastinum.

If Hodgkin lymphoma is suspected, a series of other tests should be arranged.

1. Pathology[17]
◆ Look for Reed-Sternberg cells
2. Fine-needle aspiration
◆ May be suggestive, but not adequate for diagnoses
◆ Indicated for patients with B symptoms or low blood counts
◆ B symptoms include night sweats, fevers, weight loss
3. Immunophenotyping
Classical:
◆ Positive CD30, CD15, B-cell-specific activating protein
◆ CD20 positive in 40% classical, but weak staining in minority of cells
Nodular Lymphocyte-predominant Hodgkin's:
◆ Positive CD20, negative CD30 & CD15
◆ T-cell-rich B-cell Lymphoma
◆ Positive CD20 & CD45, negative CD30 & CD15
CD20: 40% of Hodgkins

Conventional Treatment for Non Hodgkin Lymphomas
MALT TYPE LYMPHOMA

Extranodal marginal zone B cell lymphoma of the MALT type comprises up 8% of all non Hodgkin lymphomas. It is a small cell that presents in extranodal sites and was previously considered a small lymphocytic lymphoma or pseudolymphoma until it was recognized that there was an association between an infection with *H. pylori* in the gut and the appearance of these small extranodal cells. A hemopathologist can make an accurate diagnosis by the pattern of infiltration of the small lymphocytes that are monoclonal B cells and CD5-. At times, there may be a mixed cellularity due to a transformation of the small B cell infiltrates to diffuse large B cells. A dual diagnosis can be made within the same biopsy.[18]

These lesions may occur in the stomach, intestine, orbit, lung, thyroid, salivary gland, skin, soft tissues, bladder, kidney, and CNS. It can be associated with local symptoms or present as a new mass found upon routine examination. Patients with gastric lymphoma need to have studies that look for the presence or

Prognosis
Most patients with extranodal marginal B cell lymphoma MALT type have a good prognosis with a 5-year survival rate of 75%. The IPI score is a prognostic predictor in survival rate with a low score showing a 5-year survival rate of 90% and a high score dropping that survival rate to 40%.[18]

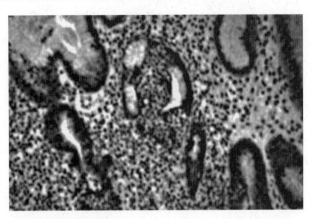

Malt Type Lymphoma
Involves the mucosa-associated lymphoid tissue (MALT), frequently of the stomach, but virtually any mucosal site can be afflicted. It is a cancer originating from B cells in the marginal zone of the MALT, and is also called extranodal marginal zone B cell lymphoma.

absence of the infective bacteria, and endoscopic studies that include ultrasound to define the extent of the disease and organ involvement. MALT lymphomas are localized to the organ of origin in 40% of cases and to the organ and regional lymph nodes in 30% of patients.[18] However, distant metastasis can occur – particularly with transformation to diffuse large B cell lymphoma. Many patients who develop this lymphoma will have an autoimmune or inflammatory process, such as Sjögren's syndrome (salivary gland MALT), Hashimoto's thyroiditis (thyroid MALT), or *Helicobacter* gastritis (gastric MALT).[19]

Surgery
Treatment specific for extranodal marginal B cell lymphoma MALT type is curable if the disease is localized. Surgery can be an effective cure in these cases.[20]

Antibiotics
There is a cofactor infection with *H. pylori*, so eradicating the bacterium will achieve remission of the lymphoma in the majority of cases. These remissions can last, but because of residual neoplastic cells, long-term monitoring for recurrence should be part of the treatment protocol.[21]

Ninety-five percent of gastric MALT lymphomas are associated with *H. pylori* infection, and those that are not usually express t(11;18).[22] The t(11;18) typically results in activation of NF-B, which acts a survival factor for the cells. Lymphomas with t(11;18) translocations are genetically stable and do not evolve to diffuse large B cell lymphoma. By contrast, t(11;18)-negative MALT lymphomas often acquire *BCL6* mutations and progress to aggressive histology lymphoma.[22]

Chemotherapy

Patients who have more extensive disease are usually treated with a single agent chemotherapeutic, such aschlorambucil. If there is a mixed cellularity at the time of diagnosis in an extensive disease presentation, then combination chemotherapies are utilized.[23]

MANTLE CELL LYMPHOMA

Mantle cell lymphoma comprises about 6% of all NHL. It has been recognized as a separate cancer only in the past decade, with its existence confirmed by a characteristic chromosomal translocation, $t(11;14)$ between immunoglobulin heavy chain gene on chromosome 14 and the *bcl-1* gene on chromosome 11. This causes an overexpression of the BCL-1 protein.[24]

Diagnosis is made by a hemopathologist based on morphology of the cell and the B cell tumor, usually showing a highly indented nucleus. There is also a characteristic expression of CD5. The most common clinical presentation is palpable lymphadenopathy with frequent systemic symptoms.[25]

Unfortunately, about 70% of patients will be in stage IV of their disease at the time of diagnosis; this means that there is usually bone marrow and peripheral blood involvement. Patients who present with lymphomatosis polyposis in the large intestine usually have mantle cell lymphoma. Evaluation for Mantle cell lymphoma is the same as NHL.[25]

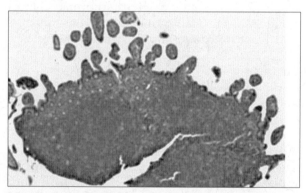

Mantle Cell Lymphoma
Subtype of B-cell lymphoma due to CD5 positive antigen-naive pregerminal center B-cell within the mantle zone that surrounds normal germinal center follicles. One of the rarest of the non-Hodgkin's lymphomas, comprising about 6% of NHL cases.

Prognosis
5-year survival rates for all patients (no matter what stage) with Mantle cell lymphoma are poor, at 25%. Patients with a high IPI score often do not survive for 5 years, while only 50% with a low IPI score survive to 5 years.[26]

Treatment

The reason for the low survival rates is that treatments for this type of lymphoma are unsatisfactory. Localized disease can be treated with combination chemo/radio therapies, while disseminated disease has been treated aggressively but with only a minority of patients achieving remission. In younger patients, more aggressive combination chemotherapy regimens are used, followed by autologous or allogeneic bone marrow transplants.[26]

FOLLICULAR LYMPHOMA

Approximately, 22% of all NHL worldwide are follicular lymphomas, with at least 30% of all NHL diagnosed in the United States.[4] This has been considered a low-grade lymphoma in the past and is typically diagnosed by a hemopathologist. The tumor is composed of small cleaved and large cells in varying proportions that are organized in a follicular growth pattern.[27]

The most common clinical presentation in follicular lymphoma is new, painless lymphadenopathy. Typically, multiple sites are involved with essentially any organ and extranodal presentations. Clinically, patients do not experience fevers, sweats, and weight loss as associated with other lymphomas: IPI scores remain low with these patients.[27]

Confirmation of diagnosis is made with B cell immunophenotyping showing a $t(14;18)$ and the abnormal expression of BCL-2 protein. Often follicular lymphoma is classified into subtypes based on cells size: those with predominately small cells; those with mixed cellularity; and those with predominately large cells. There is an associated prognostic feature to subtyping as those patients with predominantly large cell

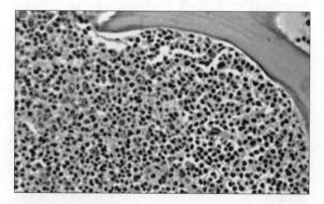

Follicular Lymphoma
The normal nodal architecture is effaced by nodular expansions of tumor cells. Nodules vary in size and contain predominantly small lymphocytes with cleaved nuclei along with variable numbers of larger cells with vesicular chromatin and prominent nucleoli.

type have a higher proliferation rate and their disease progresses more rapidly, resulting in a shorter survival rate even with chemotherapy regimens.[28]

Chemotherapy

Treatment with chemical and radiation therapies gives good response rates, with as many as 25% of patients having spontaneous remission without any intervention. Watchful waiting strategies are used in asymptomatic patients, especially in the elderly. For patients who need chemotherapy, single agent chemotherapeutics, such as chlorambucil or cyclophosphamide, are options. Combination chemotherapeutics can also be used, with the most frequent being the CHOP or CVP combinations. (CHOP = cyclophosphamide, doxorubicin, vincristine, prednisone; CVP = cyclophosphamide, vincristine, prednisone.) These therapies have helped 50% to 75% of patients achieve complete remission with a median relapse being after 2 years; 20% of patients will be complete responders and remain in remission for greater than a decade.[29]

Several new therapies have been shown to be effective in the treatment of follicular lymphoma: cytotoxic agents like fludarabine; biologic agents like interferon; monoclonal antibodies (rituximab) with or without radionucleotides; and lymphoma vaccines.[30]

DIFFUSE LARGE B CELL LYMPHOMA

This is the most common type of NHL, representing almost one third of all cases diagnosed. It is classified as an aggressive or intermediate grade lymphoma. A hemopathologist can make an accurate diagnosis with biopsied cells and proving the B cell immunophenotype is present. Other studies, such as genetic markers, s are not necessary for a diagnosis of this lymphoma, although there has been some evidence that shows that patients who overexpress the BCL-2 protein might be more likely to relapse from their cancer than those without that overexpression. Patients who have mediastinal involvement are sometimes diagnosed as a subtype with statistics of a younger median age (37 years) and more predominant in females by 66%.[28-29]

Diffuse Large B cell lymphoma can present either as lymphadenopathy with primary lymph node disease, or at extranodal sites. More than 50% of patients with this diagnosis have some extranodal involvement upon diagnosis, with the most common sites being the GI tract and bone marrow. Any organ can be affected, and a proper diagnostic biopsy becomes important for a correct diagnosis and treatment strategy. Primary diffuse B cell lymphoma of the brain has shown a diagnostic frequency due to the improved evaluation methods for this lymphoma.[28-29]

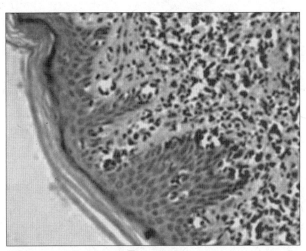

Diffuse Large B Cell Lymphoma
The neoplastic cells are heterogeneous but predominantly large cells with vesicular chromatin and prominent nucleoli.

After a careful staging evaluation, 50% of patients will be found to have stage I or II disease and 50% will have widely disseminated lymphoma. Bone marrow biopsy shows involvement by lymphoma in about 15% of cases, with marrow involvement by small cells more frequent than with large cells.[28-29]

Chemotherapy

Initial treatment for all patients with diffuse large B cell lymphoma is with a combination chemotherapy regimen. In the United States, CHOP is the most popular combination therapy, with rituximab sometimes added. Patients with stage I and II disease usually receive 3 to 4 cycles of the combination chemotherapy, which is then followed with radiation to the involved field. These results have shown to be equal if not superior to 6 to 8 cycles of combination chemotherapy yielding cure rates of 60% to 70% in stage II disease and 80% to 90% in stage I disease. In patients with stage II-IV disease, 8 cycles of combination chemo (CHOP) plus rituximab are usually used.[30,31]

Prognosis

The best predictor of prognosis is the IPI score, which was initially developed to predict outcome in patients with diffuse large B cell lymphoma. For 35% of patients with a low IPI score of under 1, 5-year survival rate is >70%; for 20% of patients with a high IPI score of 4-5, the 5-year survival rate is 20%. Other factors that affect prognosis and survival include levels of circulating cytokines, molecular features of the tumor itself, and soluble receptors.[31]

BURKITT'S LYMPHOMA/LEUKEMIA

Burkitt's lymphoma can also be classified as aleukemia. It is a rare disease in adults in the United States, with the exception of those infected with HIV. Only 1% of NHLis Burkitt's in adults, but up to 30% of childhood NHLs are Burkitt's. L3ALL (Burkitt's leukemia) makes up a small portion of childhood and adult acute leukemias. Burkitt's lymphoma is diagnosed by a hemopathologist with a high degree of accuracy.[33]

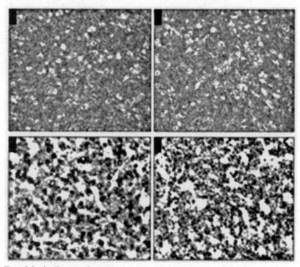

Burkitt's Lymphoma
The neoplastic cells are homogenous, medium-sized B cells with frequent mitotic figures, a morphologic correlate of high growth fraction. Reactive macrophages are scattered through the tumor and their pale cytoplasm in a background of blue-staining tumor cells give the tumor a so-called starry sky appearance.

Histopathology not only shows homogenous, medium sized cells but also a very high proliferation fraction with the presence of the t(2;8) the c-myc and light chain gene or the presence of t(8;22) c-myc and the light chain gene which are both confirmatory. Burkitt's cell leukemia is recognized by the monotonous mass of medium sized cells with round nuclei, multiple nuclei, and basophilic cytoplasm with cytoplasmic vacuoles. A positive diagnosis is made with the demonstration of B cell immunophenotype and one of the above cytogenetic abnormalities.[33]

Most patients in the USA present with peripheral lymphadenopathy or an intraabdominal mass. This disease typically progresses rapidly to metastasize in the CNS. Burkitt's is one of the most rapidly progressive human tumors. Cerebral spinal fluid should always be evaluated upon initial diagnosis.[32]

Chemotherapy

Because of its aggressive nature, treatment for Burkitt's should begin with 48 hours of diagnosis at any age. Intensive combination chemotherapies usually incorporate a high dose of cyclophosphamide. Prophylactic intrathecal chemotherapy to the CNS is mandatory. Burkitt's has a high cure rate of 70% to 80% if treatment is administered early and precisely. Once salvage therapy is needed, it is usually ineffective.[28-32]

CUTANEOUS T CELL LYMPHOMA (MYCOSIS FUNGOIDES)

This is a dermatological lymphoma with the median age of onset in the mid fifties, more common in males than females and blacks than whites.[31] It is an indolent lymphoma with patients usually experiencing years of eczema or dermatitis with a progression from a patch stage to a plague stage to the formation of cutaneous tumors. In advanced stages, this lymphoma can advance to metastasize to lymph nodes and visceral organs. Sézary's syndrome can be found in advanced stages with erythrodermal and circulating tumor cells.[34]

Treatment has a poor prognosis. Rarely does a patient in early stage localized disease attain a cure with radiotherapy (total skin electron beam irradiation). Other treatments are considered only palliative – topical glucocorticoids, topical nitrogen mustard, phototherapy, psoralen with ultraviolet A (PUVA), electron beam radiation, interferon, antibodies, fusion toxins, and systemic cytotoxic therapies.[34]

ADULT T CELL LYMPHOMA/LEUKEMIA

This disease is directly related to HTLV-1 retrovirus infection. If nationwide testing for HTLV-1 antibodies were done as a public health measure, this could lead to the disappearance of adult T cell lymphoma/leukemia. Patients who are infected can transmit the virus through blood transfusion, sexual contact, and transplacentally. Babies who acquire the HTLV-1 through breast milk are most likely to develop lymphoma; the overall risk is 2.5% but the latency averages 55 years. A shorter latency (1-3 years) is most common in people who acquire the virus as adults during sex or a transfusion.[31]

Diagnosis is made by a hemopathologist by recognizing the typical morphological picture of a T cell immunophenotype of malignant cells with the existence of antibodies to HTLV-1. Peripheral blood examination will show pleomorphic abnormal CD4+ cells with indented nuclei, called "flower" cells. Most patients present with aggressive disease that includes clinical symptoms of lymphadenopathy, hepatosplenomegaly, skin infiltrates, hypercalcemia, lytic bone lesions, and elevated LDH levels. It infiltrates the skin and manifests as lesions that can be papules, plaques, tumors, or ulcerations.[35]

Treatment is with combination chemotherapy regimens with the median survival rate of only about 7 months.[35]

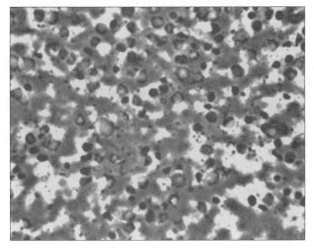

Adult T Cell Lymphoma
Peripheral blood smear showing leukemia cells with typical "flower-shaped" nucleus.

ANAPLASTIC LARGE T/NULL CELL LYMPHOMA

This lymphoma was previously diagnosed as undifferentiated carcinoma or malignant histiocytosis, but the discovery of the CD30 (Ki-1) antigen led to the identification of a new type of lymphoma. Discovery of the t(2;5) and the frequent overexpression of the anaplastic lymphoma kinase (ALK) protein has confirmed the existence of this lymphoma. It accounts for 2% of all NHL. Patients with this type of lymphoma are typically young in age (median age 33 yo) and mostly male (70%); 50% of patients present with stage I or II of the disease at the time of diagnosis. Symptoms include elevated LDH (in 50% of patients) with frequent skin manifestations.[36]

Treatment regimens used for other aggressive types of lymphomas, such as diffuse large B cell, are used. This lymphoma surprisingly has the best survival rate out of any of the aggressive lymphomas. The 5-year survival rate is >75%, with the overexpression of the ALK protein an important prognostic factor due to treatments that can target this overexpression.[37]

PERIPHERAL T CELL LYMPHOMA

This lymphoma represents 7% of all NHL cases, and makes up a group of heterogenous morphologically aggressive cancers that share a mature T cell immunophenotype. Diagnosis is made by a hemopathologist via an adequate biopsy and immunophenotyping. Most peripheral T cell lymphomas are CD4+, but a few can be CD8+, or both CD4+ and CD8+, or can be an NK cell immunophenotype. Peripheral T cell lymphomas are associated with poor IPI scores and poor outcomes. Only about 25% of patients survive past 5 years from the time of diagnosis, not treatment.[31]

Treatment regimens are the same as for other aggressive lymphomas, such as diffuse large B cell, but have a poorer response rate to these treatments. In young patients, hematopoietic stem cell transplantation is often considered as an early intervention in this population due to the poor prognosis and outcomes associated with this cancer.[39]

ENTEROPATHY-TYPE INTESTINAL T CELL LYMPHOMA

This is a rare lymphoma associated with untreated glutin sensitive enteropathy. Patients present with cachexia and sarcopenia, often with an intestinal perforation. The prognosis is poor due to a poor response to treatment. Hemophagocytic syndrome is common with the symptoms of profound anemia, ingestion of erythrocytes by monocytes, and macrophages that lead to fatality in the patient.[38]

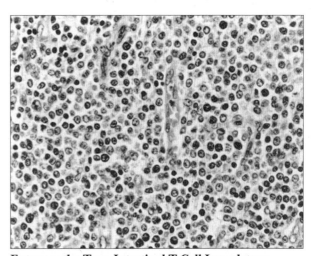

Enteropathy-Type Intestinal T Cell Lymphoma

Conventional Treatment for Lymphomas

HODGKIN LYMPHOMA

Classic Hodgkin's disease occurs in approximately 8,000 patients annually in the United States, without a noted increase in frequency. Most patients present with palpable, nontender lymphadenopathy, with the most frequent lymph nodes involved being in the neck, supraclavicular area, and the axilla. More than 50% of these patients have mediastinal adenopathy at the time of initial diagnosis. About one-third of patients present with fevers, night sweats, and/or weight loss, which are the B symptoms in the Ann Arbor staging schedule.[40]

Fever of unknown origin can often be the presenting feature of Hodgkin's lymphoma and can have unusual presentation of clinical symptoms. These include severe and unexplained pruritus, cutaneous disorders, such as erythema nodosum and ichthyosiform atrophy, paraneoplastic cerebellar degeneration, and other effects on the CNS, nephritic syndromes, immune hemolytic anemia and thrombocytopenia, hypercalcemia, and pain in the lymph nodes with ingestion of alcohol.[40]

Definitive diagnosis is made by a hemopathologist and an adequate biopsy specimen. In the United States, most patients have a nodular sclerosing Hodgkin's lymphoma. The mixed cellularity Hodgkin's or lymphocyte depletion Hodgkin's are associated with patients infected with HIV.[40]

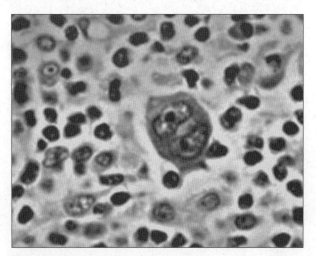

Mixed Cellularity Hodgkin Disease
A Reed-Sternberg cell is present near the center of the field; a large cell with a bilobed nucleus and prominent nucleoli giving an "owl's eyes" appearance. The majority of the cells are normal lymphocytes, neutrophils, and eosinophils that form a pleiomorphic cellular infiltrate.

To stage Hodgkin lymphoma, evaluation of the patient would include HxPE, CBC with a differential, ESR, serum chemistry panel that would include LDH, chest x-ray or CT scan (may include abdomen, pelvis), and bone marrow biopsy. Many patients should also have a PET scan or a gallium scan to document the onset of disease progress before treatment and to document remission after treatment completion.[41]

Chemotherapy

Initially, patients at all stages of Hodgkin's lymphoma are treated with chemotherapy. Patients with localized disease may receive a brief course of chemotherapy followed by radiation therapy to the nodes and sites involved.[42] Patients with more extensive disease (the B symptoms of Ann Arbor staging) receive a complete course of chemotherapy. The regimens used include doxorubicin, bleomycine, vinblastine, dacarbazine (ABVD) or mechlorethamine, vincristine, procarbazine, and prednisone (MOPP), or combination of these drugs in these two regimens. In the United States, most patients receive the ABVD. Treatments for patients with localized Hodgkin lymphoma has a high cure rate of >90%.[43]

Naturopathic Approaches to Treating Lymphomas

Naturopathic protocols for treating lymphomas are similar to therapeutic strategies for managing leukemias. Naturopathic integrative strategies outlined in previous chapters can be utilized without concern, except that melatonin should not to be used in any of the lymphomas, leukemias, or myelogenous cancers because it could affect cellular differentiation and make matters worse, immunologically speaking.

Naturopathic Therapeutic Protocol
1. Manage anemia by enhancing capacity of blood to carry oxygen and iron – B6, B12, folic acid, iron chelate
2. Avoid specific immune modulating treatments for specific cell types
3. Alleviate side effects with Glutamine
4. Counsel patients on lifestyle
5. Monitor for B-symptoms: afternoon fatigue and night sweats; weight loss; anemia (pallor etc.); fever and chills, pruritis; pain in lymph nodes after
6. First do no harm: caution melatonin

Chemotherapeutic and Naturopathic Integrated Therapies

Chemotherapeutic	Naturopathic	Daily Dose	Caution
Single agent chemotherapies: Chlorambucil Cyclophosphamide Doxorubincin Fludarabine Interferon Rituximab (with or without radioneucleuotides)	*To increase effectiveness:* Medicinal mushroom combinations are indicated for lymphomas and can be used during treatments with conventional therapies *To reduce toxicity and side effects:*[89]	Tremetes 7 and Turkey tails Ashwagandha	
Combination chemotherapies: CHOP= Cyclophosphamide Doxorubicin Vincristine Prednisone	Mucositis Nausea Vomiting Diarrhea Glutamine Honey Aloe	10 gm tid, swish & swallow	
CHOP+rituximab			
CVP= Cyclophosphamide Vincristine Prednisone			
ABVD= Doxorubicin Bleomycine Vinblastine Dacarbazine			

Mycomedicinals

Several fungi have been used traditionally as medicines for treating various cancers, including lymphoma. Recent improvement in chemical technology has allowed the isolation and purification of the relevant compounds in these medicinal mushrooms. Of specific interest are the polysaccharides, which contain demonstrable anticancer activities. Most appear to act as immune system enhancers, though some can have direct cytotoxic effects on cancer cells. Only a small number have progressed successfully to objective clinical assessment in human trials.[44-49]

Medically accepted species of mycomedicinals[44]

- *Ganoderma lucidum* (reishi or ling zhi)
- *Lentinus* (*Lentinula*)
- *Edodes* (Shiitake)
- *Phellinus linteus*
- *Porio cocos*
- *Auricularia auricula*
- *Hericium erinaceus*
- *Grifola frondosa* (Maitake)
- *Flammulina velutipes*
- *Pleurotus ostreatus* (oyster mushroom)
- *Trametes* (*Coriolus*)
- *versicolor* (turkey tails)
- *Tremella fuciformis*
- *Schizophyllum commune*
- *Cordyceps sinensis* (caterpillar fungus, not a mushroom)

Mushrooms with activity against specific cancers[45]

Breast	*Grifola frondosa, Lentinula elodes, Trametes versicolor*
Cervical/Uterine	*Agaricus blazei, Inonotus obliquus, Phellinus linteus, Schizophyllum commune, Trametes versicolor*
Colorectal	*Agaricus blazei, Grifola frondosa, Phellinus linteus*
Gastric/Stomach	*Hericium erinaceus, Phellinus linteus, Schizophyllum commune, Trametes versicolor*
Leukemia	*Cordyceps sinensis, Ganoderma lucidum, Grifola frondosa, Polysporus umbellatus, Trametes versicolor*
Liver	*Ganoderma lucidum, Grifola frondosa, Lentinula edodes, Phellinus linteus, Polysporus umbellatus, Trametes versicolor*
Lung	*Cordyceps sinensis, Ganoderma lucidum, Grifola frondosa, Polysporus umbellate, Trametes versicolor*
Lymphoma	*Cordyceps sinensis, Flammulina veluptipes*
Melanoma	*Lentinula edodes, Phellinus linteus*
Prostate	*Flammulina veluptipes, Ganoderma lucidum, Grifola frondosa, Lentinula edodes, Trametes versicolor*
Sarcoma	*Agaricus blazei, Ganoderma lucidum, Pleurotus ostreatus*

POLYSACCHARIDES

The antitumor polysaccharides isolated from mushrooms (fruit-body, submerged, cultured mycelial biomass, or liquid culture broth) are either water-soluble β-D-glucans, β-D-glucans with heterosaccharide chains of xylose, mannose, galactose or uronic acid, or β-D-glucan-protein complexes – proteoglycans.[44] Some are orally bioavailable. The main medically important polysaccharide compounds that have undergone clinical trials include lentinan from *Lentinus edodes*, schizophyllan from *Schizophyllum commune*, PSK and PSP from *Trametes versicolor*, and Grifron-D from *Grifola frondosa*. Mushroom-derived glucan and polysaccharo-peptides can act as immunomodulators. The ability of these compounds to enhance or suppress immune responses depends on a number of factors, including dosage, route of administration, timing and frequency of administration, mechanism of action, and the site of activity.[44-49]

CELLULAR EFFECTS

Several mushroom compounds have shown to potentiate the non-specific and specific immune responses. They also activate many kinds of immune cells that are important for the maintenance of homeostasis in the immune system: host cells (such as cytotoxic macrophages, monocytes, neutrophils, natural killer cells, dendritic cells) and cytokines (chemical messengers such as interleukins, interferon, colony stimulating factors) that trigger complement and acute phase responses. They can also be considered as multi-cytokine inducers able to induce gene expression of various immunomodulatory cytokines and cytokine receptors. Lymphocytes governing antibody production and cell mediated cytotoxicity (T-cells) are also stimulated. Lentinan and Schizophyllan are T-cell oriented immunopotentiators and require a functional T-cell component for biological activity by way of increasing helper T-cell production, increased macrophage production leading to a stimulation of acute phase proteins and colony stimulating factors which in turn affect proliferation of macrophages, neutrophils and lymphocytes, and activation of the complement system.[44-54] PSK and PSP (polysaccharides) are potent immunostimulators with specific activity for T-cells and for antigen-presenting cells, such as monocytes and macrophages. Their biological activity is characterized by their ability to increase white blood cell counts, interferon-γ and interleukin-2 production and delayed type hypersensitivity reactions.[44-49] This ability to effectively increase white blood cell counts helps in the integrative strategy with lymphoma/leukemia as these white cell lines are often affected in the combination chemotherapeutics creating a neutropenia that may interfere with the sequence and amount of chemotherapy to be administered.

MUSHROOM STUDIES

There have been extensive *in vivo* studies demonstrating the anticancer activity of the glucan polysaccharides and polysaccharide-peptides in animal probands. These studies strongly indicate an immunomodulating mode of action from these polysaccharides. However, in *in vitro* studies on various cancer cell lines, there is even stronger evidence for direct cytotoxic effects on the cancer cells for some, but not all, of the polysaccharides. Many of the mushroom polysaccharides have proceeded through Phase I, II, and III clinical trials, mainly in Japan and China but now in the United States.

Lentinan

L.edodes has demonstrated strong antitumor activity in a wide range of cancers, and with human clinical trials it has proven successful in prolonging survival rates, especially for patients with gastric and colorectal cancer.[45-55] Lentinan has been approved as a drug in Japan and is considered an important adjuvant treatment for several cancers.[44] Schizophyllan (*S. commune*) has proved useful for recurrent and inoperable gastric cancer, as well as increasing survival times of patients with head and neck cancers. None of these compounds show any significant side-effects.

Grifron-D

There are several on-going clinical trials with Grifron-D, GD (*G. frondosa*) on breast, prostate, lung, liver, and gastric cancers underway in Japan and in the United States showing promising results. In *in vitro* studies, GD appears to inactivate glyoxalase I, an enzyme believed to metabolize chemotherapeutic compounds used against cancer cells, thus potentially enhancing their bioavailability and possible chemoresistance.

PSK and PSP

Two compounds, PSK and PSP (derived from mycelial cultures of *T. versicolor*), have evident anticancer properties when given with conventional chemotherapeutic agents and yielding no increase in side-effects. PSK has successfully been used in Phase I, II and III clinical trials with cancers of the stomach, esophagus, nasopharynx, colon, rectum, lung, and breast cancer. PSK gave protection against the immunosuppression that normally is associated with surgery and long-term chemotherapy effecting not only the WBC line but

keeping the innate as well as acquired immune function intact. PSK continues to be used extensively in Japan as an adjunct to standard chemo/radio therapies. PSP has been extensively studied by Chinese scientists and oncologists, with little evidence of side-effects: Clinical trials have shown efficacy in gastric, esophageal and non-small cell (NSCLC) lung cancers, and PSP has been recognized as a drug by the Chinese Ministry of Public Health. A significant observation from these studies is the apparent ability of all of the above mushroom-derived polysaccharides when administered with radiotherapy and/or chemotherapy to significantly reduce the side-effects so often encountered by patients from these cytoxic strategies.[44-59] A dose response *in vitro* study showed almost complete cell death (95%) within 24 hours of exposure to maitake D-fraction ($\geq$480 mcg/ml). Combinations of maitake D-fraction in a concentration as low as 30-60 mcg/ml with 200 microM of vitamin C were just as effective as GD alone at 480 mcg/ml: all have cytoxic cell death >90%. It was found that the bioactive β-glucans from the maitake mushroom have the cytoxic effect, presumably through oxidative stress that leads to apoptosis and ultimately cancer cell death.[55] β-glucan was also demonstrated to sensitize cytotoxic cells to carmustine (BCNU) in PC-3 cells. This activity created an associated (80%) inactivation of the glutathione dependent detoxifying enzyme, glyoxalase I (Gly-I). Thus, the BCNU/beta-glucan combination may be specific to target the Gly-1 enzyme and improve current treatment efficacy.[56]

GLUTAMINE

Glutamine (GLN) not only has a preventive effect against mucositis, stomatitis, and cachexia but a therapeutic effect against cancer cells in relation to the host's defenses and ability to tolerate chemotherapy. During times of trauma and stress to the homeobalance of the system, GLN depletion has been found to occur because of GLN consumption by lymphocytes and enterocytes in an enhanced metabolic state. As a result, GLN has gained acceptance as an essential amino acid during times of stress to the system. It not only modulates the immune system function at the gut level but also promotes faster intestinal healing, significantly decreasing the severity of mucositis/stomatitis induced by chemotherapy and radiation therapy. GLN may also enhance the selectivity of antitumor drugs by sensitizing the tumor cells to the oncological therapeutics while protecting normal cells in healthy tissues. This ability to evade chemoresistance is a very important finding to add to the strategies of integrative oncology. Dosing ranges may vary depending on the status of the patient but generally the therapeutic dose is 10 g t.i.d. swish and swallow between meals.[61]

Cannabis sativa (marijuana), indica and other spp.

Marijuana has been traditionally indicated for certain conditions as a medical herbal intervention. Medical marijuana (MM) has been legalized for use in some states, with cancer diagnosis being one of the indicated disease states for legal use.

The cannabinoids are the active constituents that effect cancer pain and nausea/vomiting. THC (delta-9-tetrahydrocannabinol) is the active cannabinoid studied for its palliative effects by preventing nausea, vomiting, and pain, while stimulating appetite stimulation and enhancing mood.[61] A literature review concluded that "THC [delta-9-tetrahydrocannabinol] is superior to placebo, and equivalent in effectiveness to other widely-used anti-emetic drugs, in its capacity to reduce the nausea and vomiting caused by some chemotherapy regimens in some cancer patients."[62] A 2003 study found "Cannabinoids – the active components of cannabis sativa and their derivatives – exert palliative effects in cancer patients by preventing nausea, vomiting and pain and by stimulating appetite. In addition, these compounds have been shown to inhibit the growth of tumor cells in culture and animal models by modulating key cell-signaling pathways. Cannabinoids are usually well tolerated, and do not produce the generalized toxic effects of conventional chemotherapies."[63,64] Marinol is a prescriptive THC in a fat soluble pill form that resembles a probiotic "pearl." While this is thought of often as an alternative to medical marijuana it is usually not prescribed correctly and not as efficacious as the combusted whole herba. It is in the combustion of the whole herba that has the most medicinal benefits. Beyond its effect on digestion, appetite stimulation and anti pain and nausea uses, medical marijuana has shown that cannabinoids arrest many kinds of cancer growths through the promotion of apoptosis and anti-angiogenesis effects.[65-74] There is evidence that shows direct antitumor activity of cannbinoids, specifically the CB1 and CB2 agonists (which includes a large range of cancer types; skin, pituitary, prostate, brain gliomas and bowel). Cannabinoids have shown in both animal and human tissues to reduce tumor blood supply, metastasis, regress the tumor burden and turn on apoptosis.[75-93]

Other journals have also reported on cannabinoids' antitumoral potential. Italian research teams reported in 1998 and 2001 that the endocannabinoid anandamide, which binds to the same brain receptors as cannabis, "potently and selectively inhibits the proliferation of human breast cancer cells in vitro" by interfering with their DNA production cycle.[79-81] Cannabis has been shown in recent studies to inhibit the growth of thyroid, prostate and colorectal cancer cells.[82-84] THC has been found to cause the death of glioma cells.[85-87] And research on pituitary cancers shows cannabinoids are key to regulating human pituitary hormone secretion.[87-90]

Medical marijuana is not only indicated for the treatment of anorexia, nausea/vomiting, hence mucositis and cachexia effectively addressed with this herb. If the patient does not want to smoke the MM, it can be combusted for them in an apparatus called a vaporizer that combusts the herba and captures the released THC in the smoke that can be inhaled without any accumulation of tar from the combustion. Other methods of delivery include eating the herba or taking it as an infusion. A tea is not a very effective mode of delivery as it is not a strong hydrophilic extraction method for the fat soluble molecule, THC. The best alternative to combustion would be to make a fat soluble extraction of the herba by emulsifying it in butter or coconut milk (high fat content). Making a ghee, or clarified butter with the above mentioned carriers allows the patient to cook with the ghee to make 'cookies, cakes' or vegetable gelatin capsules to ingest the MM.

References

1. Guyton AC, Hakk JE.Textbook of Medical Physiology. 10th ed. St Louis, MO: Saunders Co;2000.

2. Moore KL, Dalley AF, AMR Aqur. 2009. Clinically Oriented Anatomy. 6th ed. Baltimore, ON: Lippincott Williams & Wilkins;2009.

3. Young RC. Harrison's Internal Medicine, online. Chapter 89, Pancreatic Cancer, Yu Jo Chua, David Cunnignham. 2010.

4. McPhee SJ, Papadakis M A. Eds. Gonzales R, Zeiger R. Online Eds. 2009. CURRENT Medical Diagnosis & Treatment, 2009. 48th ed.

5. www.medcinenet.com

6. American Joint Committee on Cancer (AJCC). AJCC Cancer Staging Manual. 6th ed. New York, NY: Springer-New York, 2002 www.springeronline.com

7. http://www.cancer.org

8. http://www.cdc.gov

9. Jaffe ES. The 2008 WHO classification of lymphomas: implications for clinical practice and translational research. Hematology Am Soc Hematol Educ Program. 2009:523-31.

10. http://medinfo.ufl.edu/~bms5191/lymphoma/staging/annarbor.html.2012.

11. http://www.cancer.org/Cancer/Non-HodgkinLymphoma/DetailedGuide/non-hodgkin-lymphoma-risk-factors. 2012.

12. Jemal A, Bray F, Center MM, et al. Global cancer statistics. CA A Cancer Journal for Clinicians. 2011;61(2):69-90.

13. Newton R, Ferlay J, Beral V, Devesa SS. The epidemiology of non-Hodgkin's lymphoma: comparison of nodal and extra-nodal sites. Int J Cancer. 1997;72(6):923-30.

14. Engels EA. Infectious agents as causes of non-Hodgkin lymphoma. Ca Epidem Biomark Prev. 2007;16(3):401-04.

15. Carulli G, Canigiani S, Volpini M, et al. Bone marrow infiltration in B-cell non-Hodgkin's lymphomas: comparison between flow cytometry and bone marrow biopsy. Recent Prog Med. 2005;96(6):284-90.

16. http://www.cancer.org/Cancer/Non-HodgkinLymphoma/DetailedGuide/non-hodgkin-lymphoma-survival-rates 2012

17. http://www.bcshguidelines.com/documents/Lymphoma_disease_app_bcsh_042010.pdf : Parker A, Bain B, Devereux S, et al. Best Practice in Lymphoma Diagnosis and Reporting. Reviewed. 2012.

18. Freedman Am Friedberg JW. Treatment of marginal zone (MALT) lymphoma. http://www.uptodate.com/contents/treatment-of-marginal-zone-malt-lymphoma 2012

19. Wohrer S, Troch M, Streubel B, et al. MALT lymphoma in patients with autoimmune diseases: a comparative analysis of characteristics and clinical course. Leuk 2007;21(8):1812-18.

20. Malek SN, Hatfield AJ, Flinn IW. MALT lymphomas. Curr Treat Opt Oncol. 2003;4(4):269-79.

21. Steinbach G, Ford R, Glober G, et al.; Antibiotic treatment of gastric lymphoma of mucosa-associated lymphoid tissue Uncontrolled Trial. Ann of Inter Med. 1999;131(2):88-95.

22. Liu H, Ye H, Ruskone-fourmestraux A, et al. T(11;18) is a marker for all stage gastric MALT lymphomas that will not respond to H. pylori eradication. Gastro. 2002;122(5):1286-94.

23. Raderer M, Paul de Boer J. Role of chemotherapy in gastric MALT lymphoma, diffuse large B-cell lymphoma and other lymphomas. Best Pract Res Clin Gastro. 2012;24(1):19-26.

24. Bentz M, Plesch A, Bullinger L, et al. t(11;14)-positive mantle cell lymphomas exhibit complex karyotypes and share similarities with B-cell chronic lymphocytic leukemia. Genes Chromo Ca. 2000;27(3):285-94.

25. Freedman AS, Aster JC. Clinical manifestations, pathologic features, and diagnosis of mantle cell lymphoma. http://www.uptodate.com/contents/clinical-manifestations-pathologic-features-and-diagnosis-of-mantle-cell-lymphoma. 2012.

26. Abbasi MR. Mantle Cell Lymphoma. Drugs, Diseases & Procedures 2012 http://emedicine.medscape.com/article/203085-overview

27. Salles GA. Clinical features, prognosis and treatment of follicular lymphoma. Hematology Am Soc Hematol Educ Program. 2007:216-225.

28. American Cancer Society. Non-Hodgkin's lymphoma. www.cancer.org/acs/groups/cid/documents/webcontent/003126-pdf.pdf. Accessed 2011

29. US Department of Health and Human Services. National Cancer Institute. What you need to know about™ non-Hodgkin's lymphoma. www.cancer.gov/cancertopics/wyntk/non-hodgkin-lymphoma.pdf. 2011

30. Hiddemann W, Kneba M, Dreyling M, et al. Frontline therapy with rituximab added to the combination of cyclophosphamide, doxorubicin, vincristine, and prednisone (CHOP) significantly improves the outcome for patients with advanced-stage follicular lymphoma compared with therapy with CHOP alone: results of a prospective randomized study of the German low-grade lymphoma study group. Blood. 2005;106(12):3725-32.

31. http://www.cancer.gov/cancertopics/types/nonhodgkin. 2012.

32. http://www.nlm.nih.gov/medlineplus/ency/article/001308.htm .2012.

33. Blum KA, Lozanski G, Byrd JC. Adult Burkitt leukemia and lymphoma. Blood 2004;104(10):3009-20.

34. http://www.cancer.gov/cancertopics/pdq/treatment/mycosisfungoides/Patient/page1#Keypoint1. 2012.

35. http://www.uptodate.com/contents/treatment-of-adult-t-cell-leukemia-lymphoma Matsuoka M, Tabinai K. 2012.

36. Jacobsen E. Anaplastic large-cell lymphoma, T-/Null-Cell Type. The ocolii 2006;11(7):831-40.

37. Agarwal S, Ramanathan U, Naresh KN. Epstein Barr virus association and ALK gene expression in anaplastic large cell lymphoma. Hum Pathol 2002;33(2):146-52.

38. Gale J, Simmonds PD, Mead GM, et al. enteropaty-type 1inntestinal T-Cell Lymphoma: clinical features and treatment of 31 patients in a single center. JCO. 2000;18(4):795.

39. Foss FM, Zinzani PL, Vose JM, et al. Peripheral T-cell lymphoma. Blood. 2011;117(25):6756-67.

40. http://www.cancer.gov/cancertopics/types/hodgkin.2 01241. http://www.cancer.org/Cancer/HodgkinDisease/ DetailedGuide/hodgkin-disease-staging .2012.

42. http://www.nlm.nih.gov/medlineplus/ency/article/000580.htm .2012.

43. Mallick I. ABVD Chemotherapy. 2008. http://lymphoma.about.com/od/treatment/qt/abvdchemo.htm

44. Smith JE, Rowan NJ, Sullivans R. Medicinal mushrooms: their therapeutic properties and current medical usage with special emphasis on cancer treatments. Cancer Research. 2007 monograph. www.icnet.uk

45. Stamets P,Yao \wa, CD. MycoMedicinals. MycoMedia Productions, division of Fungi Perfecti, LLC. 2002:1-96.

Abstract, 87th Meeting Am. Ass. Cancer Res. (AACR) special conference

46. Kidd, P. The use of mushroom glucans and proteoglucans in cancer treatment. Alt Med Rev. 2000 5(1):4-27.

47. Ghoneum, M. NK-Immunomodualtory and anti cancer properties of (MGN-3), a modified xylose from rice bran, in 5 patients with breast cancer. The interface between basic and applied research Nov. 5-8, 1995, Baltimore, MD.

48. Ghoneum, M. Enhancement of human natural killer cell activity by modified arabinoxylane from rice bran (MGN-3). Int Nat. J of Immunotherapy. 1998;14(2);89-99.

49. Mondoa, E and Kitei, M. Sugars that heal the new healing science of glyconutrients. New York, NY: Ballantine;2001.

50. Ooi VE, Liu F. A review of pharmacological activities of mushroom polysaccharides. Int J of Medicinal Mushrooms. 1999.;1:195-206.

51. Ooi VE, et al. Immunomodulation and anticancer activity of polysaccharide protein complexes. Curr Med Chem. 2000 July;7(7);710-29.

52. Koh, JH, Yu KW, Suh HJ, Choi YM, Ahn TS. Activation of macrophages ant the intestinal immune system by an orally administered decoction from cultured mycelia of Cordyceps sinensis. Biosci biotechnol Biochem. 2002. Feb 66(2):407-11.

53. Zhou S, Gao Y. The immunomodulating effects of Ganoderma lucidum(Curt:Fr) P. Karst (Ling Zhi, Reishi mushroom) Aphyllophoromycetideae. International J of Medicinal Mushrooms. 2002.4(1):1-12.

54. Sugimachi K, Maehara Y, Ogawa M, Kakegawa T, Tomita M. Dose intensity of uracil and tegafur in postoperative chemotherapy for patients with poorly differentiated gastric cancer. Cancer chemotherapy and pharmacology.1997; 40(3):233-38.

55. Fullerton SA, Samadi AA, Tortorelis DG, et al. Induction of apoptosis in human prostatic cancer cells with beta-glucan (Maitake mushroom polysaccharide). Mol Urol. 2000;4(1):7-13.

56. Finkelstein MP, Aynehchi S, Samadi AA, Drinis S, Choudhury MS, Tazaki H, Konno S. Chemosensitization of carmustine with maitake ≤-glucan on androgen-independent prostatic cancer cells: involvement of glyoxalase I. J Altern Complement Med. 2002;8:573-80.

57. Cui FJ, Li Y, Xu YY, et al. Induction of apoptosis in SGC-7901 cells by polysaccharide-peptide GFPS1b from the cultured mycelia of Grifola frondosa GF9801. Toxicol In Vitro. 2007 Apr;21(3):417-27.

58. Cui FJ, Tao WY, Xu ZH, et al. Structural analysis of anti-tumor heteropolysaccharide GFPS1b from the cultured mycelia of Grifola frondosa GF9801. Bioresour Technol. 2007 Jan;98(2):395-401.

59. Preuss HG, Echard B, Bagchi D, et al. Enhanced insulin-hypoglycemic activity in rats consuming a specific glycoprotein extracted from maitake mushroom. Mol Cell Biochem. 2007 Dec;306(1-2):105-13.

60. Noe, JE. L-glutamine use in the treatment and prevention of mucositis and cachexia: a naturopathic perspective. Integr Ca Ther. 2009;8(4):409-15.

61. Gieringer D. Review of the Human Studies on the Medical Use of Marijuana. 1996 http: //norml.org/medical/ medmj.studies.shtml. See state studies at http: //www.drug-policy.org/

62. Hall W, et al. The Health and Psychological Consequences of Cannabis Use, Canberra, Australian Government Publishing Service 189.1994. http://www.druglibrary.org/

63. Guzman M (2003) Cannabinoids: potential anticancer agents. Nat Rev Cancer. 2003;3(10):745-55.

64. Joy E. (1999) op. cit., 259. (Chapter 4 of this report contains sections on nausea, vomiting, wasting syndrome and anorexia)

65. Doblin R, Kleiman MAR. Marijuana as antiemetic medicine: a survey of oncologists' experiences and attitudes. J Clin Oncol. 1991;9:1275-90.

66. James JS. Medical marijuana: Unpublished Federal Study Found THC- Treated Rats Lived Longer, Had Less Cancer. AIDS Treatment News. 263.1997. http://www.immunet.org/

67. Guzman M (2003). Cannabinoids: Potential Anticancer Agents. Nature Reviews, Cancer. 2003;3,745 -55.

68. Blazquez C, et al. Inhibition of tumor angiogenesis by cannabinoids. FASEB J. 2003;17(3):529-31.

69. Sanchez C, et al. Inhibition of glioma growth in vivo by selective activation of the CB(2) cannabinoid receptor. Cancer Res. 2001;61(15):5784-89.

70. Casanova ML, et al. Inhibition of skin tumor growth and angiogenesis in vivo by activation of cannabinoid receptors. J Clin Invest. 2003;111(1):43-50.

71. Jacobsson SO, et al. Inhibition of rat C6 glioma cell proliferation by endogenous and synthetic cannabinoids. Relative involvement of cannabinoid and vanilloid receptors. J Pharmacol Exp Ther. 2001 Dec;299(3):951-59.

72. Galve-Roperph I, et al. Antitumoral action of cannabinoids: involvement of sustained ceramide accumulation of ERK activation. Nature Medicine. 2000;6 313-19; ACM Bulletin. "THC destroys brain cancer in animal research." http://www.acmed.org/english/2000/eb000305.html

73. Benard J.Cannabinoids, among others, send malignant tumors to nirvana. Bull Cancer. 2007;87:299-300.

74. Di Marzo V, et al. Palmitoylethanolamide inhibits the expression of fatty acid amide hydrolase and enhances the anti-proliferative effect of anandamide in human breast cancer cells. Biochem J. 2001;15(358):249-55.

75. Ruiz L, et al. Delta-9-tetrahydrocannabinol induces apoptosis in human prostate PC-3 cells via a receptor-independent mechanism. FEBS Letter. 1999;458:400-04.

76. Baek S, et al. Antitumor activity of cannabigerol against human oral epitheloid carcinoma cells. Arch Pharm Res. 1998;21:353-56.

77. Harris L, et al. Anti-tumoral Properties of Cannabinoids. The Pharmacology of Marihuana, ed. M. Braude et al., 2 vols., New York, NY: Raven Press 2: 773-776 as cited by L. Grinspoon et al., Marihuana: The Forbidden Medicine. 2nd ed. New Haven, CT: Yale University Press;1997:173.

78. Toxicology and Carcinogenesis Studies of 1trans-delta-9-tetrahydrocannabinol in F344N/N Rats and BC63F1 Mice. National Institutes of Health National Toxicology Program, NIH Publication No. 97-3362 (November 1996).

79. De Petrocellis L, et al. The endogenous cannabinoid anandamide inhibits human breast cancer cell proliferation, Proceedings of the National Academy of Sciences 1998;95 8375-80. http://www.pnas.org/cgi/content/abstract/95/14/8375

80. Pot Chemicals Might Inhibit Breast Tumors, Stroke Damage, Dallas Morning News, July 13, 1998.

81. Di Marzo V, et al. Palmitoylethanolamide inhibits the expression of fatty acid amide hydrolase and enhances the anti-proliferative effect of anandamide in human breast cancer cells. Biochem J. 2001;358(Pt 1):249-55.

82. Portella G, et al. Inhibitory effects of cannabinoid CB1 receptor stimulation on tumor growth and metastatic spreading: actions on signals involved in angiogenesis and metastasis.FASEB J. 2003;17(12):1771-73. Epub 2003 Jul 03.

83. Mimeault M, et al. Anti-proliferative and apoptotic effects of anandamide in human prostatic cancer cell lines: implication of epidermal growth factor receptor down-regulation and ceramide production. Prostate. 2003;56(1):1-12.

84. Ligresti A, et al. Possible endocannabinoid control of colorectal cancer growth. Gastroenterology. 2003;125(3):677-87.

85. Gomez del Pulgar T, et al. De novo-synthesized ceramide is involved in cannabinoid-induced apoptosis. Biochem J. 2002;363(Pt 1):183-88.

86. Gomez Del Pulgar T, et al. Cannabinoids protect astrocytes from ceramide-induced apoptosis through the phosphatidylinositol 3-kinase/protein kinase B pathway. J Biol Chem. 2002;277(39):36527-33.

87. Gonzalez S, et al. Decreased cannabinoid CB1 receptor mRNA levels and immunoreactivity in pituitary hyperplasia induced by prolonged exposure to estrogens. Pituitary. 2000;3(4):221-26.

88. Pagotto U, et al.Normal human pituitary gland and pituitary adenomas express cannabinoid receptor type 1 and synthesize endogenous cannabinoids: first evidence for a direct role of cannabinoids on hormone modulation at the human pituitary level. J Clin Endocrinol Metab. 2001;86(6):2687-96.

89. Rubovitch V, Gafni M, Sarne Y. The cannabinoid agonist DALN positively modulates L-type voltage-dependent calcium-channels in N18TG2 neuroblastoma cells. Brain Res Mol Brain Res. 2002;01(1-2):93-102.

90. Bifulco M, et al. Control by the endogenous cannabinoid system of ras oncogene-dependent tumor growth. FASEB J. 2001;15(14):2745-47.

91. Massi P, et al. Antitumor effects of cannabidiol, a nonpsychoative cannabinoid, on human glioma cell lines. JPET 212;308:838-45.

92. McAllister SD, et al. Cannabinoids selectively inhibit proliferation and induce death of cultured human glioblastoma multiforme cells. J Neurooncol. 2005 Aug;74(1):31-40.

93. Hazekamp A, et al. Evaluation of a vaporizing device (Volcano(R)) for the pulmonary administration of tetrahydrocannabinol. J Pharm Sci. 2006 Apr;24: 1308-17.

Pathophysiology

Production of female reproductive hormones and ovulation are the primary functions of the ovaries. Beginning in puberty, the follicle stimulating hormone (FSH) produced by the anterior pituitary starts the process of creating a primary follicle from the ovum stored since birth in the ovaries. These follicles under the influence of FSH become a primary oocyte by the process of proliferation and differentiation. Most of the primary follicles degenerate along with the primary oocytes within them each month, except the one that continues to develop and becomes a secondary follicle. The granulose cells start secreting estrogen and the antrum forms within the follicle.[1]

When the antrum starts to develop, the follicle is then considered a secondary follicle. The granulose cells then secrete a glycoprotein substance that forms a clear membrane called the zona pellucid around the oocyte. After about 10 days of growth, the follicle matures into a vesicular (graafian) follicle, which forms a cyst on the surface of the ovary and contains the secondary oocyte that is ready for ovulation and eventually fertilization. Ovulation is promoted by luteinizing hormone (LH) from the anterior pituitary and occurs when the mature follicle reaches the surface of the ovary and ruptures, releasing the secondary oocyte into the perineal cavity. If the secondary oocyte is not fertilized, it degenerates within a few days. After ovulation and in response to luteinizing hormone, the portion of the follicle that remains in the ovary enlarges and is transformed into the corpus luteum.[2]

The corpus luteum is a glandular structure that secretes progesterone and some estrogens. The fate of the corpus luteum depends on whether fertilization occurs. If fertilization does not take place, then the corpus luteum remains functional for about 10 days before it begins to degenerate and it ceases hormone output. If fertilization occurs, the corpus luteum persists and continues its hormone function until the placenta develops sufficiently to secrete the necessary hormones, especially progesterone. The corpus luteum ultimately degenerates, but with fertilization it remains functional for a longer period of time, causing a spike in the pregnant woman's progesterone levels.[3]

ANATOMY OF THE OVARIES

The ovaries are the primary female gonadal organs. These two glands provide tissue sacs in which eggs can develop and connect to the uterus via the fallopian tubes or ovaducts. Fingerlike projections called fimbriae (located at the opening of the ovaducts) sweep an egg released from an ovary into the tube. Each ovary is a solid, ovoid-shaped structure about the size of an almond (3.5 cm length, 2 cm width, 1 cm thick). Each is located in the ovarian fossae and one on each side of the uterus in the lateral walls of the pelvic cavity.[1-3]

The ovaries are covered with an outside layer of epithelium called the germinal or ovarian epithelium, which is actually the visceral epithelium (peritoneal) that envelopes the ovaries. The ovary has an outer cortex and an inner medulla. The cortex is dense and granular because of the multiple presence of the ovarian follicles in various stages of development. Each of these follicles contains an oocyte, which is a female germ cell. The medulla is a loose connective tissue with copious blood vessels, lymphatic vessels, and nerve fibers.[1-3]

HISTOLOGY

Ovarian cancers are histologically diverse. At least 80% originate in the epithelium; 75% of these cancers are serous cystadenocarcinoma, while the rest include mucinous, endometrioid, transitional cell, clear cell, unclassified carcinomas, and Brenner tumor. The remaining 20% of ovarian cancers originate in primary ovarian germ cells or in sex cord and stromal cells or are metastases to the ovary (most commonly, from the breast or GI tract).[3,4] Germ cell cancers usually occur in women < 30 and include dysgerminomas, immature teratomas, endodermal sinus tumors, embryonal carcinomas, choriocarcinomas, and polyembryomas. Stromal (sex cord–stromal) cancers include granulosa-theca cell tumors and Sertoli-Leydig cell tumors.[4] Ovarian cancer spreads by direct extension, exfoliation of cells into the peritoneal cavity (peritoneal seeding), especially to the greater and lesser omentum, lymphatic dissemination to the pelvis and around the aorta, or, less often, hematogenously to the liver, lungs, and brain.[5]

Female Reproductive System

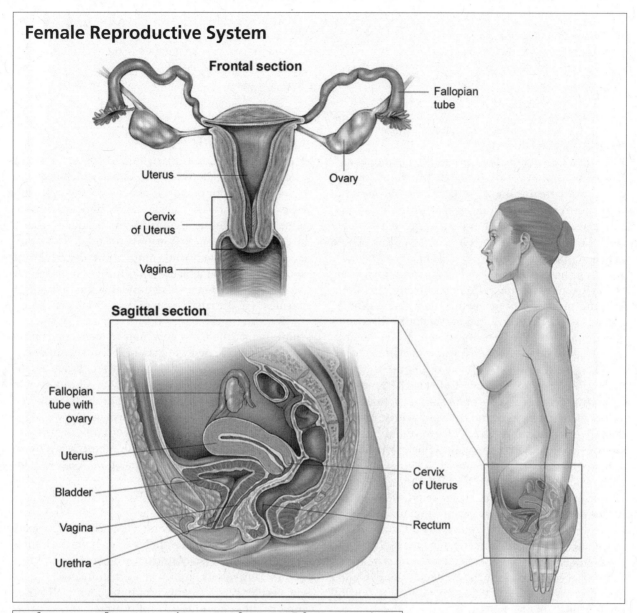

Frontal section

Fallopian tube

Uterus

Ovary

Cervix of Uterus

Vagina

Sagittal section

Fallopian tube with ovary

Uterus

Bladder

Vagina

Urethra

Cervix of Uterus

Rectum

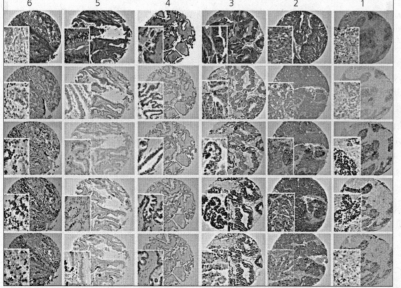

6   5   4   3   2   1

Six Kinds of Ovarian Cancer Cells

1. Serous Papillary Carcinoma

2. Carcinosarcoma

3. Endometroid Ovarian Carcinoma

4. Serous Borderline Tumor

5. Mucinous Ovarian Carcinoma

6. Clear Cell Ovarian Carcinoma

Epidemiology
PREVALENCE AND INCIDENCE

In the United States, ovarian cancer is the second most common gynecologic cancer (affecting about 1/70) and the deadliest (1% of all women die of it). It is the fifth leading cause of cancer-related deaths in women. It is estimated in 2012, in the United States, 22,280 new cases were diagnosed, and 15,550 women will die from ovarian cancer.[6] Epithelial ovarian cancer is the most common type and the leading cause of death from gynecological cancers in the USA. This type of ovarian cancer accounts for about 5% of all cancer deaths in women in the USA, with more women dying from this disease than cervical or endometrial cancers combined.[6]

Risk Factors

> **Risk factors[7]**
> - Incidence is higher in developed countries in women past 65 years of age
> - Ovarian cancer affects mainly perimenopausal and postmenopausal women
> - Nulliparity, delayed childbearing, and delayed menopause increase risk
> - Oral contraceptive use decreases risk due to overall estrogen exposure in a lifetime
> - Personal or family history of endometrial, breast, or colon cancer increases risk
> - Probably 5% to 10% of ovarian cancer cases are related to mutations in the autosomal dominant BRCA gene. XY gonadal dysgenesis predisposes to ovarian germ cell cancer.[4]

GENETIC FACTORS

Women with a positive family history of breast or ovarian cancer have a higher incidence of two susceptible gene loci: BRCA 1 and BRCA 2.[7-8] BRCA 1 is located on chromosome 17q12-21, and BRCA 2 is located on chromosome 13q12-13. Both of these are tumor suppressor genes, they are large, and they produce nuclear proteins that effect genomic integrity. Because of their large size, numerous mutations have been found in these genes, though many mutations are not even known at this time. This adds to the malignant nature of these genetic mutations.[8]

The risk of developing ovarian cancer with the mutated BRCA 1 and 2 genes is 25%. Mutated genes can be inherited by either parent, and men in families with mutated BRCA genes have a higher incidence of prostate cancer and breast cancer.[9] This is what is referred to as the triad of cancer: breast, prostate and ovarian cancers. Questioning the family history of a patient with this triad may give clues into the mystery of the genetic mutations associated within families of origin. A fourth factor is adenocarcinoma of the colon, or colorectal cancer.

Assessment
SYMPTOMS

Because ovarian cancer is insidious and hides well in the earlier stages, most women with ovarian cancer are asymptomatic and may experience only mild symptoms of GI upset or pelvic pressure. Ovarian cancer is often fatal because it is usually in an advanced stage when diagnosed, while if caught in earlier stages it could potentially be curable. Symptoms are usually absent in the early stage and nonspecific in advanced stages until ascites and other physical symptoms of widely metastatic disease occur.[10]

Detection in women with early stage disease is usually incidental upon annual gynecological bimanual examination. An adnexal mass, often solid, irregular, and fixed, may be discovered. Pelvic and rectovaginal examinations typically detect diffuse nodularity on one or both ovaries. A few women present with severe abdominal pain secondary to torsion of the ovarian mass.[11]

Most women with advanced ovarian cancer present with nonspecific symptoms (dyspepsia, bloating, early satiety, gas pains, and low backache). Later symptoms include pelvic pain, anemia, cachexia, and abdominal swelling due to ovarian enlargement and ascites usually is concurrent.[12] Germ cell or stromal tumors may have functional effects due to their action on hormone production (hyperthyroidism, feminization, virilization.[13]

DIAGNOSIS

Diagnosis is definitive with histopathologic analysis. Staging is surgical. Evaluation usually includes ultrasonography, CT or MRI, and measurement of tumor markers (cancer antigen 125).[14]

If cancer is suspected, transvaginal ultrasonography is done first as a screening diagnostic tool. Ultrasonography allows differentiation between ovarian masses that are benign or potentially malignant. Color doppler imaging further enhances the specificity of ultrasound diagnosis.[14] Findings that suggest cancer include:[14]

- Solid component to the ovary or growth on the ovary
- Surface changes on the gland

Staging and Survival in Gynecologic Malignancies

Stage	Ovarian	5-Year Survival, %	Endometrial	5-Year Survival, %	Cervix	5-Year Survival, %
0	—		—		Carcinoma in situ	100
I	Confined to ovary	90	Confined to corpus	89	Confined to uterus	85
II	Confined to pelvis	70	Involves corpus and cervix	73	Invades beyond uterus but not to pelvic wall	65
III	Intraabdominal spread	25–50	Extends outside the uterus but not outside the true pelvis	52	Extends to pelvic wall and/or lower third of vagina, or hydronephrosis	35
IV	Spread outside abdomen	1–5	Extends outside the true pelvis or involves the bladder or rectum	17	Invades mucosa of bladder or rectum or extends beyond the true pelvis	7

(Adapted from McPhee SJ, et al. CURRENT Medical Diagnosis and Treatment 2009. New York, NY: 2009)[4]

- Size > 6 cm
- Irregular shape
- Low vascular resistance on transvaginal Doppler flow studies

A pelvic mass, plus ascites, usually indicates ovarian cancer, and CT or MRI is usually done before surgery to determine the extent of the cancer and whether a surgical oncologist can debride the bulky tumor burden without neoadjuvant chemotherapy or radiation to shrink the tumor burden. Histologic analysis is mandatory for adnexal masses unless they appear benign.

Benign-appearing masses include benign cystic teratomas (dermoid cysts), follicular cysts, or endometriomas. For masses that appear benign, ultrasonography is repeated after 6 weeks.

If women are not surgical candidates, samples are obtained by needle biopsy for masses or by needle aspiration for ascitic fluid.

Screening asymptomatic women using ultrasonography and serum CA 125 measurements can detect some cases of ovarian cancer but has not been shown to improve outcome, even for high-risk subgroups.[15]

Tumor Markers

Tumor markers, including the β subunit of human chorionic gonadotropin (β-hCG), LDH, α-fetoprotein (AFP), inhibin, and cancer antigen (CA 125), are also measured. CA 125 (> 35 units) is elevated in 80% of advanced epithelial ovarian cancers, but only by 50% in early ovarian cancer. CA 125 may be mildly elevated in endometriosis, pelvic inflammatory disease, pregnancy, fibroids, peritoneal inflammation, or nonovarian peritoneal cancer. A mixed solid and cystic pelvic mass in postmenopausal women, especially if CA 125 is elevated, suggests ovarian cancer.[16]

Staging and Grading
SURGICAL STAGING[17]

Suspected or confirmed ovarian cancer is staged surgically. Laparotomy is now the primary surgical procedure used to establish the correct diagnosis and accurate staging. An abdominal midline incision that allows adequate access to the upper abdomen is required if widely metastatic disease is found. All peritoneal surfaces, hemidiaphragms, and abdominal and pelvic viscera are inspected and palpated. Washings from the pelvis, abdominal gutters, and diaphragmatic recesses are obtained, and multiple

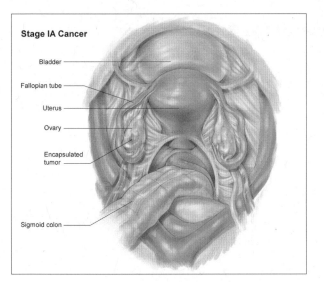

Stage IA Cancer

Bladder

Fallopian tube

Uterus

Ovary

Encapsulated
tumor

Sigmoid colon

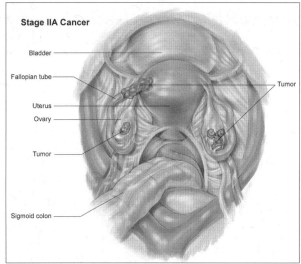

Stage IIA Cancer

Bladder

Fallopian tube

Uterus

Ovary

Tumor

Tumor

Sigmoid colon

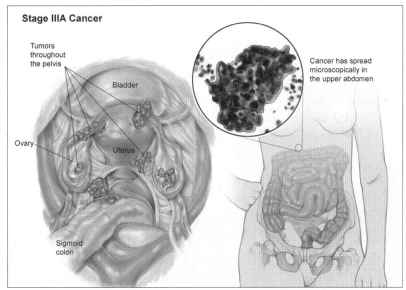

Stage IIIA Cancer

Tumors
throughout
the pelvis

Bladder

Ovary

Uterus

Cancer has spread
microscopically in
the upper abdomen

Sigmoid
colon

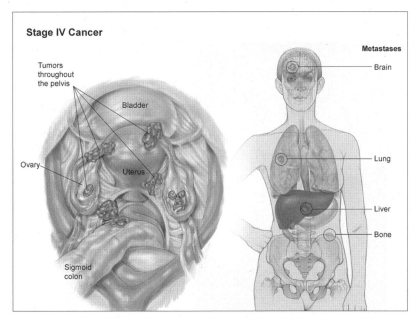

Stage IV Cancer

Tumors
throughout
the pelvis

Bladder

Ovary

Uterus

Sigmoid
colon

Metastases

Brain

Lung

Liver

Bone

Surgical Staging of Ovarian Carcinoma: Stage & Description[16]

Stage	Description
I	Limited to the ovaries
IA	Limited to one ovary; no tumor on the external surface, and capsule intact
IB	Limited to both ovaries; no tumor on the external surface, and capsules intact
IC Stage IA or IB	With tumor on the surface of one or both ovaries, with capsule ruptured, or with ascites or peritoneal washings containing malignant cells
II	Involving one or both ovaries with pelvic extension or metastases
IIA	Extension or metastases to the uterus, fallopian tubes, or both
IIB	Extension to other pelvic tissues
IIC Stage IIA or IIB	With tumor on the surface of one or both ovaries, with capsule ruptured, or with ascites or peritoneal washings containing malignant cells
III	Histologically confirmed peritoneal metastases outside the pelvis, superficial liver metastases, positive retroperitoneal or inguinal lymph nodes, or tumor limited to the true pelvis but with histologically verified malignant extension to the small intestine or omentum
IIIA Gross tumor	Limited to the true pelvis with negative lymph nodes but with microscopic tumor outside pelvis histologically confirmed
IIIB	Histologically confirmed abdominal peritoneal metastases that extend beyond the pelvis and are < 2 cm in diameter and negative lymph nodes
IIIC	Abdominal peritoneal metastases that extend beyond the pelvis and are > 2 cm in diameter, positive retroperitoneal or inguinal lymph nodes, or both
IV	Distant metastases, including parenchymal liver metastases; if pleural effusion is present, cytologic test results must be positive to signify stage IV

Prognosis
The 5-year survival rates with treatment are:[18]
70 to 100% with stage I
50 to 70% with stage II
15 to 35% with stage III
10 to 20% with stage IV
Prognosis is worse when tumor grade is higher or when surgery cannot remove all visibly involved tissue; then, prognosis is best when the involved tissue can be reduced to < 1 cm in diameter. With stages III and IV, recurrence rate is about 70%.

biopsies of the peritoneum in the central and lateral pelvis and in the abdomen are done. For early-stage cancer, the infracolic omentum is removed, and pelvic and para-aortic lymph nodes are sampled. Cancers are also graded histologically from 1 (least aggressive) to 3 (most aggressive).[18]

Conventional Treatment for Ovarian Cancer

Conventional treatment includes hysterectomy, bilateral salpingo-oophorectomy, and excision of as much involved tissue as possible, with peritoneal washings, and, unless the cancer is localized, chemotherapy and radiation therapy.[19]

SURGERY

Hysterectomy and bilateral salpingo-oophorectomy are usually indicated. An exception is nonepithelial or low-grade unilateral epithelial cancer in young patients; fertility can be preserved by not removing the unaffected ovary and uterus. All visibly involved tissue is surgically removed if possible. If it cannot be removed completely, removing as much as possible (cytoreductive surgery) improves the efficacy of other therapies. Cytoreductive surgery usually includes infracolic omentectomy, sometimes with rectosigmoid resection (usually with primary reanastomosis), radical peritoneal stripping, resection of diaphragmatic peritoneum, or splenectomy.[20]

POST-OPERATIVE CHEMOTHERAPY

- Stage IA or B/grade 1: epithelial adenocarcinoma requires no postoperative therapy
- Stage IA or B/grade 2 or 3 cancers and stage II cancers: require six courses of chemotherapy, typically paclitaxel (Taxol) and carboplatin.[21]
- Stage III or IV cancer: requires six courses of similar chemotherapy. Intraperitoneal chemotherapy or high-dose chemotherapy with bone marrow transplantation is under study. Radiation therapy is used infrequently.[22]
- Germ cell cancer or stage II or III stromal cancer: require a combination chemotherapy, usually bleomycin, cisplatin, and etoposide[23]

Residual Tumor

Even if chemotherapy results in a complete clinical response (normal physical examination, normal serum CA 125, and negative CT scan of the abdomen and pelvis), about 50% to70% of patients with stage III or IV cancer will have recurrent or residual tumor.[23] Of patients with persistent elevation of CA 125, 90% to 95% have residual tumor or recurrent disease.[23] If cancer recurs or progresses after effective chemotherapy, chemotherapy is restarted using different strategies due to chemoresistance. Other useful drugs include topotecan, liposomal doxorubicin (Adriamycin), docetaxel (Taxotere), vinorelbine (Navelbine), gemcitabine (Gemzar), hexamethylmelamine, and oral etoposide (Etopohos Vepesid).[25]

Naturopathic Approaches to Treating Ovarian Cancer

Naturopathic Therapeutic Protocol
1. Decrease Inflammation
2. Detoxify
3. Scavenge Reactive Oxygen Species (ROS)
4. Counsel Patients

1. DECREASE INFLAMMATION
Herbal COX-2 Inhibitors

Cox-1 and Cox-2 pro-inflammatory initiating enzymes when overexpressed cause an autocrine stimulation of the aromatase gene by tumor cells. This is due to the conversion of arachidonic acid to pro-inflammatory prostaglandins in series 2 (PGE2). Once the PGE2 series is turned on, it stimulates the aromatase enzymes, which increases peripheral aromatization of sterols to estrogens. This can lead to increased estrogen production endogenously by the system. Progression of ovarian cancer is accompanied by the increased expression of estrogens. By inhibiting the Cox-2 pathway specifically, the beneficial effects include an inhibition of angiogenesis, decreased cancer cell growth and invasion, pro-apoptotic effects, and the inhibition of PGE2 associated aromatase induction.[25]

Curcumin longa

Curcumin has been studied as a chemotherapy enhances and for chemoresistance reversal. A series of naturally occurring as well as synthetic structural analogs of the dietary constituent curcumin (turmeric) from the plant *Curcuma longa radix* was examined in order to determine its activity as an anti-inflammatory by elucidating which portions of the molecule are critical for the ability to induce Phase 2 detoxification enzymes. This upgrade of the Phase 2 detoxification systems would make these compounds chemoprotective. The researchers found that all "curcuminoids elevate the specific activity of quinone reductase in both wild type and mutant cells defective in either the aryl hydrocarbon (*Ah*) receptor or cytochrome P4501A1 activity.[26] This indicates that neither binding to this receptor, nor metabolic activation by P4501A1 are required for the signaling process originating from this family of electrophiles and ultimately resulting in Phase 2 enzyme induction."

Skullcap

In one trial, *Scutellaria baicalensis* (Chinese skullcap) was compared to a known pharmaceutical COX-2 inhibitor celecoxib (Celebrex) for suppressed proliferation cell nuclear antigen expression and PGE2 synthesis. Skullcap inhibited COX-2 expression, whereas celecoxib inhibited COX-2 activity directly. A 66% reduction in tumor mass was observed. *Scutellaria baicalensis* selectively and effectively inhibits cancer cell growth *in vitro* and *in vivo* and can be an effective chemotherapeutic enhancing agent. Inhibition of PGE2 synthesis via suppression of COX-2 expression may be responsible for its anticancer activity.[27]

Zyflamend

This compound has been studied for its role in anti-angiogenesis, as a COX-2 inhibitor, and for inducing apoptosis. In one study, Zyflamend suppressed NF-κ B activation induced by TNF. The report concluded that "the expression of NF-κ B-regulated gene products involved in anti-apoptosis (inhibitor-of-apoptosis protein 1/2, Bcl-2, Bcl-xL, FADD-like interleukin-1β converting enzyme/caspase-8 inhibitory protein, TNF receptor-associated factor-1, and surviving) and angiogenesis (vascular endothelial growth factor, cyclooxygenase-2, intercellular adhesion molecule, and matrix metalloproteinase-9) was also down-regulated by Zyflamend. This correlated with potentiation of cell death induced by TNF and chemotherapeutic agents. Overall, our results indicate that Zyflamend suppresses osteoclastogenesis, inhibits invasion, and potentiates cytotoxicity through down-regulation of NF-κ B activate and lipid peroxidation and free radical generation."[28] Curcumin also inhibits the generation of reactive oxygen species (ROS) in a concentration-dependent manner. This effect has been demonstrated in vivo with oral dosing.[29]

Vitamin E and Vitamin C

Natural vitamin E (a-tocopherol) and vitamin C (ascorbate), independently and in combination with each other, have been shown to decrease the production of reactive oxygen species in human spermatocytes exposed to H_2O_2.[30] The pretreatment of hepatocytes with tocopherol succinate (TS) dramatically enriched cells and mitochondria with alpha-tocopherol and provided these membranes with complete protection against ethyl methanesulfonate (EMS)-induced oxidative damage. TS pretreatment suppressed EMS-induced cellular ROS production generated from mitochondrial complex I and III sites.[31] It has also been found that vitamin C supplementation in chronic hemodialysis patients can reduce the lymphocyte intracellular ROS production, as well as up-regulate hOGG1 gene expression for repair.[32]

2. DETOXIFY

Detoxification with natural therapies is a strategy to use before and after chemotherapy rounds and when patients are on breaks from active therapy. This can be achieved by altering carcinogen metabolism. These botanicals and nutrients may be of benefit in preventing recurrence and in decreasing chemoresistance in cancer cells.

These agents should not be used during active conventional treatment unless they have been proven not to interfere with the conventional treatment expected outcomes. Therefore, they should be used before, between, and after courses of conventional treatments are completed.

Allium sativum

Garlic contains flavonols (such as quercitin and kaempferol), sulfur compounds (such as diallyl-sulfide), and glutathione. These compounds are antimutagens and increase the activity of glutathione S-transferase.[33] Quercitin increases the glucuronosyl transferase enzymes and glutathione and glutathione-2-transferase, which results in detoxification of dietary carcinogens. The dose equating to this action is as little as 1 to 3 cloves daily.[34]

Garlic also acts as a chemopreventive by inhibiting the genetic damage to the cell, increasing metabolic detoxification, scavenging reactive radicals, and enhancing time for DNA to repair, while inhibiting oncogene expression and restoring tumor suppressor gene function (p53). Once a cell has become initiated into the promotion of a cancer cell, then garlic can restore normal cell differentiation by modulating signal transduction pathways, inhibiting polyamine metabolism, and altering calcium influx, while inhibiting arachidonic acid metabolism. Once the cancer cell has become dysplastic, garlic still works chemopreventively by stimulating the body's own immune surveillance and still inhibits angiogensis and induces apoptosis.[35]

Camellia sinensis

Green tea has powerful polyphenols that not only act as exogenous antioxidants but also aid in detoxifying the carcinogenic effects of chemical carcinogens, such as benzenes.[36] The dry leaf of the green tea contains 30% to 35% polyphenols: catechins (C), epicatechins (EC), epicatechin-3-gallate (ECG), epigallocatechin (EGC), and epigallocatechin-3-gallate (EGCG). Catchins, ECG, and EGCG have all demonstrated antimutagenic effects against bacterial mutagens *in vivo*, and it is the EGCG that counters the carcinogenic effects of benzenes.[36]

Silybum marianum

Milk thistle has been studied extensively for its action in detoxification of the liver and rejuvenation of hepatocytes. Milk thistle contains a flavonoid complex called silymarin, which includes another constituent called silybinin. Orally administered, silymarin significantly elevates phase II activity *in vivo*, particularly the glutathione-S-transferase activity, which aids in the detoxification of chemical carcinogens.[37] Orally administered, silymarin has shown a reduction in colon, skin, and tongue carcinogenesis.[38] Orally administered, silybinin also showed a significant increase in phase II glutathione-S-transferase and also activity in the quinine reductase activity in a dose and time dependent manner *in vivo*.[39]

Schisandra chinensis

Wu Wei Zi is a hepatoprotective and adrenal adaptogenic tophorestorative that has been used for centuries in traditional Chinese herbal medicine. It is best indicated for anxiety, insomnia, palpitations, and forgetfulness due to excess stress as an anxiolytic and sedative herb. Orally administered, schisandra berry has been shown to increase hepatic reduced glutathione (r-GSH) with an increased activity in glutathione reductase and glutathione-S-transferase. Pretreatment with schisandra showed protection in rats against aflatoxin and the toxic-heavy metal cadmium, as well as chloride toxicity.[40]

Glycyrrhiza glabra

Licorice root has been used as a medicinal botanical in TCM for more than 3000 years to improve health, support detoxification, and aid in recovery. Modern use for this medically indicated herbal is to aid in detoxification, as an adrenal adaptogen, and as a potent phytoestrogen and GI demulcent. It is a very strong antiviral as well as an anti-inflammatory, anti-atherogenic, and anticarcinogenic stimulant. Glycyrrhizic acid and its aglycone, glycyrrhetic acid, combined with plentiful polyphenols, have antimutagenic activity.[41] These constituents also increased glucuronidation, thus aiding in the detoxifying xenobiotics in the liver.[42]

Curcuma longa

Curcumin has a long historical use in traditional Ayurvedic medicine as an anti-inflammatory agent, as a wound healer, and as an agent to promote health and longevity.[26] It is used abundantly in the culinary tradition of the culture. The root contains curcumin, which has been and continues to be investigated as a chemopreventive. One mechanism of action is to induce the phase II detoxification enzymes, especially the glutathione transferases and quinine reductase, while inhibiting procarcinogen activity in the phase I enzymes, such as cP450 1A1, *in vivo*.[26]

Selenium

This essential trace mineral has been shown to inhibit intestinal, prostate, lung, and liver cancer development and associated mortality from that cancer in both animal and human models. Selenium is one of the most powerful chemopreventive elements in the human diet, but the mechanism of action is still not fully understood. There is a direct correlation between low levels and a decrease in the expression of genes involved in the detoxification pathway, thus reducing the pathways influence.[43]

Amino Acids

N-acetyl-cysteine, glycine, sulfate, methionine, and taurine are all amino acids that play an important role in phase II detoxification pathway activities. Methylation is a phase II pathway activity that adds methyl groups to toxic compounds. These methyl groups come from S-adenosylmethionine, which is synthesized from methionine. In order to synthesize these methyl groups, choline, vitamin B-12, B-6, and folic acid are required. There also must be an inborn ability for the biochemistry of the system to take dietary folic acid and change it into its three active methylated forms to be used in this methylation/donor process.[44]

Glucuronidation is a phase II activity that adds glucuronic acid to toxic compounds. Sulfate conjugation is the major conjugation pathway for amine neurotransmitters and steroid hormones to be detoxified out of the system; but this sulfate conjugation system is also used for drugs and other xenobiotics, especially phenolic compounds. Glycine conjugates intermediary metabolites to form hippuric acid.[45]

Glutathione, a tripeptide, is composed of glutamic acid, cysteine, and glycine. The conjugation of glutathione with intermediary biotransformed xenobiotics from phase I results in the excretion of mercapturic acids, the most deadly precarcinogens. Acetylation adds an acetyl group to a cP450 metabolite, which then is ready for excretion. Most phase II conjugation pathways require vitamin B-6, B-12, folic acid, and a variety of the other B vitamins in order to flux and work properly.[45]

3. SCAVENGE REACTIVE OXYGEN SPECIES (ROS)

CoQ10 (Ubiquinone) and Adriamycin (Doxorubicin)

CoQ10 reduces free radical formation induced by doxorubicin.[67] Adriamycin-induced cardiomyopathies have also been prevented by concomitant supplementation with CoQ10. Studies with both animals and humans have found that pretreating with coenzyme Q10, at levels of 100 mg per day, reduces cardiac toxicity caused by doxorubicin.[46,47] CoQ10 is used with vitamin E to protect patients from chemotherapy-induced cardiomyopathies. CoQ10 is nontoxic even at high dosages and has been shown to prevent liver damage from the drugs Mitomycin C and 5-FU.[47]

Dose: CoQ10 at 100 mg per day is the desired dose while on active chemotherapies. Once those therapies are on a break between sequences and rotations of 4 weeks, post treatment dosage can be 300-400 mg up to b.i.d. or t.i.d. as indicated. A combination of CoQ10, L-carnitine, magnesium taurate, and cardiac herbal tonics has been successful in treating cardiomyotoxicity and insufficient cardiac effusion rates that promoted discontinuation of active chemotherapy. Within a matter of weeks the effusion rates were improved up past the 50% range and active treatment could then be resumed.

Melatonin and Ovarian Cancer

In the medical literature, there are more than 600 specific publications on melatonin and cancer, making melatonin the most thoroughly studied hormone in human clinical trials. Melatonin is a pineal secretory product with antioxidant properties. More than 50% of those studies evaluated exogenous melatonin treatment and cancer patients clinically. Common findings include:

- Melatonin acts as a biological response modifier in cancer patients.[48]
- Melatonin protects against cisplatin-induced nephrotoxicity in rats.[49]
- Melatonin blocks the mitogenic effects of tumor promoting hormones and growth factors.[50]
- Concomitant administration of melatonin with radiation treatment (TMX) induces regression in refractory to TMX alone.[51]
- Melatonin reverses LHRH resistance in cancer.[52]
- Melatonin down-regulates 5-lipoxygenase gene expression.[53]

Some physicians initially thought that ovarian cancer patients should not take melatonin, but a study in *Oncology Reports* by the leading Italian researcher of melatonin in 1996 demonstrated that high doses of melatonin were indicated and may be beneficial in treating ovarian cancer. In this study, 40 mg of melatonin were given nightly, along with low doses of IL-2, to 12 advanced ovarian cancer patients who had failed chemotherapy. While no complete response was seen, a partial response was achieved in 16% of patients, and a stable disease was obtained in 41% of the cases.[54] This preliminary study suggested that melatonin is not contraindicated in advanced ovarian cancer patients. It is still not known what the effects of melatonin are in leukemia, lymphoma, and myelogenous cancers; therefore, these patients should use melatonin with caution or not at all.

Dosage: Studies in dosing and toxicity have shown that the therapeutic dose for adults in the treatment of cancer is 10-40 mg, preferably taken at the hour of sleep.

Tamoxifen Cautions

- Avoid using Indole-3-carbinol with tamoxifen because it may have harmful estrogenic effects and can increase the speed at which the tamoxifen is metabolized. Some studies show that it may increase estrogen metabolism toward carcinogenic and anticarcinogenic metabolites.
- Consider using DIM with tamoxifen and Indole-3-carbinol with Arimidex for these potentiated effects.
- Avoid quercitin with tamoxifen.
- Check estrogen clearance with urine estradiol and estrone metabolites.

Chemotherapeutic and Naturopathic Integrated Therapies

Chemotherapeutic	Naturopathic	Daily Dose	Caution
Cisplatin/Carboplatin	*To increase effectiveness:* NAC[55]	200-600 g qd-tid	Follow 3-4 day rule with use (discontinue 1-2 days before chemotherapy, day of and 1-2 days after chemotherapy): Contraindicated to use with Coumadin, warfarin, and other blood thinning or anti-platelet aggregators due to synergistic effects
	Ginkgo biloba[56]	120-240 mg qd[57]	Again follow safety guidelines with use during active chemotherapy
	Silymarin[58]	600-900 mg in standardized doses May be indicated up to 500 mg tid [59]	
	Selenium[60]	400-800 mcg qd[61]	
Cisplatin	*To increase effectiveness:* Quercitin[62] Silymarin[63] Curcumin[64] Vitamin A[65] Vitamin C[66] Vitamin D[67]	100-300 mg qd-tid 600-900 mg qd 500-1000 mg qd-tid 10,000-50,000 IU qd TBT 2000-5000 IU qd	Caution with quercitin, silymarin, and curcumin on days receiving chemotherapy
	To reduce toxicity: Silymarin[68] Selenium[69] Ginkgo biloba [70]	600-900 mg qd 400-800 mcg qd 120-240 mg qd	Avoid NAC and high dose vitamin B-6 above 200 mg q.d.
Doxorubicin (Adriamycin)	*To increase effectiveness:* Green tea[71] Quercitin[72]	5-10 cups 100-300 mg qd-tid	Caution with NAC, glutathione, and curcumin
	To reduce toxicity: CoQ10[73] L-Carnitine[74] Vitamin A[75] Vitamin C[76] Vitamin E[77]	100 mg qd 100-1000 g qd 10,000-50,000 IU TBT 400-1200 IU qd	

References

1. Guyton AC, Hall JE. 2000. Textbook of Medical Physiology. 10th ed. St Louis, MO: WB Saunders Co;2000.

2. Moore, KL, AF Dalley, and AMR Aqur. Clinically Oriented Anatomy. 6th ed. Lippincott Williams & Wilkins;2009.

3. Young, RC. Harrison's Internal Medicine, online. Chapter 93 Gynecologic Malignancies.

4. McPhee S, Papadakis MA. Eds. Gonzales R, Zeiger Online Eds. 2009. 40th edition. CURRENT Medical Diagnosis & Treatment; 2009.

5. Young, Robert C. Chapter 93. Gynecologic Malignancies: Ovarian Cancer. CURRENT Medical Diagnosis & Treatment. 2009. 4th ed.

6. http://seer.cancer.gov/statfacts/html/ovary.html. 2012.

7. http://www.cancer.org/Cancer/OvarianCancer/Detail edGuide/ovarian-cancer-risk-factors Jan. 22, 2012.

8. McLemore M, Miaskowski C, Aouizerat BE, et al. Epidemiologic and eneretic factors Associated with Ovarian Cancer. Cancer Nurs 2009;32(4):281-290.

9. Fearon ER, Vogelstein B. Tumor Supressor Gene Defects in Human Cancer, Chapter 5. Holland-Frei Cancer Medicine. 5th ed. Bast RC, Kufe DW, Pollock Re, et al eds. Hamilton ON: BC Decker;2000.

10. http://www.cdc.gov/cancer/ovarian/basic_info/symp toms.htm Sept. 2010

11. http://www.ovarian.org/symptoms.php. 2012.

12. Goff BA, Mandel LS, Melancon CH, et al. Frequency of symptoms of ovarian cancer in women presenting to primary care Clinics. JAMA. 2004;291(22):2705-12.

13. Koulouris CR, Penson RT. Ovarian stromal and germ cell tumors. Semin Onco. 2009;36(2):126-36.

14. http://www.medicinenet.com/ovarian_cancer/article.htm . 2012.

15. http://www.cancer.org/Cancer/OvarianCancer/Detailed Guide/ovarian-cancer-staging . 2012.

16. http://ovariancancer.about.com/od/testsdiagnosis/a/tumor_markers.htm .Vasilev S 2008.

17. Trimbo B, Timmers P, Percorelli S, et al. Surgical staging and treatment of early ovarian cancer: long term analysis from a randomized trial. J Natl Can Inst. 2010;102(13):982-87.

18. http://www.cancer.org/Cancer/OvarianCancer/Detai ledGuide/ovarian-cancer-survival-rates Jan. 2012.

19. Roett MA, Evans P. Ovarian cancer: an overview. Am Fam Phys. 2009;80(6):609-16.

20.http://www.mskcc.org/cancer-care/adult/ovarian/treatment. 2012.

21. Akinkugbe A, Uguru VE, Mordi VPN. Post-operative chemotherapy for ovarian carcinoma: a prospective study with cyclophosphamide. Int J Gyn & Ob. 1985;23(6):499-504.

22. Covens A, Carey M, Bryson P, et al. Systematic review of first line chemotherapy for newly diagnosed postoperative patients with Stage II, III, or IV epithelial ovarian cancer. Gyn Onco. 2002;85(1):71-80.

23. Rubin SC, Thoma R, Armstong KA, et al. Ten Year follow up of ovarian cancer patients after second look lapratomy with negative findings. Ob &Gyn. 1999;93(1):21-24.

24. Markam M, Walker JL. Intraperitoneal chemotherapy of ovarian cancer: a review with a focus on practical aspects of treatment. JCO. 2006;24(6):988-94.

25. Alschuler LN, Gazella KA. Alternative Medicine Magazine's Definitive Guide to Cancer: An Integrated Approach to Prevention, Treatment, and Healing (Alternative Medicine Guides). Berkley, CA: Ten Speed Press, 2005.

26. Albena T.Dinkova-Kostova and Paul Talalay. Relation of structure of curcumin analogs to their potencies as inducers of Phase 2 detoxification enzymes. Carcinogenesis. 1999;20(5):911-14.

27. Zhang D, Wu j, et al. Inhibition of cancer cell proliferation and prostaglandin E2 Synthesis by Scutellaria Baicalensis. CANCER RESEARCH 2003 July 15;63: 403743.

28. Santosh K. Sandur, Kwang Seok Ahn, et al. Zyflamend, a polyherbal preparation,inhibits invasion, suppresses osteoclastogenesis, and potentiates apoptosis through down-regulation of NF-_ B activation and NF-_ B-Regulated gene products. Nutrition and Cancer. 2007 May;http://www.informaworld.com/smpp/title~content=t775653687~db=all~tab =issueslist~branches=57 - v5757(1): 78 -87.

29. Somasundaram et al. Dietary curcumin inhibits chemotherapy-induced apoptosis in models of human breast cancer. Cancer Res., 2002;62:3868-65.

30. Donnelly ET, et al. The effect of ascorbate and alpha tocopherol supplementation in vitro on DNA integrity and hydrogen peroxide induced DNA damage in human spermatozoa. Mutagenesis. 1999;14(5): 5055-12.

31. Zhang, et al. Chem Biol Interact. 2001 Dec;138(3):267-84.

32. Tarng DC, Liu TY, Huang TP. Protective effect of vitamin C on 8-hydroxy-2'-deoxyguanosine level in peripheral blood lymphocytes of chronic hemodialysis patients Kidney Int. 2004;66;:820-31.

33. Dorant E, van den Brandt PA, Goldbohm RA. Allium vegetable consumption, garlic supplement intake, and female breast carcinoma incidence. Breast Cancer Res Treat. 1995;33(2):163-170.

34. Van der Logt EMJ Peters WHM. Induction of rat hepatic and intestinal UDP-glucouronosyltransferases by naturally occurring dietary anticarcinogens. Carcinogenesis. 2003 Oct; 24(10):1651-56.

35. Wataru Y, Hiromichi S, et al. Expression of epidermal growth factor receptor in human gastri and colonic caricinomas. Cancer Res. 48:137-41.

36. Kuroda Y, Hara Y. Antimutagenic and anticarcinogenic activity of tea polyphenols. Mutat Res. 1999;436;69-97.

37. Yanaida Y, Kohno H, Yoshida K, et al. Dietary silymarin

suppresses 4-nitroquinoline 1-oxide-induced tongue carcinogenesis in male F344 rats. Carcinogenesis 2002;23(5):787-94.

38. Katiyar SK.Slymarin and skin cancer prevention: anti-inflammatory, antioxidant and immunomodulatory effects (review). Int J Oncol. 2005 Jan;26(1):169-76.

39. Zhao J, Agarwal, R. Tissue distribution of silibinin, the major active constituent of silymarin, in mice and its association with enhancement of phase II enzymes: implications in cancer chemoprevention. Carcinogenesis. 1999 Nov;20(11):2101-08.

40. Ip SP, Mak DH, Li PC, Poon MK, Ko KM. Effect of a lignan-enriched extract of Schisandra chinensis on aflatoxin B1and cadmium chloride-induced hepatotoxicity in rats. PharmacolToxicol 1996:78:413-16.

41. Wang ZY, Nixon DW. Licorice and cancer. Nutr Cancer. 2001;39(1):1-11.

42. Moon A, et al. Effect of Glycyrrhiza glabra roots and glycyrrhizin on the glucuronidation in rate. 3:2.115-119.

43. Rao L, Puschner B, et al. Gene expression profiling of low selenium status in mouse intestine: transcriptional activation of genes linked to DNA damage, cell cycle control and oxidative stress. J Nutr. 2001;131:3175-81.

44. http://balancedconcepts.net/liver_phases_detox_paths.pdf

45. MacDonald Baker S, Bennett P, Bland JS, et al. Textbook of Functional Medicine. David S. Jones, ed. Gig Harbor WA: Publisher; 2006.

46. Folkers K. 1985; Gaby AR. 1987; Anonymous. Nutr Rev 1988;46:1367; Beyer RE. Biochem Cell Biol 1992 70(6):390-403.

47. Ogura R, Toyama H, Shimada T, Murakami M. The role of ubiquinone (Coenzyme Q10) in preventing Adriamycin-induced mitochondrial disorders in rat heart. J Appl Biochem 1979,1:325.

48. Neri B, De Leonardis V, Gemelli MT, et al. 1998. Melatonin as biological response modifier in cancer patients. Anticancer Res, 1998;18:1329-32.

49. Lissoni P, Bucovec R, Bonfanti A, et al. 2001.Thrombopoietic properties of 5-methoxytryptamine plus melatonin versus melatonin alone in the treatment of cancer-related thrombocytopenia. J Pineal Res 2001;30:123-26.

50. Thomsen LL, Miles DW, Happerfield L, Bobrow LG, Knowles RG, Moncada S. Nitric oxide synthase activity in human breast cancer. Br J Cancer. 1995;72:41-44.

51. Lissoni P, Barni S, Meregalli S, et al. 1995. Modulation of cancer endocrine therapy by melatonin: a phase II study of tamoxifen plus melatonin in metastatic breast cancer patients progression under tamoxifen alone. Brit J Cancer. 1995;71:854-56.

52. Fossa SD, Woehre H, Kurth KH, et al. Influence of urological morbidity on quality of life in patients with prostate cancer Eur Urol. 1997. 31:(Suppl 3):3-8.

53. Vasilescu S, Ptushkina M, Linz B, Muller PP, McCarthy

JE. 1996. Mutants of eukaryotic initiation factor eIF-4E with altered mRNA cap binding specificity reprogram mRNA selection by ribosomes in Saccharomyces cerevisiae. J Biol Chem. 1996, 271:7030-37.

54. Lissoni P, Brivio O, Brivio F, Barni S, Tancini G, Crippa D, Meregalli S. Adjuvant therapy with the pineal hormone melatonin in patients with lymph node relapse due to malignant melanoma. J Pineal Res. (IT)1996 Nov;21(4):239-42.

55. Smyth JF, Bowman A, Perren T, et al. Glutathione reduces the toxicity and improves quality of life of women diagnosed with ovarian cancer treated with cisplatin: results of a double-blind, randomised trial. Ann Oncol. 1997;8:569-73.

56. Cascinu S, et al. Neuroprotective effect of reduced glutathione on cisplatin-based chemotherapy on advanced gastric cancer: a randomized double-blind placebo-controlled trial. J Clin Oncol. 1995;13(1): 26-32.

57. Pirotzky E, Guilmard C, Sidoti C, Ivanow F, Principe P, Braquet P.1990 Platelet-activating factor antagonist, BN-52021 protects against cis-diamminedichloroplatinum nephrotoxicity in the rat. Ren Fail. 1990;12(3):171-76.

58. Bokemeyer C, Fels LM, Dunn T, Voigt W, Gaedeke J, Schmoll HJ, Stolte H, Lentzen H. Silibinin protects against cisplatin-induced nephrotoxicity without compromising cisplatin or ifosfamide anti-tumour activity. Br J Cancer. 1996 Dec;74(12):2036-41.

59. Gaedeke J, et al. Cisplatin nephrotoxicity and protection by silibinin. Nephrol Dial Transplant. 1996;11: 55-62.

60. Hu YJ, Chen Y, Zhang YQ, et al. The protective role of selenium on the toxicity of cisplatin-contained chemotherapy regimen in cancer patients. Biol Trace Elem Res. 1997 Mar;56(3):331-41.

61. Hofmann J, Fiebig HH, Winterhalter BR, Berger DP, Grunicke H. 1990. Enhancement of the antiproliferative activity of cis-diamminedichloroplatinum(II) by quercetin. Int J Cancer. 1990 Mar 15;45(3):536-39.

62. Scambia G, De Vincenzo R, Ranelletti FO, Panici PB, Ferrandina G, D'Agostino G, Fattorossi A, Bombardelli E, Mancuso S. Antiproliferative effect of silybin on gynaecological malignancies: synergism with cisplatin and doxorubicin. Eur J Cancer. 1996 May;32A(5):877-82.

63. Navis I, Sriganth P, Premalatha B. 1999. Dietary curcumin with cisplatin administration modulates tumour marker indices in experimental fibrosarcoma. Pharmacol Res. 1999 Mar;39(3):175-79.

64. Kobayashi, Y., K. Kariya, K. Saigenji & K. Nakamura, 1994. "Enhancement of anti-cancer activity of cisdiamineddichloroplatinum by the protein-bound polysaccharide of Coriolus versicolor QUEL (PS-K) in vitro. Cancer Biotherapy. Winter; 9(4)351-58.

65. Barata JD, D'Haese PC, Pires C, Lamberts LV, Simoes J, De Broe ME. Low-dose (5 mg/kg) desferrioxamine treatment in acutely aluminium-intoxicated haemodialysis patients using two drug administration schedules. Nephrol Dial Transplant. 1996 Jan;11(1):125-132.

66. Fukaya H, Kanno H. 1999. Experimental studies of the protective effect of ginkgo biloba extract (GBE) on cisplatin induced toxicity in rats]. Nippon Jibiinkoka Gakkai Kaiho. Jul 1999;102(7):907-917.

67. Sugiyama T, Sadzuka Y, Tanaka K, Sonobe T. Inhibition of glutamate transporter by theanine enhances the therapeutic efficacy of doxorubicin. Toxicol Lett. 2001 Apr 30;121(2):89-96.

68. Sugiyama S, Yamada K, Hayakawa M, et al. Approaches that mitigate doxorubicin-induced delayed adverse effects on mitochondrial functions in rat hearts; Liposome-encapsulated doxorubican or combination therapy with antioxidant. Biochem Mol Biol Int. 1995;36:1001-07; 1995.

69. Neri B, Neri GC, Bandinelli M. Differences between carnitine derivatives and coenzyme Q10 in preventing in vitro doxorubicin-related cardiac damages. Oncology. 1988; 45:242-26.

70. Antunes LM, Takahashi CS. Effects of high doses of vitamins C and E against doxorubicin-induced chromosomal damage in Wistar rat bone marrow cells. Mutat Res. 1998 Nov 9;419(1-3):137-43.

71. Faure H, Coudray C, Mousseau M, Ducros V, Douki T, Bianchini F, Cadet J, Favier A. 5-Hydroxymethyluracil excretion, plasma TBARS and plasma antioxidant vitamins in adriamycin-treated patients. Free Radic Biol Med. 1996;20(7):979-83.

Pathophysiology

The pancreas is about 6 inches long and looks something like a pear lying on its side. The wider end (head) is located near the center of the abdomen next to the upper part of the small intestine (duodenum). The main part (body) of the pancreas stretches behind the stomach, and the narrow end (tail) is on the left side, next to the spleen.

EXOCRINE AND ENDOCRINE FUNCTIONS

As part of the digestive system, the pancreas performs two essential functions: exocrine and endocrine . It produces digestive juices and enzymes that help break down proteins, carbohydrates, and fats so that food can be digested in the small intestine; this is the exocrine function. It secretes the hormones insulin and glucagon that regulate the way the body metabolizes sugar (glucose); this is the endocrine function.[1-2]

Most of the pancreas is composed of cells that produce digestive enzymes and juices. Pancreatic juices flow into the main pancreatic duct, which leads into the small intestine (duodenum). The pancreatic duct joins up with the tube leading from the gallbladder to form the common bile duct, which then empties into the small intestine. The pancreas also contains small "islands" of cells that secrete the hormones insulin and glucagon, along with somatostatin.[1-2]

ADENOCARCINOMAS

Most pancreatic tumors originate in the duct cells or in the cells that produce digestive enzymes (acinar cells).[3] Called adenocarcinomas, these tumors account for nearly 95% of pancreatic cancers.[3] Tumors that begin in the islet cells (endocrine tumors) are much less common. When they do occur however, they may cause the affected cells to produce too much hormone. For example, tumors in glucagon cells (glucagonomas) might cause excess amounts of glucagon to be secreted, while tumors in insulin cells (insulinomas) may lead to an overproduction of insulin. Tumors can also develop in the ampulla of Vater, the place where bile and pancreatic ducts empty into the small intestine. Called ampullary cancers, these tumors often block the bile duct, leading to jaundice. Because even a small tumor can obstruct the bile duct, signs and symptoms of ampullary cancer usually appear earlier than do symptoms of other pancreatic cancers.[4]

More than 90% of all pancreatic cancers are ductal adenocarcinomas of the exocrine pancreas. These tumors occur twice as frequently in the pancreatic head compared to the rest of the organ, and tend to be aggressive, often only found when the presenting signs and symptoms show and then the cancer is usually locally inoperable or found after distal metastases have already occurred.[5]

Epidemiology
PREVALENCE AND INCIDENCE

Pancreatic cancer, primarily ductal adenocarcinoma, accounts for about 30,500 cases and 29,700 deaths in the United States annually. Most pancreatic cancers are exocrine tumors that develop from ductal and acinar cells.[6] Adenocarcinomas of the exocrine pancreas arise from duct cells 9 times more often than from acinar cells; 80% occur in the head of the gland. Adenocarcinomas appear at the mean age of 55 years of age and occur 1.5 to 2 times more often in men.[6]

Neuroendocrine tumors account for 2% to 5% of pancreatic neoplasms. Cystic neoplasms account for only 1% of pancreatic cancers, but they are important because they are often mistaken for pseudocysts. A cystic neoplasm should be suspected when a cystic lesion in the pancreas is found in the absence of a history of pancreatitis.[7] At least 15% of all pancreatic cysts are neoplasms. Whereas serous cystadenomas (which account for 32% to 39% of cystic pancreatic neoplasms and also occur in patients with von Hippel–Lindau disease) are benign, mucinous cystic neoplasms (defined by the presence of ovarian stroma) (10% to 45%), intraductal papillary mucinous neoplasms (21% to 33%), solid pseudopapillary neoplasms (< 5%), and cystic islet cell tumors (3% to 5%) may be malignant, although their prognoses are better than the prognosis of adenocarcinoma of the pancreas, unless the neoplasm is locally advanced.[4]

Anatomy of the Pancreas

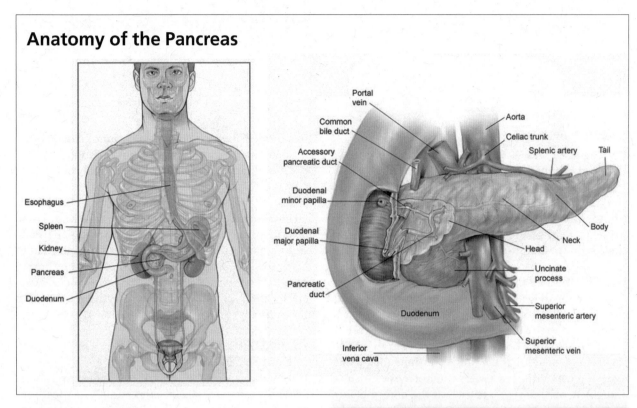

Histopathology

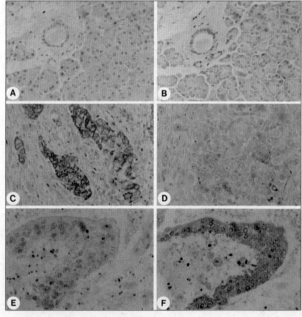

A-B Normal Pancreas Cells
C-F Pancreatic Cancer Cells

RISK FACTORS[9]

- Smoking: Smokers are 2-3x more likely to develop pancreatic cancer than nonsmokers. This is probably the greatest known risk factor for pancreatic cancer, with smoking associated with almost one in three cases of pancreatic cancer.
- Alcohol: Heavy alcohol use.
- Diabetes: Having diabetes may increase the risk of pancreatic cancer. Insulin resistance or high insulin levels may also be risk factors for pancreatic cancer. Metabolic syndrome, which is hallmarked by insulin resistance, will also present a higher risk of developing this disease.
- History of chronic pancreatitis.
- Heredity: There is an increased incidence of pancreatic cancers in families with an intermediate family member with diagnosed pancreatic cancer. The chances of developing pancreatic cancer increase if there are intermediate relatives that have hereditary chronic pancreatitis. Hereditary pancreatitis (HP) is a rare genetic condition marked by recurrent attacks of pancreatitis which is a painful inflammatory condition of the pancreas.
- Race: Black men and women have a higher risk of pancreatic cancer.
- Gender: More men than women develop pancreatic cancer.
- Excess weight: People who are very overweight or obese may have a greater risk of developing pancreatic cancer than do people of normal weight.
- Diet: A diet high in animal fat and low in fruits and vegetables may increase the risk of pancreatic cancer.
- Chemical exposure: People who work with petroleum compounds, including gasoline and other chemicals, have a higher incidence of pancreatic cancer than people not exposed to these chemicals.

GENETICS

About 7% to 8% of patients with pancreatic cancer have a family history of pancreatic cancer in a first-degree relative, compared with 0.6% of control subjects. Point mutations in codon 12 of the K-ras oncogene are found in 70% to 100%. Inactivation of the tumor suppressor genes INK4A on chromosome 9, TP53 on chromosome 17, and MADH4 on chromosome 18 were found in 95%, 75%, and 55% of pancreatic cancers, respectively. Mutation of the paladin gene is reported to be common.[10]

Pancreatic cancer can also occur as part of several hereditary syndromes, including hereditary pancreatitis, familial atypical multiple mole melanoma, Peutz–Jeghers syndrome, ataxia-telangiectasia, familial breast cancer (BRCA-2), and hereditary nonpolyposis colorectal cancer. Polymorphisms of the genes for methylene tetrahydrofolate reductase and thymidylate synthase have been reported to be associated with pancreatic cancer.[11]

Epigenetics

Researchers don't know exactly what damages DNA in the majority of cases of pancreatic cancer, but it is known that a small percentage of people develop the disease as a result of a genetic predisposition. These people who have a close relative, such as a parent or sibling, with pancreatic cancer have a higher risk of developing pancreatic cancer themselves. Additionally, a number of genetic diseases have been associated with an increased risk of pancreatic cancer, including familial adenomatous polyposis, nonpolyposis colon cancer, familial breast cancer associated with the BRCA2 gene, hereditary pancreatitis, and familial atypical multiple mole-melanoma syndrome, which is a very serious type of skin cancer. This means that people who have a hereditary predisposition to develop these cancers are also more likely to develop pancreatic cancer.[12]

However, only about 10% of pancreatic cancers result from an inherited tendency. A greater number are caused by environmental or lifestyle factors, such as smoking, diet, and chemical exposure.[11]

Assessment
SYMPTOMS AND SIGNS

Symptoms occur late, and by the time of diagnosis, approximately 90% of patients have locally advanced tumors that have involved the retroperitoneal structures and have spread to regional lymph nodes or metastasized to the liver or lung. Most patients have severe upper abdominal pain, which usually radiates to the back. The pain may be relieved by bending forward or assuming the fetal position (much like a gall bladder attach), but this usually means that the cancer has already spread beyond the pancreas into surrounding structures and is metastatic. More than 70% of patients have the presenting complaint of pain with weight loss.[13]

Adenocarcinomas of the head of the pancreas produce obstructive jaundice (often causing pruritus) in

---

SYMPTOMS OF PANCREATIC CANCER[14]

Upper abdominal pain
Pain may radiate to the middle or upper back. Pain is a common symptom of advanced pancreatic cancer. Abdominal pain occurs when a tumor presses on surrounding organs and nerves. Pain may be constant or intermittent and is often worse after you eating or lying down.

Loss of appetite and unintentional weight loss
Unintended weight loss is a common sign of pancreatic cancer. Weight loss occurs in most types of cancer because cancerous (malignant) cells deprive healthy cells of nutrients while increasing the metabolic "spin" of the system. This is especially true in pancreatic cancer, which also affects the ability to digest (digestive enzyme production) as well as respond to foods with the hormones of digestion (insulin and glucagon).

Yellowing of the skin and the whites of the eyes (jaundice, icterus)
About half of people with pancreatic cancer develop jaundice, which occurs when bilirubin, a breakdown product of worn-out blood cells, accumulates in the blood. Normally, bilirubin is eliminated in bile, a fluid produced by the liver and housed in the gallbladder. But if a pancreatic tumor blocks the flow of bile, excess pigment from bilirubin may turn the skin and the whites of the eyes yellow. In addition, the urine may be dark brown and the stools white or clay-colored. Although jaundice is a common sign of pancreatic cancer, it is more likely to result from other conditions, such as gallstones or hepatitis in the liver.

Itching
In the later stages of pancreatic cancer, the patient may develop severe itching when high levels of bile acids, another component of bile, accumulates in the skin.

Nausea and vomiting
In advanced cases of pancreatic cancer, the tumor may block a portion of the digestive tract, usually the upper portion of the small intestine (duodenum), causing nausea and vomiting.

Digestive problems
When cancer prevents pancreatic enzymes from being released into the intestine, it is hard to digest foods, especially those high in fat content. Eventually, this may lead to significant weight loss, as much as 25 pounds or more, as well as malnutrition. Diarrhea sometimes is an early symptom of the developing pancreatic cancer.

80% to 90% of patients. Cancer in the body and tail may cause splenic vein obstruction, resulting in splenomegaly, gastric and esophageal varices, and GI hemorrhages. The cancer causes diabetes in 25% to 50% of patients, leading to symptoms of glucose intolerance and showing symptoms of polyuria and polydipsia.[15]

PHYSICAL EXAMINATION

In early stages of disease, patients may not have any significant abnormalities detectable on physical examination. Jaundice may be a presenting feature in some cases; in these patients, a palpable, nontender gallbladder (Courvoisier's sign) may be palpated under the right costal margin. Patients with more advanced disease may have an abdominal mass (a periumbilical mass is the Sister Joseph's sign) hepatomegaly,

splenomegaly, or ascites. The left supraclavicular lymph node (Virchow's node) may be involved with tumor, or widespread peritoneal disease may be palpable on rectal examination in the pouch of Douglas.[15]

LABORATORY TESTS

Diagnosis is confirmed by CT scan, but routine laboratory tests should also be obtained.[16]

- Elevation of alkaline phosphatase and bilirubin indicate bile duct obstruction or liver metastases. There may be mild anemia.
- Glycosuria, hyperglycemia, and impaired glucose tolerance or true diabetes mellitus are found in 10% to 20% of cases.
- Pancreas-associated antigen CA 19 9 may be used to follow patients diagnosed with pancreatic carcinoma and to screen those at high risk. However,

this test is not sensitive or specific enough to be used for population screening.

- Elevated levels should drop with successful treatment; subsequent increases indicate progression. Amylase and lipase levels are usually normal.

PANCREATIC CANCER TUMOR MARKERS

Serological markers for pancreatic cancer may be classified as serum enzymes, tumor related antigens, and ectopic hormone production. Ribonuclease and amylase may be measured in the serum and have been correlated with pancreatic cancer. They are not clinically significant for the diagnosis of pancreatic neoplasm, but maybe helpful in differentiation from malignancy and chronic pancreatitis. Generally, amylase is elevated with pancreatitis but may also be elevated with malignancy, which is not a differential diagnostic marker.[17-20]

- CA 19-9: Developed from a human colorectal cancer cell line but most sensitive for the detection of pancreatic cancer. A reported sensitivity of 70% and specificity of 87%. Notable is that there is no difference in sensitivity between local and metastatic disease. CA 19-9 is best used conjunctively with CEA.[18,20]
- CEA has been found to be present in pancreatic cancer but has a low sensitivity and generally is not used.[20]
- CA 125: While primarily an ovarian cancer marker, it has been noted that pancreatic cancer has been found to have estrogen receptor sites. Thus, the CA 125 would not be a marker used to help in diagnosis, but rather one used to follow the therapeutic gains of treatment modalities.[17]
- Her2/neu: Pancreatic cancer is known to over express growth factor receptors. The gene HER2 is present in duct and acinar cells of normal pancreas and over expressed in pancreatic cancer.

Other serum tumor markers:

- CA 50
- DUPAN-2
- SPAN-1
- POA (pancreatic oncofetal antigen)

These antigens are less sensitive than CA 19-9, but when used in combination may improve the assessment of treatment response.[19-20]

Genetic Markers

P53 tumor suppressor gene mutations are also associated with pancreatic cancers:

- The 53-kd nuclear phosphoprotein product of the p53 gene is thought to control the activation

of transcription and to allow the cell to progress from G0/G1 to S phase. Overexpression of this protein due to mutations of the p53 gene is the most frequent type of genetic alteration in human cancer.[21]

- These mutations have potential cooperation with c-K-ras mutations in cellular transformation. The ras oncogene is the largest group of oncogenes associated with human neoplasia.[22]
- From 75% to 90% of pancreatic tumors contain c-K-ras mutations and have a high specificity for pancreatic cancer. There is a very low incidence of ras mutations in biliary, hepatic, gastric, and esophageal cancers. This specificity helps in the differentiation of pancreatic cancer from other upper abdominal masses, including chronic pancreatitis.[22]

IMAGING AND SCOPING PROCEDURES

A number of related scoping procedures may also be used in diagnosing pancreatic cancer and examining the biliary tract.

CT and MRI

The preferred tests are an abdominal helical CT or MRI of the pancreas (MRCP). If CT or MRCP demonstrates unresectable or metastatic disease, a percutaneous needle aspiration of an accessible lesion might be considered to obtain a tissue diagnosis. If CT demonstrates a potentially resectable tumor or no tumor, MRCP or endoscopic ultrasound may be used to stage the disease progression or detect small tumors not visible with CT. Patients with obstructive jaundice may have ERCP as the first diagnostic procedure.[23]

An MRI provides images similar to those obtained with CT. An advantage over CT is that it does not involve exposure to x-rays. Its drawbacks include being more expensive than CT and taking longer to perform than other imaging methods do. Its major use is in providing images of the biliary tract, termed magnetic resonance cholangiopancreatography (MRCP). The quality of the image produced can reduce the need for more invasive tests, in which dye is directly injected into the biliary and pancreatic ducts.[23]

Endoscopic retrograde cholangiopancreatography (ERCP)[24]

In this test, an endoscope (a flexible viewing tube) is passed through the mouth, esophagus, and stomach and into the duodenum (the first segment of the small intestine). A fine tube is inserted through the endoscope and into the biliary tract. A radiopaque dye is then injected into the bile ducts, and x-rays are taken of the biliary tract and pancreatic duct and its tributaries. This test causes inflammation of the pancreas (pancreatitis) in 3% to 5% of the people who undergo it.[24]

Biliary Tract

Computed tomography (CT) and ultrasound scanning are used most commonly to view the biliary tract. If additional imaging is needed, several diagnostic procedures may be used. In these procedures, a radiopaque dye (a dye visible on x-rays) is injected in the biliary tract, then x-rays are taken. These procedures can detect blockages and other abnormalities in the biliary tract.[25]

In percutaneous transhepatic cholangiography, **a** radiopaque dye is injected through the skin directly into a small bile duct in the liver. The radiopaque dye then flows through the biliary tract. In operative cholangiography, a radiopaque dye is injected directly into the biliary tract during gallbladder surgery.

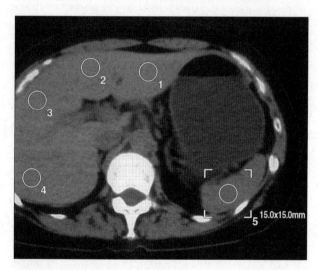

CT Scan of Pancreatic Cancer
Axial CT image with i.v. contrast. Macrocystic adenocarcinoma of the pancreatic head (plus sign clicks are surrounding the tumor in this CT image).

Staging and Grading

Following staging and grading, conventional treatment is surgical resection and adjuvant chemotherapy and radiation therapy.

TNM SYSTEM

The American Joint Committee on Cancer (AJCC) TNM system is used to describe the stages of cancer in the exocrine pancreas:[6]

- **T** describes the size of the primary tumor(s), measured in centimeters (cm), and indicates whether the cancer has spread within the pancreas or to nearby organs.
- **N** describes the spread to nearby (regional) lymph **n**odes.
- **M** indicates whether the cancer has **m**etastasized (spread) to other organs of the body. The most common sites of pancreatic cancer spread are the liver, lungs, and peritoneum – the space around the digestive organs.

Numbers or letters appear after T, N, and M to provide more details about each of these factors:

- The numbers 0 through 4 indicate increasing severity.
- The letter X means "cannot be assessed" because the information is not available.
- The letters "is" mean "carcinoma in situ," which means the tumor is contained within the top layers of pancreatic duct cells and has not yet invaded deeper layers of tissue.

TNM Staging[6]

- **TX:** The main tumor cannot be assessed.
- **T0:** No evidence of a primary tumor.
- **Tis:** Carcinoma in situ (very few tumors are found at this stage)
- **T1:** The cancer has not spread beyond the pancreas and is smaller than 2 cm (about ? inch) across.
- **T2:** The cancer has not spread beyond the pancreas but is larger than 2 cm across.
- **T3:** The cancer has spread from the pancreas to surrounding tissues near the pancreas but not to major blood vessels or nerves.
- **T4:** The cancer has extended further beyond the pancreas into nearby large blood vessels or nerves.

N categories[6]

- **NX:** Regional lymph nodes cannot be assessed.
- **N0:** Regional lymph nodes (lymph nodes near the pancreas) are not involved.
- **N1:** The cancer has spread to regional lymph nodes.

M categories[6]

- **MX:** Spread to distant organs cannot be assessed.
- **M0:** The cancer has not spread to distant lymph nodes (other than those near the pancreas) or to distant organs, such as the liver, lungs, or brain.
- **M1:** Distant metastasis is present.

Stage Grouping[26]

After the T, N, and M categories of the cancer have been determined, this information is combined to assign a stage, which is expressed in Roman numerals I through IV. The process of assigning a stage number based on TNM stages is called stage grouping. For example:

- **Stage 0 (Tis, N0, M0):** The tumor is confined to the top layers of pancreatic duct cells and has not invaded deeper tissues. It has not spread outside of the pancreas. These tumors are sometimes referred to as pancreatic carcinoma in situ or pancreatic intraepithelial neoplasia III (PanIn III).
- **Stage IA (T1, N0, M0):** The tumor is confined to the pancreas and is less than 2 cm in size. It has not spread to nearby lymph nodes or distant sites.
- **Stage IB (T2, N0, M0):** The tumor is confined to the pancreas and is larger than 2 cm in size. It has not spread to nearby lymph nodes or distant sites.
- **Stage IIA (T3, N0, M0):** The tumor is growing outside the pancreas but not into large blood vessels. It has not spread to nearby lymph nodes or distant sites.
- **Stage IIB (T1-3, N1, M0):** The tumor is either confined to the pancreas or growing outside the pancreas but not into nearby large blood vessels or major nerves. It has spread to nearby lymph nodes but not distant sites.
- **Stage III (T4, Any N, M0):** The tumor is growing outside the pancreas into nearby large blood vessels or major nerves. It may or may not have spread to nearby lymph nodes. It has not spread to distant sites.
- **Stage IV (Any T, Any N, M1):** The cancer has spread to distant sites.

Grade

Although not formally part of the TNM system, other factors are also important in determining prognosis or outlook.[49] The grade of the cancer (how abnormal the cells look under the microscope, indicating how aberrant the cells have become) is sometimes listed on a scale from G1 to G4, with G1 cancers looking the most like normal cells and having the best outlook.[26]

Extent of Resection

For patients who have surgery, another important factor is the extent of the resection – whether or not all of the tumor is removed and clean margins are obtained. This is sometimes listed on a scale from R0 (where all visible and microscopic tumor was removed) to R2 (where some visible tumor could not be removed).[27]

Resectable, Locally Advanced (Unresectable), and Metastatic[28]

From a practical standpoint, how far the cancer has spread in this organ often cannot be determined accurately without surgery because of the pancreas lies retroperitoneal. That is why doctors often use a simpler staging system, which divides cancers into groups based on whether or not it is likely they can be removed surgically. These groups are called resectable, locally advanced (unresectable), and metastatic. These terms can be used to describe both exocrine and endocrine pancreatic cancers.

Resectable

If the cancer is only in the pancreas (or has spread just beyond it) and the surgeon can remove the entire tumor, it is called resectable.

Locally Advanced (Unresectable)[30]

If the cancer has not yet spread to distant organs but it still can't be completely removed with surgery, it is called locally advanced. Often the reason the cancer cannot be removed is because too much of it is present in nearby blood vessels. Since the cancer cannot be removed entirely by surgery, it is also called unresectable. For these tumors, surgery would only be done to relieve symptoms or problems like a blocked bile duct or intestinal tract.

Metastatic

When the cancer has spread to distant organs, it is called metastatic. Surgery may still be done, but the goal would be to relieve symptoms, not to cure the cancer.[31]

5-YEAR SURVIVAL BY STAGE[29]

The 5-year survival rate refers to the percentage of patients who live at least 5 years after their cancer is diagnosed. Of course, some people live much longer than 5 years. Five-year rates are used as a standard way of discussing prognosis. Five-year relative survival rates compare the survival of people with the cancer to the survival for people without the cancer. Since some patients will die of causes other than cancer, this is a way to look only at deaths from the particular cancer. The 5-year relative survival rate is a more accurate way to describe the outlook for patients with a particular type and stage of cancer. Remember that these numbers are based on patients who were diagnosed at least 5 years ago. Improvements in treatment since that time may have improved survival for those diagnosed more recently.

Prognosis

Pancreatic cancer, especially in the body or tail, has a poor prognosis. Five-year survival rates range from 2% to 5%. If the patient has cancer in the head of the pancreas and it can be resected, this can result in longer survival rates. The poorest prognostic features are jaundice and lymph node involvement. It has been suggested that for people who have a positive family history of pancreatic cancer, screening exams with helical CT or endoscopic ultrasound should begin 10 years before the age of onset at which the family member was diagnosed with pancreatic cancer.[32]

5-year relative survival for exocrine pancreatic cancer
Overall, about 20% of people with pancreatic cancer live at least 1 year after diagnosis, while less than 4% will be alive after 5 years.[32]

Stage IA:	37%
Stage IB	21%
Stage IIA	12%
Stage IIB	6%
Stage III	2%
Stage IV	1%

5-year relative survival for endocrine pancreatic cancer
Pancreatic neuroendocrine cancers are not staged like cancers of the exocrine pancreas. Instead, the statistics are broken down into different stages: localized (only in the pancreas), regional (spread to nearby lymph nodes or tissues), and distant (spread to distant sites, such as the liver). The relative 5-year survival for all patients taken together is 42%.[33]

Localized	87%
Regional	70%
Distant	24%

Conventional Treatment for Pancreatic Cancer

In 30% of patients, abdominal surgical exploration may be necessary when cytologic diagnosis cannot be made or resection is to be attempted. A laparoscopy may detect tiny peritoneal or live metastases in patients without jaundice, with localized tumor in the head of the pancreas, thus avoiding resection in 4% to 13% of patients.[27] A Whipple's procedure (also known as a radical pancreaticoduodenal resection) is indicated for pancreatic cancer that is limited to only the head of the pancreas, periampullary zone, and duodenum (T1, N0, M0). Survival rates based on 5 years statistics show that in this group of patients rates can range from 20% to 40% if there is negative resection margins and no lymph node involvement.[30]

Adjuvant or neoadjuvant chemotherapy is generally with gemcitabine and fluorouracil and may be combined with radiation therapy appears to benefit the survival rates for those who have unresectable tumors. This chemoradiation is considered palliative for pancreatic cancer that is confined to the pancreas. Chemotherapy alone has had disappointing outcomes in metastatic pancreatic cancer.[31]

Endoscopic stenting of the bile duct to relieve jaundice is usually performed and a plastic stent is used if the patient's anticipated survival is less than 6 months while a metal stent is used if the patient is anticipated to survive more than 6 months.[28]

Naturopathic Approaches to Treating Pancreatic Cancer

Naturopathic Therapeutic Protocols

1. Maintain proper appetite and digestive functions
2. Ensure adequate proteins and calories in the diet
3. Prevent and treat common side effects
4. Counsel patients

Naturopathic therapies are specific to the diagnosis. Naturopathic physicians need to bear in mind the affect of treatment on all bodily functions. The goals of the integrative treatment plan are to maintain proper digestive function, provide adequate proteins and calories in the diet, and prevent and treat common side effects: mucositis, anorexia, cachexia, dysgeusia, and malnutrition.

1. MAINTAIN PROPER APPETITE AND DIGESTION FUNCTIONS

The most common problem in pancreatic cancer patients is nausea and vomiting with a loss of appetite. This cancer induces anorexia and cachexia as the cancer cells invade the tissue. To compound this problem, chemotherapy or radiation therapy may cause mucositis, dysgeusia, diarrhea, and changes in taste. Some patients experience a residual metallic taste in their mouths; others find that things taste too sweet; and most often the smell of food decreases the appetite or causes nausea and/or vomiting. Some of these effects can be attributed to mucositis post chemoradiation intervention, while others are the result of the cancer location and interference.

Mucositis and cachexia can affect the outcome of patients with pancreatic cancer. Mucositis is an intestinal mucosal damage of the gastrointestinal tract – mouth, throat, stomach, intestines, rectum, and anus – that is caused directly by chemotherapies and radiotherapies.[34] Cancer cachexia is a significant biochemical event, which is characterized by weight loss, fatigue, and indicative of depletion of skeletal muscle GLN – a hypercatabolic state.[35]

Dysgeusia includes nausea, vomiting, loss of appetite, dysbiosis, mucositis, anorexia and cachexia with sarcopenia, all as side effects of the lack of digestion. The inability to digest what they eat not only leads to the above mentioned affects, but also becomes discouraging for the patients mental status. Several nutraceuticals and herbal medicines have been studied and found effective in restoring appetite and reversing of dysgeusia.

L-Glutamine

L-glutamine, a non-essential amino acid, is effective in preventing and treating mucositis and cachexia. Studies have shown that by a simple 'swish and swallow' application of glutamine (GLN), the side effects of mucositis and cachexia can be treated and prevented. The side effects of mucositis are nausea, vomiting, diarrhea, stomatitis (mouth ulcers), and changes in taste. It is easy to see how mucositis can lead to cachexia and sarcopenia in this population. Add to this list a loss of appetite (anorexia), and negative outcomes can accumulate quickly for this patient population. Glutamine can be integrated into conventional chemotherapy and radiation therapy to improve positive outcomes and survival rates.[36]

As one study concluded, "cytotoxic chemotherapies and radiotherapies are most effective against rapidly dividing cells. As a consequence of this mechanism, these conventional treatment interventions may also damage host tissues that contain rapidly dividing cells. The cells of the GI tract are the most rapidly proliferating cells in the human body.[34] These intestinal cells absorb large amounts of GLN and metabolize nearly all the absorbed dietary GLN in addition to extracting circulating GLN from other tissues. Mucositis – that is, inflammation of the mucous membranes lining the digestive tract from the mouth to the anus – is a common toxic side effect of cancer chemotherapy and radiotherapy and it can involve any part of the digestive tract. As mentioned earlier, it was found in a pilot study that GLN can significantly decrease the severity and duration of mucositis/stomatitis induced by chemotherapy and radiation treatments, which is a significant side effect in this patient population and an important cause of increased morbidity in patients being treated for cancer."[36]

Dosage: The oral dosing range in adult patients for therapeutic effect on mucous membranes is 20 to 30 g in daily divided doses (which increases enterocyte contact), swished and swallowed, starting from the first round of conventional chemotherapy and/or radiotherapy until at least 2 weeks post therapy. The inability of lower doses to affect mucositis/stomatitis has been previously shown in clinical trials. Cachexia is the ultimate issue with mucositis/stomatitis and loss of appetite. In addition, cachexia is a secondary event from the high metabolism associated with cancer disease. Once a patient becomes cachexic, the body is using its own muscle mass as a protein source, causing sarcopenia. The oral route of GLN administration is inexpensive and convenient and the only treatment of stomatits known to reverse or 'cure' these mouth ulcers as well as prevent them along with the other mucositis effects on the gastrointestinal tract. For an in depth meta-analysis of L-Glutamine research and its use please refer to the authors published research. www.jodyenoe.com/publications.

2. ENSURE ADEQUATE PROTEINS AND CALORIES IN THE DIET

Follow the dietary therapy guidelines described in the chapter on naturopathic modalities, specifically the discussion of calorie restricted diets, which are not recommended in treatment of pancreatic cancer, and high protein diets, which are. Encourage patients to follow a macronutrient-rich diet that is high in proteins, low in high-glycemic carbohydrates, high in fiber, low in monosaturated fats but high in omega-3 fatty acids. Focus on anticancer foods that are rich in phytochemicals and antioxidants.

Add digestive enzymes, full spectrum, with each meal.

3. PREVENT AND TREAT COMMON SIDE EFFECTS

The common side effects of pancreatic cancer, besides loss of appetite and digestive function, can be treated effectively with specific botanical medicines.

Zingiber officinale

About 70% of cancer patients who receive chemotherapy complain of nausea and vomiting. As one study of ginger and nausea noted, "there are effective drugs to control vomiting, but the nausea is often worse because it lingers. …Nausea is a major problem for people who undergo chemotherapy and it has been a challenge for scientists and doctors to understand how to control it."[37] Ginger root has been studied for decades for its use against nausea and vomiting associated with cancer and cancer therapies. It also has been used successfully to aid in the reversal of anorexia and dysbiosis, as recently presented at ASCO (American Society of Oncologists' conference).[38]

At the Community Clinical Oncology Program Research Base at the Wilmot Cancer Center in Rochester, the largest randomized study of ginger as a treatment for nausea has been conducted. This Phase II/III placebo-controlled, double-blind study included 644 cancer patients who received at least three chemotherapy treatments. They were divided into four arms that received placebos, 0.5 gram of ginger, 1 gram of ginger, or 1.5 grams of ginger along with antiemetics (antivomiting drugs, such as Zofran, Kytril, Novaban, and Anzemet.) Patients took the ginger supplements 3 days prior to chemotherapy and 3 days following treatment. Patients reported nausea levels at various times of day following their chemotherapy, and those who took the lower doses had a 40% reduction.[38] Ginger is readily absorbed in the body and has long been considered a remedy for stomach aches. "By taking the ginger prior to chemotherapy treatment, the National Cancer Institute-funded study suggests its earlier absorption into the body may have anti-inflammatory properties."[38]

This rhizome has components of volatile oils, phenols, and alkaloids. The phenols – ginergerol, zingerone and shagoal – are the chemical constituents most likely to have the antinausea effect. This effect is achieved by their activity as a visceral antispasmodic and carminative that is highly antiemetic. Ginger root has been classically used as a tonic stomachic and digestive aid for sub-acid gastritis, dyspepsia, and anorexia. As a silalgogue, it stimulates the flow of saliva, while raising the tone of the intestinal musculature, thus aiding in perastalsis. The ginerols and shagoals are strong antiemitics and are still very active in the powdered root product.[39]

Mint Family
Nepeta spp. (Catnep, catmint) and *Metha spp.* peppermint and spearmint have been used as aperitifs and cordials throughout history to aid in digestion and elimination. Often these two mints can have a strong and pungent flavor, which, for a cancer patient, may be too strong or stimulating.[40]

However, catnep is a mild herb in the mint family that has no taste or flavor but acts as a carminative relaxant for the digestive tract. Its constituents include volatile oils, carvacrol, citronellal, nerol, geraniol, pulegone, thymol, nepetalic acid, tannins, and iridoids, including epideoxyloganic acid and 7-deoxyloganic acid.[41] Catnep eases any stomach upsets, dyspepsia, flatulence, and colic, as well as nausea and vomiting associated with cancer and conventional cancer treatment strategies. It is a classic remedy for the treatment of diarrhea in children, not only efficacious but safe.[42] Its sedative action on the nerves adds to its generally relaxing properties and helps this tea to have a quieting nervous system effect as well as a carminative for nausea.[42]

Dosage: Taken as an infusion with a 1 tablespoon of dried herb to 1 cup of water, sweeten with honey if desired (honey has its own antimucositis effect) and taken 30-15 minutes prior to desired time of eating a meal. Take at room temperature as often hot or cold sensations arc acccntuatcd with mucositis/stomatitis.

Other Naturopathic Interventions
Naturopathic therapies and strategies discussed in other chapters of this textbook can also be applied to the integrative treatment of pancreatic cancer.

- Melatonin, MCP, herbal COX-2 inhibitors, and PGE2 modifiers are indicated in pancreatic cancer.
- In conjunction with these strategies, a multi-spectrum digestive enzyme that includes bile and HCL acids is specifically indicated for pancreatic cancer.
- Digestive enzymes, deglycyrrhated licorice root (to act as a demulcent in the GI tract) and antinausea herbal medicines will improve not only the digestive function, reduce side effects but also enhance quality of life and thus, enhance their mental attitude and ultimately their outcome in their fight against this cancer.

Chemotherapeutic and Naturopathic Integrated Therapies[85]

Chemotherapeutic	Naturopathic	Daily Dose	Caution
Gemcitabine Fluorouracil (usually combined with radiation therapy)	*To increase effectiveness:*		
	Digestion is the system most compromised in pancreatic cancer	Eat frequent small meals with dose dense proteins	
	Digestive enzymes (including pancreatin, full spectrum enzymes, HCL, and ox bile acids) Enteric coated	With meals and snacks if nausea and vomiting increase, use plant-based digestive enzymes without acids	Dose adjust for days not eating much, or solid foods vs. days eating more normally
	DGL and other demulcents both in capsule and rhizinate forms for dysgenias	Probiotics full spectrum at 25-50 billion CFUs, on an empty stomach between meals and with meds if indicated	
	To reduce toxicity and side effects: L-glutamine Catnip tea Medicinal marijuana Ginger root capsules	Use at top doses as previously recommended	

References

1. Guyton, AC, Hall JE Textbook of Medical Physiology. 10th ed. St Louis, MO: WB Saunders Co.;2000.

2. Moore, KL, AF Dalley, AMR Aqur.Clinically Oriented Anatomy 6th Ed. Baltimore, MD: Lippincott Williams & Wilkins;2009.

3. Young, RC. Harrison's Internal Medicine, online. Chapter 89, Pancreatic Cancer, Yu Jo Chua, David Cunningham.

4. McPhee SJ. Papadakis MA, Eds. Gonzales R, Zeige R. Online Eds. 2009. CURRENT Medical Diagnosis & Treatment. 48th ed.

5. www.medcinenet.com

6. American Joint Committee on Cancer (AJCC). AJCC Cancer Staging Manual, 6th ed. New York, NY:Springer-New York;2002. www.springeronline.com

7. Macari M, Finn ME, Bennett GL, Cho KC, et al. Differentiating pancreatic cystic neoplasms from pancreatic pseudocysts at MR imaging: value of perceived internal debris. Radio 2009;25(1):77-84

8. http://www.pancreatic.org/site/c.htJYJ8MPIwE/b.891917/k.5123/Prognosis_of_Pancreatic_Cancer.htm. 2012.

9. http://www.cancer.org/Cancer/PancreaticCancer/DetailedGuide/pancreatic-cancer-risk-factors. 2012.

10. http://emedicine.medscape.com/article/280605-overview Dragovich T. Pancreatic Cancer. Drugs, Diseases & Procedures. 2011.

11. http://www.cancer.net/patient/All+About+Cancer/Genetics/The+Genetics+of+Pancreatic+Cancer American Society of Clinical Oncologists website Cancer.Net Jan. 2012

12. Ang L, Omura N, Seung-Mo H, et al. Epigenetic silencing of transcription factor SIP1 in pancreatic cancer cells is associated with elevated expression and blood serum levels of microRNAs miR200a,b. Cancer Res. 2010;70(13):5226-37.

13. http://www.scientificamerican.com/article.cfm?id=experts-pancreatic-cancer-gene-upshaw Wenner M. What makes pancreatic cancer so deadly? Scientific American, 2008.

14. http://pathology.jhu.edu/pc/BasicSymptom.php?area=ba Johns Hopkins Medicine; The Sol Goldman Pancreatic Cancer Research Center. 2012.

15. http://www.mayoclinic.com/health/pancreatic-cancer/DS00357/DSECTION=symptoms. 2011.

16. http://www.cancer.net/patient/Cancer+Types/Pancreatic+Cancer?sectionTitle=Diagnosis ASCO Cancer.Net 2011 Pancreatic Cancer diagnosis Laboratory Testing.

17. http://www.tc-cancer.com/tumormarkers.html 2012.

18. http://cancer.about.com/od/pancreaticcancer/p/CA19tumormarker.htm Fayed L. CA 19-9 Tumor Marker Test Profile. 2006.

19. Okusaka T, Yamada T, Maekawa M. Serum tumor markers for pancreatic cancer: the dawn of new era? JOP. 2006;7(4):332-36.

20. Zhou W, Sokoll LJ, Bruzek DJ, et al. Identifying markers for pancreatic cancer by gene expression analysis. Ca Epidem Biomar Prev. 1998;7(2):109-12.

21. Slebos RJ, Hoppin JA, Tolbert PE, et al. K-ras and p53 in pancreatic cacner: association with medical history, histopathology, and environmental exposures in a population based study. Ca Epidem Biomar Prev 2000;9(11):1233-32.

22. http://www.surgery.usc.edu/divisions/tumor/pancreas-diseases/web%20pages/pancreas%20cancer/genetic%20changes%20in%20pancCA.html Genetics of Pancreatic Cancer, University of Southern California Center for Pancreatic and Biliary Diseases, Department of Surgery. 2012.

23. http://pancreasmd.org/ed_imaging_mrcp.html The Pancreas Center 2012

24. http://www.medicinenet.com/ercp/article.htm ERCP endoscopic retrograde cholangio-Pancreatography. 2012.

25. http://www.webmd.com/cancer/pancreatic-cancer/pancreatic-cancer-diagnosis. 2012.

26. http://www.cancer.org/Cancer/PancreaticCancer/DetailedGuide/pancreatic-cancer-staging. 2012.

27. Diener MK, et al. A systematic review and meta-analysis of pylorus-preserving versus classical pancreaticoduodenectomy for surgical treatment of periampullary and pancreatic carcinoma. Ann Surg. 2007 Feb;245(2):187-200.

28. Ghaneh P et al. Biology and management of pancreatic cancer. Gut. 2007 Aug;56(8):1134-52.

29. Hassan MM, et al. Risk factors for pancreatic cancer: case-control study. Am J Gastroenterol. 2007 Dec;102(12):2696-707.

30. Rodriguez JR et al. Branch-duct intraductal papillary mucinous neoplasms: observations in 145 patients who underwent resection. Gastroenterology. 2007 Jul;133(1):72-79.

31. Sultana A et al. Meta-analyses of chemotherapy for locally advanced and metastatic pancreatic cancer. J Clin Oncol. 2007 Jun 20;25(18):2607-15.

32. http://seer.cancer.gov/statfacts/html/pancreas.html National Cancer Institute Surveillance Epidemiology and End Results. 2012.

33. Pansulto F, Nasoni S, Falconi M, et al. Prognostic factors and survival in endocrine tumor patients: comparison between gastronintestinal and pancreatic localization. Endo Relat Ca. 2005;12(4):1083-92.

34. Nausea From Chemotherapy. Science Daily. Retrieved June 14, 2010, from http://www.sciencedaily.com/releases/2009/05/090514221920.htm

35. Kern KA, Norton JA. Cancer achexia. JPEN 1988;12(3):286-98.

36. Noe, JE. L-Glutamine use in the treatment and prevention of mucositis and cachexia: a naturopathic perspective. Integrative Cancer Ther. 2010 Jan; 8(4): 409-15.

37. http://www.urmc.rochester.edu/news/story/index.cfm?id=2491 Ryan JL. Ginger Quells Cancer Patient' Nausea From chemotherapy. 2009.

38. Ryan JL. Treatment of Chemotherapy induced nausea in cancer patients. Eur Onco 2010;6(2):14-16.

39. http://cms.herbalgram.org/expandedE/Ginger-root.html Expanded Comission E Monograph on Ginger Root. 2012.

40. Labrioloa D. Complementary cancer therapies: combining traditional and alternative approaches for the best possible outcome. 2009.

41. http://plants.usda.gov/java/profile?symbol=NECA2 USDA Plant Profile Nepeta cataria L. 2012.

42. http://www.okanogan1.com/botany/herbal/herbal-db.pdf The Herbal Database listing herbs, spices and medicinal plants. 2008.

43. Gieringer D. Review of the Human Studies on the Medical Use of Marijuana.1996. http: //norml.org/medical/medmj.studies.shtml. See state studies at http: //www.drug-policy.org/

44. HallW, et al. The Health and Psychological Consequences of Cannabis Use, Canberra, Australian Government Publishing Service 189;1994. http://www.druglibrary.org/

45. Guzman M. Cannabinoids: potential anticancer agents. Nat Rev Cancer. 2003;3(10): 745-55.

46. Joy E. op. cit., 259. (Chapter 4 of this report contains sections on nausea, vomiting, wasting syndrome and anorexia)

47. Doblin R, Kleiman MAR. Marijuana as antiemetic medicine: a survey of oncologists' experiences and attitudes. J Clin Oncol. 1991;9:1275-90.

48. James JS. Medical Marijuana: Unpublished Federal Study Found THC- Treated Rats Lived Longer, Had Less Cancer. 1997. AIDS Treatment News. 263. http://www.immunet.org/

49. Guzman M (2003). Cannabinoids: potential anticancer agents. Nature Reviews. 2003;3:745 -55.

50. Blazquez Cet, al. Inhibition of tumor angiogenesis by cannabinoids. FASEB J. 2003;17(3): 529-31.

51. Sanchez C, et al. Inhibition of glioma growth in vivo by selective activation of the CB(2) cannabinoid receptor. Cancer Res. 2001;61(15): 5784-89.

52. Casanova ML, et al. Inhibition of skin tumor growth and angiogenesis in vivo by activation of cannabinoid receptors. J Clin Invest. 2003;111(1): 43-50.

53. Jacobsson SO, et al. Inhibition of rat C6 glioma cell proliferation by endogenous and synthetic cannabinoids. Relative involvement of cannabinoid and vanilloid receptors. J Pharmacol Exp Ther. 2001 Dec;299(3): 951-59.

54. Galve-Roperph I, et al. Antitumoral action of cannabinoids: involvement of sustained ceramide accumulation of ERK activation. Nature Medicine. 2000;6:313-19; ACM Bulletin. "THC destroys brain cancer in animal research." http: //www.acmed.org/english/2000/eb000305.html

55. Benard J. Cannabinoids, among others, send malignant tumors to nirvana. Bull Cancer. 2000;87:299-300.

56. Di Marzo V et al. Palmitoylethanolamide inhibits the expression of fatty acid amide hydrolase and enhances the anti-proliferative effect of anandamide in human breast cancer cells. Biochem J. 2001;15(358):249-55.

57. Ruiz L, et al. Delta-9-tetrahydrocannabinol induces apoptosis in human prostate PC-3 cells via a receptor-independent mechanism. FEBS Letter. 1999;458: 400-404.

58. Baek S, et al. Antitumor activity of cannabigerol against human oral epitheloid carcinoma cells. Arch Pharm Res. 1998;2:353-56.

59. Harris L, et al. Anti-tumoral properties of cannabinoids. The pharmacology of Marihuana, ed. M. Braude et al. 2 vols., New York, NY: Raven Press;1976(2): 773-76; as cited by L. Grinspoon et al. Marihuana: The Forbidden Medicine. 2nd ed. New Haven, CT: Yale University Press;1997:173.

60. Toxicology and carcinogenesis studies of 1trans-delta-9-tetrahydrocannabinol in F344N/N Rats and BC63F1 mice. National Institutes of Health National Toxicology Program, NIH Publication No. 97-3362; November 1996.

61. De Petrocellis L, et al. The endogenous cannabinoid anandamide inhibits human breast cancer cell proliferation, Proceedings of the National Academy of Sciences 1998;95: 8375-80. http: //www.pnas.org/cgi/content/abstract/95/14/8375.

62. Pot chemicals might inhibit breast tumors, stroke damage. Dallas Morning News, July 13, 1998.

63. Di Marzo V, et al. Palmitoylethanolamide inhibits the expression of fatty acid amide hydrolase and enhances the anti-proliferative effect of anandamide in human breast cancer cells. Biochem J. 2001;358(Pt 1):249-55.

64. Portella G, et al. Inhibitory effects of cannabinoid CB1 receptor stimulation on tumor growth and metastatic spreading: actions on signals involved in angiogenesis and metastasis.FASEB J. 2003;17(12):1771-73. Epub 2003 Jul 03.

65. Mimeault M, et al. Anti-proliferative and apoptotic effects of anandamide in human prostatic cancer cell lines: implication of epidermal growth factor receptor down-regulation and ceramide production. Prostate. 2003;56(1):1-12.

66. Ligresti A et al. Possible endocannabinoid control of colorectal cancer growth. Gastroenterology. 2003;125(3):677-87.

67. Gomez del Pulgar T, et al. De novo-synthesized ceramide is in-volved in cannabinoid-induced apoptosis. Biochem J. 2002;363(Pt 1):183-88.

68. Gomez Del Pulgar T, et al.Cannabinoids protect astrocytes from ceramide-induced apoptosis through the phosphatidylinositol 3-kinase/protein kinase B pathway. J Biol Chem. 2002;277(39):36527-33. Epub Jul 19.

69. Gonzalez S, et al. Decreased cannabinoid CB1 receptor mRNA levels and immunoreactivity in pituitary hyperplasia induced by prolonged exposure to estrogens. Pituitary. 2000;3(4):221-26.

70. Pagotto U. Normal human pituitary gland and pituitary adenomas express cannabinoid receptor type 1 and synthesize endogenous cannabinoids: first evidence for a direct role of cannabinoids on hormone modulation at the

human pituitary level. J Clin Endocrinol Metab. 2001;86(6):2687-96.

71. Rubovitch V, Gafni M, Sarne Y. The cannabinoid agonist DALN positively modulates L-type voltage-dependent calcium-channels in N18TG2 neuroblastoma cells. Brain Res Mol Brain Res. 2002;101(1-2):93-102.

72. Bifulco M, et al. Control by the endogenous cannabinoid system of ras oncogene-dependent tumor growth. FASEB J. 2001;15(14): 2745-7. Epub Oct 29.

73. Massi P, et al. Antitumor effects of cannabidiol, a nonpsy-choative cannabinoid, on human glioma cell lines. JPET. 2004;308:838-45.

74. McAllister SD, et al. Cannabinoids selectively inhibit proliferation and induce death of cultured human glioblastoma multiforme cells. J Neurooncol. 2005 Aug;74(1):31-40.

75. Hazekamp A. Evaluation of a vaporizing device (Volcano(R)) for the pulmonary administration of tetrahydrocannabinol. J Pharm Sci. 2006;95(6):1308-17.

Pathophysiology

Prostate cancer typically grows slowly over a long period time, spanning decades of a patient's life before ultimately leading to mortality from the cancer. From the first appearance of a precancerous lesion, to an invasive lesion, to a metastatic lesion that results in symptoms and eventually mortality – this all usually takes tens of years to complete.

Most prostate cancers are detected on the basis of elevations in the prostate specific antigen (PSA), not by digital rectal examination (DRE). Prostate cancer may present as focal nodules or areas of induration within the prostate gland itself, but this is usually a later finding in the progression of the disease. However, the DRE, which is the routine clinical screening examination, coupled with PSA levels, may not detect the cancer in its early developmental stages.[1]

Obstructive voiding is usually associated with benign prostatic hyperplasia (BPH), which also affects men in the same age group as prostate cancer. When prostate cancer grows into a large, extensive lesion, then it can obstruct voiding and cause other urinary retention problems. If the cancer spreads to local lymph nodes, there can be lower extremity lymphedema. If it spreads to the skeletal system, which is the most common site of metastatic disease, pathologic fractures may occur, clinically presenting as back pain.[2]

Prognosis

Prognosis for most patients with prostate cancer, especially when localized or regional, is very good. Prognosis for elderly men with prostate cancer differs little from age-matched men without prostate cancer. For many patients, long-term local control, even cure, is possible. Potential for cure, even when cancer is clinically localized, depends on the tumor's grade and stage. Without early treatment, patients with high-grade, poorly differentiated cancer have a poor prognosis. Undifferentiated prostate cancer, squamous cell carcinoma, and ductal transitional carcinoma respond poorly to the usual control measures. Metastatic cancer has no cure; median life expectancy is 1 to 3 years, although some patients live for many years beyond this.[4]

CELLULAR STRUCTURES

The prostate gland is located between the bladder and rectum, wrapping around the urethra in men. The gland itself consists of three types of cells, surrounded by a dense, fibrous capsule:[3]

1. Glandular cells, which produce a milky fluid that liquefies semen
2. Smooth muscle cells, which contract during sex and squeeze the fluid into the urethra
3. Stroma cells, which form the structure of the prostate. The stroma is composed of branching tubuloalveolar glands arranged in lobules, including a compartment of fibroblasts and smooth muscle cells. The acni compartment includes epithelial, basal, and neuroendocrine cells, with the compartments separated by a basement membrane.

Surrounding the prostate are the periprostatic and dorsal vein complexes, responsible for erectile function of the penis. The urinary sphincter is also associated with the prostate, and this sphincter is responsible for passive urinary control.[3]

PSA AND PAO

Prostate specific antigen (PSA) and prostate acid phosphatase (PAP) are produced in the epithelial cells and can be measured as a marker for overall prostate health. Prostate epithelial cells and stromal cells express androgen receptors and depend on these androgens for normal growth and development. The major circulating hormone in males is the androgen testosterone, which is converted by 5α-reductase enzyme to dihydrotestosterone (DHT) in the gland itself. The periurethral part of the gland is what increases in size with male puberty and can also increase in size after the age of 55, where nonmalignant cells grow in this transition zone surrounding the urethra. Most cancers develop in the peripheral zone and often can be palpated in this location by DRE.[5-6]

Anatomy of the Prostate

- Bladder
- Rectum
- Prostate
- Urethra
- Testis

- Ureteric orifice
- Bladder
- Prostate
- Corpus spongiosum & bulbospongiosus muscle

Risk factors[7]

- Age: About 80% of these tumors are discovered in men older than 65.
- Percentage: One in six men will develop invasive cancer of the prostate during his lifetime.
- Family history: Men with several close relatives who have prostate cancer, or whose relatives are younger than 60 at diagnosis, are at greater risk.
- Race: African-American men are twice as likely to develop the disease as Caucasian men,
- Cadmium exposure: This typically occurs in people who work as chemists, loggers, farmers, textile workers, painters, and rubber tire workers, and to people who smoke commercial cigarettes.
- Altered hormone levels: Both female and male sex hormones may be altered.
- High-fat diets: Especially if the diet includes charred red meats (α-linoleic acid or polycyclic aromatic hydrocarbons).

Epidemiology

INCIDENCE AND PREVALENCE

Adenocarcinoma of the prostate is the most common non-dermatologic cancer in men > 50 in the United States. In 2012, in the United States about 241,700 prostate cancer cases were diagnosed and approximately 28,170 men died from their disease.[8] In recent years, deaths from prostate cancer have decreased with the increased correlated use of PSA markers to detect cancer earlier in men. Incidence increases with each decade of life; autopsy studies show prostate cancer in 15% to 60% of men age 60 to 90, with incidence increasing with age. Median age at diagnosis is 72, and > 75% of prostate cancers is diagnosed in men > 65. The highest risk group is Afro-American men in the United States.[8]

Sarcoma of the prostate is rare, occurring primarily in children. Undifferentiated prostate cancer, squamous cell carcinoma, and ductal transitional carcinoma also occur. Hormonal influences contribute to adenocarcinoma, but almost certainly not to other types of prostate cancer. Prostatic intraepithelial neoplasia (PIN) is precancerous histologic change. It may be low- or high-grade; high-grade is considered a precursor of invasive cancer.[9]

RISK FACTORS

Genetic

The risk of being diagnosed with prostate cancer increases by 2x if one first-degree relative is affected by the cancer, and by 4x if two first degree relatives are affected. The current estimate is that 40% of early onset and 5% to 10% of all prostate cancers are hereditary.[10]

In age-matched ethnic groups, black males compared to white males have both a greater number of precancerous cells, prostatic intraepithelial neoplasia (PIN), and larger tumor size, which has been shown to be related to higher endogenous levels of testosterone. Other genetic effects in this population include higher polymorphic variants of the androgen receptor gene, the CYP 450 C17 gene, and the 5α-reductase type II (SRD5A2) gene, all leading to a higher incidence of prostate cancer in the black male proband.[11]

Environmental

The incidence of clinical disease varies perhaps because of environmental factors, including diet and lifestyle.[12]

Inflammation

Although the cause of prostate cancer remains unknown, this cancer is a multistep process that often

Prostate Flow Chart[13]

Men > 50 or African Americans > 45 or + Family History

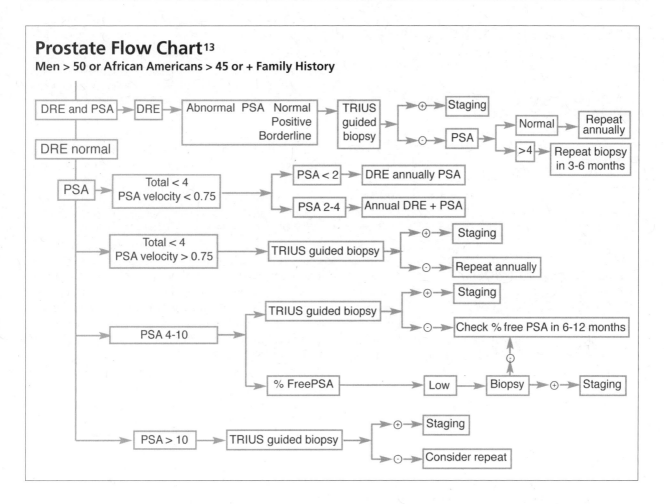

develops in or by an area of inflammation. One of the earliest changes noted in prostate cancer is the hypermethylation of the GSTP1 gene promoter, which once turned on leads to the loss of the gene that functions to detoxify carcinogens.[14] Inflammation is the second step in the development of the aberrant cancerous cell, with many prostate cancer growths found adjacent to a proliferative-inflammatory atrophic (PIA) site. There can be no inflammation without oxidative and free radical damage, which leads to the development of the aberrant cancer cell.[15]

Screening for prostatic cancer[16]

Test	Sensitivity	Specificity	Positive Predictive Value
Abnormal PSA (> 4 ng/mL)	0.67	0.97	0.43
Abnormal DRE	0.50	0.94	0.24
Abnormal PSA or DRE	0.84	0.92	0.28
Abnormal PSA and DRE	0.34	0.995	0.49

Adapted by permission, from Kramer BS et al. Prostate cancer screening: what we know and what we need to know. Ann Intern Med. 1993 Nov 1;119(9):914–23.

CLINICAL STAGE DIAGNOSIS

At each step of the evaluation, the practitioner should assess whether further diagnostics are needed to monitor or treat the prostate. The patient remains at this state of his current diagnosis until an indicator changes and moves him into a different category or state. At each evaluation stage, ask if the patient has now developed prostate cancer, or if he has prostate cancer, ask if the disease has perpetuated and extended. Because prostate cancer develops over a long period, clinical state diagnosis is especially effective.[16]

For example, a patient with localized prostate cancer who has had all cancer removed surgically remains in the state of localized disease as long as the PSA remains undetectable. The time within a state becomes a measure of the efficacy of an intervention, though the effect may not be assessable for years. As many men with active cancer are not at risk for developing metastases, symptoms, or death, the states model allows a distinction between *cure* – the elimination of all cancer cells, the primary therapeutic objective when treating most cancers – and cancer *control*, in which the tempo of the illness is altered and symptoms controlled until the patient dies of other causes.

These can be equivalent therapeutically from a patient standpoint if the patient has not experienced symptoms of the disease or the treatment needed to control it. Even when a recurrence is documented, immediate therapy is not always necessary. Rather, at the time of diagnosis, the need for intervention is based on the tempo of the illness as it unfolds in the individual, relative to the risk-to-benefit ratio of the therapy being considered.[16]

DIGITAL RECTAL EXAMINATION

Prostate screening tests currently used as standard of care practices include annual DRE and PSA testing with the follow up of a transrectal ultrasound (TRUS)

if further diagnostic evaluation is warranted. TRUS should not be used as a first-line screening tool because of its low specificity rate, which leads to a higher biopsy rate and minimal improvement of detection when compared to DRE and PSA testing.[17]

The DRE should be a regular part of yearly physical exams for men beginning at age 40. Sometimes stony hard induration or nodules are palpable. Induration and nodularity suggest cancer, but must be differentiated from granulomatous prostatitis, prostatic calculi, and other prostate disorders. Extension of induration to the seminal vesicles and lateral fixation of the gland suggest locally advanced prostate cancer. Prostate cancers detected by DRE tend to be large, and > 50% extend through the capsule. Once extended through the capsule, prostate cancer is considered to be in a metastatic disease state.[18]

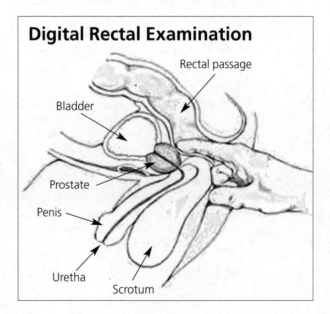

Digital Rectal Examination

Rectal passage

Bladder

Prostate

Penis

Uretha

Scrotum

PROSTATE SPECIFIC ANTIGEN

PSA should be tested annually because there is over a 50% chance of a normal PSA level showing a pathological implication within one years' time. PSA is a prostate specific antigen not a prostate cancer specific antigen. It is a kallikrein-like serine protease that causes liquefaction of seminal coagulum that can be produced by both nonmalignant and malignant epithelial cells. It can be elevated by infection, as in prostatitis and BPH, as well as by prostate cancer. A prostate biopsy can increase PSA levels by 10x for up to 8 to 10 weeks. It has a half life of 2 to 3 days in the serum and should be undetectable if the prostate is removed.[19]

A rate change in the PSA over time can be indicative of a cancerous prostate. Even if the PSA levels remain in normal ranges, a rise within these normal parameters over time can indicate prostate cancer. A rate of change >0.75ng/ml per year is considered a change that would be associated with the growth of prostate cancer. Even if the DRE is normal, the elevation in PSA is sufficiently sensitive and specific to warrant further investigation with a TRUS and biopsy.[16]

PSA Reference Ranges

According the Current Medical Diagnosis and Treatment Manual,[2] new age specific reference ranges for PSA have been established, based on a previously normal serum PSA of <4ng/ml:

- Men 40-49 years of age <2.5 ng/ml
- Men 50-59 years of age <3.5 ng/ml
- Men 60-69 years of age <4.5 ng/ml
- Men 70-79 years of age <6.5 ng/ml

Age-specific Reference Ranges

PSA concentration is directly related to the man's age, and establishing these age-specific reference ranges with increases to sensitivity of the test itself means that fewer older men would undergo biopsy and more younger men with cancer would be detected and undergo evaluation and treatment earlier. Men 50 and over should have an annual prostate specific antigen (PSA) test. African-American men and men with a family history of prostate cancer should begin PSA testing at age 45.[20]

Free and Bound PSA

Another screening model to detect cancer earlier in men is the use of free and bound PSA because men with prostate cancer have a lower percentage of free serum PSA. Men with free fractions of PSA exceeding 25% are unlikely to have prostate cancer, while those with free fractions of less than 10% of PSA result in about a 50% chance of having prostate cancer.[21]

TRANSRECTAL ULTRASOUND AND BIOPSY

A true diagnosis of prostate cancer is determined by a transrectal ultrasound guided needle biopsy. Directly visualizing the prostate assures that all areas of the gland are sampled by biopsy. Usually a minimal of six separate samples of cores are taken, three from the right and three from the left, as well as the transitional zone in a separate biopsy if indicated. Men who have abnormal PSA levels but negative biopsy results are advised to undergo a repeat biopsy. Each sample, or core, of the biopsy is examined for the presence of cancer, and, if found, the amount of cancer is then quantified by the length and extension of the tumor into that individual core sample. How much of the core that is involved is paramount to the diagnosis of prostate cancer.[22]

TRUS guided biopsy is the standard method for the detection and diagnosis of prostate cancer. The specimen cores preserve the glandular architect, thereby permitting the accurate grading and staging of the cancer. Prostate biopsy specimens are taken from the apex of the gland, mid portion, and base on each half of the gland, which is divided by the sulcus. Areas of local tumor invasion and transitional cell zones can also be sampled to ensure proper diagnosis. If abnormalities of the seminal vesicles are seen, samples of these structures should be specifically biopsied to identify local tumor invasion. TRUS is also used for staging of prostate cancer. These cancer sites typically appear as hypoechoic areas on the ultrasound.[22]

Ultrasound complications and limitations
- Difficulty penetrating bony structures
- US waves do not pass through air

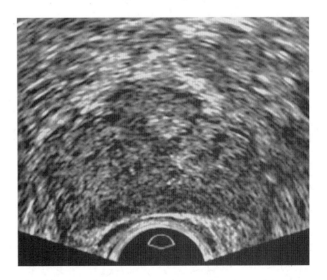

TNM staging system for prostate cancer[23]

T: Primary tumor

Tx	Cannot be assessed
T0	No evidence of primary tumor
T1a	Carcinoma in 5% or less of tissue resected; normal DRE
T1b	Carcinoma in more than 5% of tissue resected; normal DRE
T1c	Detected from elevated PSA alone; normal DRE
T2a	Tumor in 1/2 of one lobe
T2b	Tumor in >1/2 of one lobe
T2c	Tumor in both lobes
T3a	Extracapsular extension
T3b	Seminal vesicle involvement
T4	Adjacent organ involvement

N: Regional lymph nodes

Nx	Cannot be assessed
N0	No regional lymph node metastasis
N1	Metastasis in one or more regional lymph nodes

M: Distant metastasis

Mx	Cannot be assessed
M0	No distant metastasis
M1a	Metastasis to non-regional lymph node(s)
M1b	Metastasis to bone(s)
M1c	Metastasis to other site(s) with or without bone disease

Adapted from Greene FL, et al (eds). AJCC Cancer Staging Manual. 6th ed. New York, NY: Springer, 2002.

IMAGING STUDIES

After a diagnosis of prostate cancer is reached, further diagnostic imaging studies may be used to assess the extent of the disease and to follow the progression of the cancer. Magnetic resonance imaging (MRI) of the prostate allows for evaluation of the cancerous lesion and surrounding lymph nodes. The detection of both penetration through the capsule of the prostate and invasion of the seminal vesicles is about equal to that of a TRUS. Computed tomography (CT scan) plays a small role because of its inability to accurately identify and stage prostate cancer, although it is used to detect regional metastasis to the lymph and intra abdominal metastasis. Radionuclide bone scan is superior to the conventional plain skeletal radiographs in detecting bony metastases.[24] Most prostate cancer metastases are multiple, not singular, and are usually found in the axial skeleton. The more advanced and extensive the disease the more likely advanced local lesions into the skeleton will be found. Patients who have clinical symptoms of bone pain, high grade of the disease or continual elevations in PSA should also have cross section imaging done with the scan either with CT or MRI.[25]

TESTOSTERONE LEVELS

Testosterone levels, both free and bound, should be taken and monitored as part of the diagnostic work up for suspected prostate cancer.[26]

Staging and Grading
FIVE GRADES[27]

The majority of prostate cancer arises in the periphery of the prostate gland, called the peripheral zone. A small percentage comes from the central zone (5% to 10%) and the transition zone (20%). The Gleason grading system is used where a primary "grade" is given to the architectural pattern of the cancerous glands that occupy the largest area of the specimen, while a secondary grade is given to the next to the largest area where the cancer is found.

Grading is based on architecture rather than histological criteria, giving a possibility of five grades. Adding up the scores of the primary and secondary patterns gives the total that equates to the Gleason score. This score then correlates to the tumor size, volume, and pathological state, as well as a prognosis. The higher the score, the worse prognosis.

TNM STAGING[23]

The TNM staging (**T** for tumor, **N** for lymph nodes, and **M** for metastasis) categorizes the cancer not only by what is palpable on DRE but also by abnormal PSA levels (T1c). TNM works well for those cancers that are palpable but confined to the gland and not extending through the capsule of the gland (T2); and for those cancers that have extended outside of the capsule surrounding the gland (T3 and T4). Key indications are the growth of the tumor itself, whether it has invaded the capsule or not, whether lymph nodes and seminal vesicles are involved, and to what extent there is metastasis.

RADIONUCLEOTIDE BONE SCAN

The radionucleotide bone scan can be used if there is metastatic disease to see if there has been any osseous spread. Although this test is sensitive, it is not very specific, and areas can show increased activity (or uptake) and not be metastatic disease. Fractures, arthritis, and other conditions can all light up the scan and be a false positive finding. However, there is no one good test that can look at all of these parameters and fully define the extent of the disease.[28]

Diagnostic protocol

◆ Grading: based on the resemblance of tumor architecture to normal glandular structure, grading helps define the aggressiveness of the tumor and takes into account thehistologic heterogeneity in the tumor.

◆ Combined assessment: Gleason score, clinical stage, DRE, and PSA together predict pathologic stage and prognosis better than any of them alone.

◆ Gleason score: The most prevalent pattern and the next most prevalent pattern are each assigned a grade of 1 to 5, and the 2 grades are added (total score: 2 to 4 = well differentiated, 5 to 7 = moderately differentiated, and 8 to 10 = undifferentiated).

◆ Localized tumors: Gleason score helps predict the likelihood of capsular penetration, seminal vesicle invasion, and any spread to lymph nodes.

◆ Both acid phosphatase (PAP) and PSA levels decrease after treatment and increase with recurrence, but PSA is the most sensitive marker for monitoring cancer progression and response to treatment.

◆ Androgens are measured as a cofactor in the influence of the denaturing of the prostate cell. Testosterone (free and bound), androsteinodione, and dihydrotestosterone should all be included in the evaluation of the prostate patient.

Integrative Therapy Strategies

TREATMENT BY CLINICAL STATE

The time from the appearance of chronic inflammatory changes on the prostate cell creating a preneoplastic transformation to that of an invasive lesion that will result in clinical symptoms and eventually death can span decades in its progression. For this reason, you can monitor the state of the progression and determine when a patient changes from one disease state to another. This strategy allows fluctuation of treatment protocols to match the patient's current clinical state of disease. At each assessment the decision to offer treatment or change treatment strategies is based on the risk of the cancer to the patient compared to the probability of developing of symptoms or dying from the disease.[29]

Therefore, men with active cancer but are not at risk of developing metastases versus men with active metastatic disease can be assessed across the continuum and a distinction can be made between cure, control, and chronic disease. This risk-to-benefit strategy allows for each individual to be assessed independently within the nature of his disease, even when a recurrence happens and immediate treatment may not be warranted depending on the other parameters of the disease progression.[30]

Clinically Localized Disease Factors[31]

After staging the prostate cancer, patients with non-metastatic disease that is localized to the gland and not extending outside of the capsule should be treated based on several factors:

- Clinical symptoms
- Probability of the tumor becoming more aggressive and metastatic
- Probability of the tumor being cured by a single modality or with a multi-treatment approach
- Age because the older male usually has a less aggressive cancer cell that does not progress and may not become metastatic in his life time
- PSA, grade and extent of tumor, coexisting disorders, and life expectancy

---

ACTIVE SURVEILLANCE

While most patients, regardless of age, prefer definitive therapy, watchful waiting may be appropriate for asymptomatic patients > 70 with localized prostate cancer, particularly if it is well or moderately well differentiated and low volume, or if life-limiting disorders coexist. In these patients, risk of death due to other causes is greater than that due to prostate cancer. This approach requires periodic DRE, PSA measurement, and monitoring of symptoms. If symptoms worsen, treatment is required. In elderly men, watchful waiting results in the same overall survival rate as prostatectomy; however, patients who had surgery had a significantly lower risk of distant metastases and disease-specific mortality.[32]

Active surveillance is the term now used for this watchful waiting strategy. Ongoing diagnostic repeat testing allows a "waiting" period until the tumor shows progression. In some instances, this treatment is the most appropriate as the tumor progression does not actively correlate to the age and morbidity or mortality of the patient. This practice was founded on studies that revealed elderly men with well differentiated tumors showed no clinical significance between watchful waiting and treatment probands.[32]

RADICAL PROSTATECTOMY

Radical prostatectomy (removal of prostate with adnexal structures and regional lymph nodes) is probably best for patients < 70 with a tumor confined to the prostate. Prostatectomy is appropriate for some elderly patients, based on life expectancy, coexisting disorders, and ability to tolerate surgery and anesthesia.[33]

The goal of removing the gland completely is to excise all of the cancer with clear surgical margins, while maintaining continence and erectile function by sparing the autonomic nerves in the neurovascular bundle. Nerve-sparing radical prostatectomy reduces the likelihood of erectile dysfunction but cannot always be done, depending on tumor stage and location.[33]

New techniques have been created to meet these treatment goals: robotics and laparoscopic surgery. Despite the effectiveness these technologies, the skill and experience of the surgeon is paramount to the outcome of the surgery.[33]

Complications include urinary incontinence (about 5 to 10%), bladder neck contracture or urethral stricture (about 7% to 20%), erectile dysfunction (about 30% to 100% – heavily dependent on age and current function), and fecal incontinence (1% to 2%). Major complications occur in > 25%, more often in elderly patients.[34]

In a series treated at an academic center, 6% of patients had mild stress urinary incontinence (SUI) (requiring 1 pad/day), 2% moderate SUI (>1 pad/day), and 0.3% severe SUI (requiring artificial urinary sphincter). At 1 year, 92% were completely continent. In contrast, the results in a Medicare population treated at multiple centers showed that at 3, 12, and 24 months following surgery, 58%, 35%, and 42% (respectively) wore pads in their underwear, and 24%, 11%, and 15% reported "a lot" of urine leakage.[35]

> **Cryotherapy**
> Cryotherapy (destruction of prostate cancer cells by freezing with cryoprobes, followed by thawing) is less well established; long-term outcomes are unknown. Adverse effects include bladder outlet obstruction, urinary incontinence, erectile dysfunction, and rectal pain or injury.[36]

NEOADJUVANT HORMONAL BLOCKADE THERAPIES

Neoadjuvant hormonal blockade therapies have been shown to improve outcomes of surgery for high-risk cell types. Several large trials have shown that androgen depletion before surgery showed effects on serum PSA by 96% and prostate tumor volume decreased by 34% with an increase of clear margins from 17% to 41%. However, these neoadjuvant hormonal therapies did not show an improvement in PSA relapse free survival and are not used by all practitioners.[37]

RADIATION THERAPY

Radiation is applied to the prostate either by external beam, radioactive seeds or cathodes, or with a combination of several strategies.

External Beam Radiation (EBRT)

Modern external beam techniques follow a three-dimensional conformal treatment protocol that uses intensity modulated radiation therapy (IMRT). This minimizes the exposure of surrounding healthy tissues while maximizing the dose of radiation to the cancer cells. IMRT can safely deliver doses approaching 80 Gy to the prostate; data indicate that the rate of local control is higher, especially for high-risk patients.[38]

This strategy has allowed the delivery of higher doses of radiation to the affected cells with fewer side effects and better outcomes. Side effects still occur with IMRT: mucositis, some decrease in erectile function at least 40%, radiation proctitis, cystitis, diarrhea, fatigue, and, possibly, urethral strictures, particularly in patients with a prior history of transurethral resection of the prostate.[39]

Brachytherapy

This therapy involves direct implantation of radioactive sources into the prostate gland. It is based on the idea that direct deposits of radiation energy to the tissues affected by cancer will deliver intense radiation to the prostate while minimizing the exposure of the surrounding healthy tissues. Radioactive seeds or cathodes are implanted according to a customized template based on CT and US assessment of the tumor and its location within the gland. Most radiation oncologists reserve implantation for those patients with good or intermediate prognostic factors. Implantation is performed transperineally with real time imaging without an "open" procedure.

Brachytherapy also decreases erectile function, although it may be delayed and patients may be more responsive to phosphodiesterase type 5 (PDE5) inhibitors than patients whose neurovascular bundles are resected or injured during surgery. Urinary frequency, urgency, and, less often, retention are common but usually subside over time. Other adverse effects include increased bowel movements; rectal urgency, bleeding, or ulceration; and prostatorectal fistulas.[40]

ORCHIECTOMY

Metastatic disease in the non-castrated male is reliant on non-castrated levels of testosterone and imaging studies. The patient can be newly diagnosed or have a recurrence of his disease after treatment. Symptoms of metastatic disease include bone pain and coagulopathies with advanced disease dependant on which other organ system is involved. Over 90% of male hormones originate from the testes and the other 10% are synthesized in the adrenal glands.[41]

The gold standard for hormone blockade is orchiectomy, but it is the least acceptable therapy to patients, which has resulted in the development of medical strategies of hormone blockade. These therapies are divided into agents, those that lower testosterone and antiandrogens that bind to the androgen receptor to block signaling.[42]

TESTOSTERONE LOWERING STRATEGIES

Gonadotropin releasing hormone (GnRH) analogues, estrogens, and progesterone are hormones manipulated in the effort to lower testosterone. DES (diethylstilbestrol) was once used in this therapeutic approach but has not been in recent strategies due to the risk of vascular complications (edema, phlebitis, emboli, and stroke). GnRH analogues, such as leuprolide and goserelin acetate, create a chemical castration by affecting the feedback loops to the pituitary gland.[42] At first a rise in luteinizing hormone (LH) and follicle stimulating hormone (FSH) is seen, which is then followed by the downregulation of receptors in the

Hormones Involved in Prostate Cancer[12]

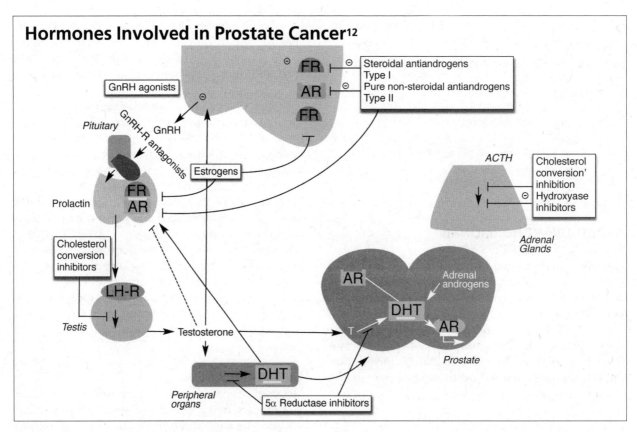

pituitary gland resulting in a chemical castration via the decreased amounts of male androgens produced.[42] The systemic effects are much like those that women experience during menopause: hot flashes/flushes, fatigue, muscle weakness and loss of mass, personality changes, anemia, depression and reduced bone density. Vitamin D-3 and calcium supplementation may prevent bone loss, but the GnRH analogues have led to alterations in body metabolism, resulting in glucose intolerance and metabolic syndrome and osteoporosis.[43]

ANTIANDROGEN THERAPY

Antiandrogen therapy is usually administered in conjunction with GnRH analogues, initially used to lower the rise in testosterone with the onset of analogue therapy. This combination of androgen blockade and a GnRH analogue produces chemical castration.[44] Nonsteroidal antiandrogens are used, such as flutamide (Eulexin), bicalutamide (Casodex), and nilutamide (Nilandron). These pharmaceutical agents bind to androgen receptors, block receptor site activity, and promote hormone creation/secretion. According to large randomized comparison studies, this combination strategy shows only a modest improvement in survival rates (<10%), and it is recommended in practice that most patients be treated with the antiandrogen therapy only for the first 2 to 4 weeks of GnRH analogue treatment.[45]

For short-term palliation, one or more drugs may be used, including antiandrogens, chemotherapy drugs (mitoxantrone, estramustine, taxanes), corticosteroids, and ketoconazole. Docetaxel plus prednisone is a common combination. Local radiation therapy is usually palliative for patients with symptomatic bone metastases.[46]

CHEMOTHERAPY

Cytotoxic and biologic drugs (genetically designed vaccines, antisense therapy, monoclonal antibodies), angiogenesis inhibitors (thalidomide, endostatin), and matrix metalloproteinase inhibitors are being studied and may provide palliation and prolong survival, but their superiority over corticosteroids alone has not been proved. For high-grade tumors that extend beyond the prostatic capsule, several treatment protocols exist. Chemotherapy, with or without hormonal therapy, is used before surgery in some protocols and along with radiation in others. Chemotherapy regimens vary by center and trial.[47]

Naturopathic Approaches

The naturopathic approach to treating prostate cancer and supporting conventional prostate cancer treatments is fourfold, grounded in our knowledge of cell biology and inflammatory pathways.

CASTRATION-RESISTANT DISEASE[48]

Although surgical castration is the gold standard in hormone blockade strategies, castration-resistant disease can manifest in many ways. Usually a rise in PSA levels post castration is the indication that alerts the patient and physician to a resistant disease process. Rising PSA levels and progression to metastasis in the bone may manifest without any other symptom of the diseases progression. The rising PSA is an indication of continued signaling through the androgen biofeedback receptor axis loop. This significant androgen production from the adrenal gland is upregulated by the tumor and shows adaptive and selective changes to promote the progression of tumor growth.

Castration-resistant disease does not necessarily mean that the tumor is hormone refractory. Exogenous estrogens are rarely used because they have a risk of cardiovascular and thromboembolic complications. There is no standard therapy for hormone-refractory prostate cancer.

Ketoconazole (Nizoral) is used to inhibit adrenal androgen synthesis and has been found to be effective in these cases. Other hormones that may also have some of this antiandronergic activity are the estrogens, progestins, and glucocorticoids. Cytotoxic chemotherapeutic strategies, such as mitoxantrone (novatrone), were first utilized in metastatic disease as palliation therapy for pain, showing a reduction in pain with less use of narcotics and less fatigue. Docetaxel (Taxotere) replaced the first-line strategy of mitoxantrone around 2004 due to a trial showing its superiority in measurable disease regression and improvement of preexisting disease.

Naturopathic therapeutic goals and order

1. Inhibit 5-apha reductase
2. Inhibit COX-2
3. Initiate apoptosis
4. Promote antiproliferative agents

To achieve these therapeutic goals, naturopathic medicine employs the modalities of clinical nutrition, botanical medicine, and immunotherapy (psychoneuroendoimmunology and endoimmunology).

1. INHIBIT 5-ALPHA REDUCTASE

5-alpha Reductase converts testosterone to DHT, which increases prostatic cell proliferation while also increasing the size of the gland. By inhibiting 5-alpha reductase, DHT is decreased, thereby decreasing prostatic cell proliferation and progression of the cancer.

Serona repens

Saw palmetto inhibits 5-alpha reductase, the enzyme that converts testosterone to DHT, inhibiting both type I and II isoenzymes and acting selectively on prostate cells. It is important to use a product that is standardized to 80% to 90% fatty acids of saw palmetto berries for this selective activity. Other actions of saw palmetto are to increase apoptosis in prostate epithelial cells, while also decreasing epidermal growth factor, thus affecting two different strategies of cancer progression.[49]

The anti-inflammatory action of saw palmetto shows that it inhibits both the cyclooxygenase and lipoxygenase pathways, which both produce proinflammatory prostaglandins that induce cancer cell activity. COX-2 inhibition is part of an exciting area in naturopathic medicine research in cancer prevention and treatment.

Dosage: 85%-95% Betasitosterol 320 mg q.d.to t.i.d.

2. INHIBIT COX-2

COX-2 catalyzes the conversion of arachidonic acid to pro-inflammatory prostaglandins (PG) series 2. These PGs increase tumor cell proliferation, resistance to apoptosis, and angiogenesis. Naturopathic therapeutics aimed at COX-2 inhibition show potential as chemopreventive strategies. Herbal Cox-2 inhibitors have been closely scrutinized by conventional allopathic researchers for their activity in prostate cancer.

Glycyrrhiza uralensis

Through its isoliquiritigenin constituent, licorice root decreases activity of COX-2, which results in decreased PGE-2 and nitric oxide. This constituent is not found in deglycyrrhated licorice products.[50]

Dosage: Solid extract, 1/4 tsp. q.d. to t.i.d.

Phyllanthus amarus

Studies have shown that *in-vitro* application of this extract inhibits induction of iNOS, COX-2, and TNF-alpha.[51]

Dosage: 100-400 g q.d. to t.i.d.

Zingiber officinalis

In-vitro human synoviocytes, obtained during primary knee replacement from osteoporosis patients, when incubated with ginger extract demonstrated significantly suppressed production of TNF-alpha COX-2 expression. NF-kappaB was also suppressed, suggesting that ginger blocks transcription of COX-2.[52] Dosage: 50-100 g q.d. to t.i.d.

Multiple herb extract

Zyflamend™ is a multiple herbal extract with a base in ginger root. One study reported that Cox-1 and Cox-2 enzyme activities decreased with Zyflamend by 45% to 80% with PGE2 production decreased by 91%. Apoptosis was induced in cell lines after a 72-hour treatment period. Cox-2 enzyme activity was inhibited with decreased signaling through PKCdelta and STAT3.[53]

Scutellaria baicalensis

Oral administration of *Scutellaria baicalensis* to mice inoculated with these cells caused inhibition of COX-2 expression, whereas celecoxib inhibited COX-2 activity directly. No inhibition was seen in mice inoculated with a nontumorigenic cell line, indicating a selective inhibition of COX-2 in tumor cells. A 66% reduction in tumor mass was also observed in these mice.[54] Dosage: 250-500 g t.i.d.

3. INITIATE APOPTOSIS

Specific nutraceuticals induce programmed cell death via various mechanisms, such as p53 induction.

- Vitamins can induce differentiation and apoptosis in cancer cells. A mixture of antioxidant vitamins is more effective than individual vitamins. In contrast to cancer cells, normal cells never undergo apoptosis after conventional treatment with vitamins with the exception of the retinoids. Dosage: Vitamin D3 2000-10,000 q.d.[55]
- **N-Acetyl-Cysteine (NAC)** elevates p53 activity and apoptosis in cancer cells but not in healthy cells. Dosage: 200-600 mgq.d. to t.i.d.[56]
- **Curcumin** induces apoptosis in sarcoma, colon, kidney, and hepatocellular cancers, but not in normal cells. Curcumin also induces apoptosis in a p53-independent manner, and at the higher concentrations, induces capase gene expression. Dosage: 500-1000 mg q.d. to t.i.d.[57]
- **Silybinin** (a constituent found in milk thistle) was found to significantly inhibit bladder transitional cancer cell lines while also inducing apoptosis. These effects were due to the activation of capase-3 and modulation of the cyclin cascade. Dosage: 250-500 mg q.d. to t.i.d.[58]

- **Quercitin** has shown to be able to block epidermal growth factor receptor signanglin pathways leading to the induction of apoptosis. Dosage: 100-300 mg q.d. to t.i.d.[59]
- **Cimicifuga** interrupts VEGF formation by inducing capases and thus apoptosis in MCF-7 cell lines.[60]
- **Green Tea extract EGCG** increases apoptosis in cancer cells, interrupts VEGF formation by interrupting survival signals which result in capases activation and subsequent cell death. Dosage: 5-10 cups q.d.[61]
- **Scutellaris baicalensis** (Chinese skullcap) also induces capsase function to result in apoptosis. Dosage: 100-500 mg q.d. to t.i.d.[62]

4. PROMOTE ANTIPROLIFERATIVE AGENTS

These nutraceuticals arrest the cell cycle, which stops the promotion of the cancer cells and inhibit growth factors, including epidermal growth factor, insulin-like growth factor, and basic fibroblast growth factor.

Curcumin longa

Turmeric root has been investigated for its anticancer activities, specifically the constituent diferuloylmethane. Curcumin has ben shown to induce Phase 2 detoxification enzymes, especially the glutathione transferases and quinine reductase, while inhibiting procarcinogen activating Phase 1 enzymes such as CP450 1A1.[63] While it has been shown that curcumin aids in apoptosis, it is also specific in sensitizing the prostate cells to radiation treatment (chemoprevention), making them more susceptible to apoptosis and death by the treatment.[64] Curcumin in combination with radiation treatment showed inhibition of TNF-alpha-mediated NFkappaB activity, resulting in bcl-2 protein down-regulation.[64]

Numerous other studies have shown several specific mechanisms in which curcumin inhibits prostate cancer cell growth; activates genes that turn on apoptosis and self destruction of the cancer cell; reprogram the prostate cancer cells to inhibit their metastatic capacity to the bone, the primary site of prostate cancer cell metastasis.[65] Other research has shown that curcumin can act as a chemopreventative agent and significantly decrease the recurrence of prostate cancer.[66]

SELECT TRIAL[67]

This trial was designed by the National Institutes of Health to look at the long-term effects of selenium taken in combination with vitamin E. These studies show that selenium potentiates the vitamin E-induced inhibition of prostate cancer cells in vitro by affecting the reduction of the percentage of cancer cells in the S phase. The SELECT trial was stopped with the conclusion stating that these nutraceuticals produced no significant effect on cancer cells, contrary to previous studies.

RESULTS: As of October 23, 2008, median overall follow-up was 5.46 years (range, 4.17-7.33 years). Hazard ratios (99% confidence intervals [CIs]) for prostate cancer were 1.13 (99% CI, 0.95-1.35; n = 473) for vitamin E, 1.04 (99% CI, 0.87-1.24; n = 432) for selenium, and 1.05 (99% CI, 0.88-1.25; n = 437) for selenium + vitamin E vs 1.00 (n = 416) for placebo. There were no significant differences (all P>.15) in any other prespecified cancer end points. There were statistically non-significant increased risks of prostate cancer in the vitamin E group (P = .06) and type 2 diabetes mellitus in the selenium group (relative risk, 1.07; 99% CI, 0.94-1.22; P = .16) but not in the selenium + vitamin E group. CONCLUSION: Selenium or vitamin E, alone or in combination at the doses and formulations used, did not prevent prostate cancer in this population of relatively healthy men.

5. PROSTATE SPECIFIC NATUROPATHIC INTERVENTIONS

Other nutraceuticals and botanical medicines have a significant effect on prostate cancer, which may be taken individually or, in some cases, synergistically.

Lycopene

This red carotenoid, found in abundance in tomatoes and watermelon, has shown an inverse relationship between the dietary intake of lycopene and the risk of prostate cancer. A study evaluating the genomic effects of lycopene in men with localized prostate cancer showed that the lycopene supplemented patients had major reductions in many of the DNA factors that usually favor prostate cancer cell propagation.[68] It was also found in the lycopene supplemented proband that not only the prostate cancer cells but also the hyperplastic prostatic tissue showed an increase in apoptosis. This produced a significant effect in the reduction of DNA damaged tissues with only 3 weeks of lycopene supplementation yielding almost a 3x increase of the lycopene in the prostatic cells.[68] In another study that looked at lycopene supplementation in men before radical prostatectomy, the pathology post-operative compared to control subjects found astounding results. These results not only showed significant improvement in clear surgical margins and extra-prostatic tissues, but also a reduction in tumor size and a reduction in PSA levels.[69]

Vitamin D

This vitamin has been studied extensively as a chemo-preventative and anti-recurrence supplement. In 1998 researchers showed that vitamin D can reduce prostate cancer cell growth in humans using calcitriol at doses of 20-100 IU daily with dosing strategies going as high as 20 IU per kg of body weight.[70] In a phase II clinical trial using up to 12 mcg (480 IU) with dexamethasone in androgen independent prostate cancer showed significant decreases in levels of PSA, as well as antitumor effects.[71]

Human prostate cells contain receptors for 1alpha,25-dihydroxyvitamin D, the active form of vitamin D. Prostate cancer cells respond to vitamin D(3) with increases in differentiation and apoptosis, and decreases in proliferation, invasiveness and metastasis.[72]

These findings strongly support the use of vitamin D-based therapies for prostate cancer as a second-line therapy if androgen deprivation fails.[72] The association between either decreased sun exposure or vitamin D deficiency and the increased risk of prostate cancer at an earlier age with a more aggressive progression indicates that adequate vitamin D nutrition should be a priority for men of all ages.[72]

Vitamin E

According to a 2000 study reported in the Journal of the National Cancer Institute, men with the highest blood levels of gamma tocopherol were 5x less likely to get prostate cancer.[73] Over a 7-year period, Johns Hopkins School of Public Health did a large group of over 10,000 men looking at vitamin E and prostate cancer risk. This study showed that alpha tocopherol and selenium reduced prostate cancer risk in the men who had high levels of gamma tocopherol in their blood.[74] Researchers have that vitamin E induces cell differentiation, inhibits cancer cell growth while promoting cancer cell apoptosis and is very selective in the inhibition of cancer cell growth. Specifically, vitamin E inhibits protein kinase C, the expression of oncogenes, and phosphorylation and transactivation

Nutraceutical and Botanical Medicines for Treating Prostate Cancer

Therapy	Therapeutic Dose	Anticancer Action
Serona repens	85%-95% Betasitosterol 320 mg qd-tid	Improves testosterone excretion to estrogen, binds at receptor site, anti-inflammatory
Soy Isoflavones	60-300 g qd	Improves estrogen excretion to 2 BH estrone, COX-2 inhibitor
Camellia sinensis (green tea) and Vitamin E	5-10 cups qd	Antioxidant, COX-2 inhibition, apoptosis, chemopreventative,
Vitamin E	400-1200 IU	Antioxidant, COX-2 inhibition, works best with Selenium
Selenium	200-600 mcg qd	Antioxidant, DNA/RNA repair, apoptosis
Vitamin D3	2000-10,000 qd	Pro Hormone, apoptosis, antiproliferate, antimetastatic
Lycopene	10-50 mg qd-tid	Antioxidant, DNA/RNA repair, apoptosis
Curcumin longa	500-1000 mg, qd-tid	COX-2 inhibitor, chemosensitization, inhibits cell growth, antimetastatic, chemopreventative
Glycyrrhiza uralensis	Solid extract ¼ tsp qd-tid	Apoptosis, COX-2 inhibitor, hormone blockade, antitestosterone
Phyllanthus amarus	100-400 g qd-tid	Apoptosis, COX-2 inhibitor, hormone clearance
Zingiber officinalis	500-1000 mg qd	Apoptosis, COX-2 inhibitor, chemopreventative
N-Acetyl-Cysteine (NAC)	200-600 g qd-tid	Apoptosis, chemosensitization, chemopreventative
Silybinin/Silymorin	250-500 mg qd-tid	Apoptosis, COX-2 inhibitor, chemosensitization
Quercitin	100-300 mg qd	Blocks EGFR, COX-2 inhibitor, chemosensitization
Cimicifuga	50-500 mg	Chemosensitization, COX-2 inhibitor
Scutellaris baicalensis	100-300 mg qd	Chemosensitization, COX-2 inhibitor, apoptosis
Green Tea extract EGCG	100-250 mg 5-10 cups non-decafinated tea or equivalent to equal 50-100 g polyphenic activity tid	Lowers VEGF, chemosensitization, COX-2 inhibitor

of cancer cells while stimulating the proliferation of healthy cells.[75]

Selenium

This essential trace mineral has been shown to inhibit prostate cancer cells both in humans and animal studies. Its mechanism of action is still under investigation, although it is likely to be one of the most powerful chemopreventative agents found naturally in the human diet in pumpkin seeds, brazil nuts, and other foods. Low status of selenium results in an associated increase in the risk and progression of prostate cancer, resulting from a decrease in the expression of genes involved in detoxification.[76]

Camellia sinensis

Green tea, white tea, and black tea all come from the plant *Camellia sinensis*. Green tea contains a polyphenol called epigallocatechin-3-gallate (EGCG). Green tea polyphenols are found in the dry tea leaf and include catechins and epicatechins, including epicatechin (EC), epicatechin-3-gallate (ECG), epigallocatechin (EGC), and epigallocatechin-3-gallate (EGCG). Catechins, EGCG, and ECG all have demonstrated antimutagenic effects against mutagens *in vivo*.[77]

Green tea polyphenols capture and detoxify free radicals at various stages of the promotion of cancer. These polyphenols also affect free radicals produced from exposure to radiation and catechins. Specifically, these catechins suppress formation of free radicals and reduce hydroxyl radicals. This antioxidant effect has been demonstrated in humans using urinary and WBC markers of oxidative stress.[78] EGCG can induce apoptosis in prostate cancer cells via regulation of the p53 and NF-kappaB genes; decrease DNA mutagenicity; and even repair damaged DNA while decreasing angiogenesis. This effect has been demonstrated by EGCG's influence on the excision-repair system.[79]

Oral intake of green tea polyphenols by mice that were transfected with prostate cancer resulted in a reduced level of insulin-like growth factor (IGF) as well as inhibition of markers of angiogenesis/metastasis, which include vascular endothelial growth factor (VEGF), urokinase plasminogen activator, and matrix metalloproteinases 2 and 9.[61] Oral consumption of these green tea polyphenols inhbited prostate cancer development in the mice that were transfected by the mechanisms listed above. Rats exposed to heterocyclic amines demonstrated significantly reduced mutagenicity and an increased DNA repair in hepatocytes when fed green tea.[80] EGCG was also shown to counter the carcinogenic effects of chemical carcinogens, such as benzenes, which have been shown to be strong mutagenic chemicals that induce cancer cell turn on and growth.[79]

Green tea is noted to have an inhibitory action on almost all the steps of carcinogenesis. A meta-analysis of all cohort and case-controlled studies assessing breast cancer incidence and breast cancer recurrence resulted in seven significant reports. The pooled relative risk for the highest levels of green tea consumption on the risk of developing breast cancer was 0.79 (95% CI with a p=0.064). The highest level of tea consumption was typically greater than 5 cups daily and showed a pooled relative risk of 0.56 (95% CI with a p=0.0041) for stage I and II disease.[81] Green tea consumption of 3 grams as a tea 3x a day for 7 days resulted in significant decreases in oxidative DNA damage and damage to lipid peroxidation and free radical generation.[78]

Green Tea and Vitamin E

Antioxidants may be antagonistic during radiation treatment. One study looked at mice with induced tumors undergoing radiation therapy without green tea or vitamin E, with both verum arms and with either of the active arms. The data was significant to show that tumor growth was 10% slower in the EGCG verum group as compared to the 3% slower growth in the Vitamin E group.[82]

However, together EGCG and vitamin E protected normal tissues from severe XRT related soft tissue reactions. Also in the dual arm probands intramural apoptosis concentrations increased 8.3 fold and 1.3 fold increases when compared to controls. Tumor cell invasiveness was decreased by 25% with EGCG and vitamin E compared to the control. Although both appear to be concentrated in tumors, the mechanism and significance is still unknown. Anti-angiogenic RNA expression in the EGCG tumor may explain the slower tumor growth. Both EGCG and vitamin E significantly slow tumor growth by increasing apoptosis and decreasing cell proliferation. Vitamin E and EGCG did significantly decrease radiation reaction in normal tissues, but did not reach statistical significance in increasing radiation resistance in implanted tumors.[82]

Soy Isoflavones

The isoflavones found in soy have been studied specifically in respect to prostate cancer. The isoflavone daidzein is converted by the intestinal bacteria into equol. It is these levels of concentrated equol that can arrest prostate cancer cell lines in the G0/G1 phase of cell cycle reproduction.[83] Interestingly, Asian men convert diadzein to equol more effectively than North American men, which may be associated with the small intestinal flora ecology difference between the two, associated with the differences in diets.

The other major isoflavone component in soy is Genistein. Genistein has an antiproliferative action and produces cell cycle arrest in human prostate cancer cell lines, with a decreased growth of prostate cancer tissue in a dose dependant manner.[84] Genistein also works as a regulator of the androgen receptor, modulating multiple cellular pathways that are mediated by the androgen receptor and prostate carcinogenesis. Genistein also potentiates radiation inhibition on tumor growth: when combined with radiation it caused a significantly greater inhibition of tumor growth (87%) compared to radiation (73%) or genistein alone (30%).[84]

Researchers have looked at fermented soy with *Basidiomycetes* spp. as a prostate treatment. The premise of this is that isoflavones are poorly absorbed in glycosylated forms and better absorbed in an active aglycone isoflavone. Growth of cells was inhibited by 72 hours of treatment with induction of apoptosis detected in cells with +p53.[85] In mice whose diets consisted of 2% of this fermented isoflavone, tumor growth was suppressed. The best results both *in vivo* and *in vitro* was with the wild type p53 which activated both cell cycle suppression and apoptotic signaling.[85] The conclusion was that fermented soy can be an effective chemopreventative strategy for both prostate and bladder cancers.

Following this idea of chemoprevention and early intervention in prostate cancer, isoflavones were looked at in early stage prostate cancer patients. The patients were supplemented with 60 mg of soy isoflavones and were followed for changes in hormonal and proliferative risk factors that are implicated in prostate cancer promotion; 76 patients with Gleason scores of 6 or below, between the ages of 50 and 80, were randomized for supplementation or placebo for 12 weeks. PSA changes and steroid hormone levels were analyzed at baseline and post intervention. In this group, 59 of the patients completed the 12-week intervention with serum-free testosterone being reduced or showing no change: 61% in the isoflavone treated group compared to 33% in the placebo group. Serum PSA levels were decreased or unchanged in 69% of the isoflavone group compared to 55% in the placebo group, while 19% of the isoflavone group reduced total PSA levels by 2 points or more during the 12-week period. This suggests that supplementation with soy isoflavones in early stage prostate cancer alters surrogate markers of proliferation, such as serum PSA and free testosterone.[86]

In Asian countries, the estimated isoflavone mean daily intake is between 10 and 50 mg per day. In the cancer patients the recommended intake is 35 to 60 grams of soy protein daily.[87] It is not clear whether the benefits are due to the protein source found in soy or its isoflavones, daidzein and genistein, or a combination. The best approach is to include soy as a food, especially fermented foods like tempeh. Tofu, edamame, and soy milk are recommended over taking soy isolate supplements. Look for soy products that use a non-genetically modified seed in their production.

References

1. Scher, HI. 2009. Harrison's Online Chapter 91, Benign and Malignant Diesease of the Prostate Harrison's Principles of Internal Medicine. 17th ed. New York, NY: McGraw-Hill Co.

2. Meng, MV. Chapter 39 Cancer: Prostate Cancer. McPhee J, Papadakis M, Gonzales R, Zeiger R. Online (eds.) 2009. CURRENT Medical Diagnosis & Treatment Online. New York, NY:McGraw-Hill Co. Moore KI, Dalley AF, AMR Aqur. Clinically Oriented Anatomy, 6th ed. Baltimore, MD: Lippincott; 2009.

3. http://www.cancer.gov/cancertopics/pdq/treatment/prostate/Patient/page1 National Cancer Institute PDQ 2012.

4. Prensner JR, Rubin MA, Wei JT, Chinnaiyan AM. Cancer biomarkers beyond PSA: the next generation of prostate cancer biomarkers. Sci Transl Med 2012;4(127):127rv3ht.

5. Shih WJ, Collins J, Mitchell B, Wierzbinski B. Serum PSA and PAP mearsurements discriminating patients with prostate carcinoma from patients with nodular hyperplasia. J Natl Med Assoc. 1994;86(9):667-70.

6. http://www.cancer.org/Cancer/ProstateCancer/DetailedGuide/prostate-cancer-risk-factors Prostate Cancer. 2012.

7. http://seer.cancer.gov/statfacts/html/prost.html Prostate Cancer SEER stat facts sheets. 2012.

8. http://www.prostate-cancer.org/pcricms/node/124. 2012.

9. Haiman CA, Marchand LL, Yamamato J, et al. A common genetic risk factor for colorectal and prostate cancer. Nature Genetics. 2007;39:954-56.

10. http://www.cancer.gov/cancertopics/pdq/genetics/prostate/HealthProfessional/page3 Polymorphisms and Prostate Cancer susceptibility; National Cancer Institute PDQ 2012

11. Ekman P, Gronberg H, Matsuyama H, et al. Links between genetic and environmental factors and prostate cancer risk. Prostate 1999;39(4):262-68.

12. Fauci AS, Kasper DL, Braunvald E, et al. Harrison's Principles of Internal Medicine, 17th ed.: http://www.accessmedicine.com. New Yor, NY: McGraw-Hill.

13. De Marzo AM, Meeker AK, Zha S, et al. Human prostate cancer precursors and pathobiology. Urology 2003;62(5 suppl):55-62.

14. Palapattu GS. Carcinogenesis and inflammation: emerging insights. Carcinogenesis. 2005;26(7):1170-81.

15. Kramer BS, et al. Prostate Cancer screening: what we know and what we need to know. Ann Intern Med 1993;119(9):914-23.

16. Kantoff PW, Taplin ME. Clinical presentation, diagnosis, and staging of prostate cancer. UpToDate 2012. http://www.uptodate.com/contents/clinical-presentation-diagnosis-and-staging-of-prostate-cancer

17. http://www.cancer.gov/cancertopics/pdq/screening/prostate/HealthProfessional/page3 Prostate Cancer Screening PDQ; National Cancer Institute 2012.

18. Okotie OT, Roehl KA, Han M, et al. Characteristics of prostate cancer detected by digital rectal examination only. Urology 2007;70(6):1117-20.

19. http://www.cancer.gov/cancertopics/factsheet/detection/PSA National Cancer Institute Prostate specific antigen test Fact Sheet. 2012.

20. Connolly DJ, Black A, Murray LJ, et al. Population based age specific reference ranges for PSA. ASCO Prostate Cancer Symposium Proceedings. 2007.

21. http://www.cancer.gov/cancertopics/screening/understanding-prostate-changes/page5 Understanding Prostate changes: A health guide for men. National Cancer Institute 2012.

22. Carroll P and Shinohara K. Transrectal Ultrasound guided prostate biopsy. http://www.cancer.gov/cancertopics/screening/understanding-prostate-changes/page5 2012.

23. American Joint Committee on Cancer (AJCC). 2012. AJCC Cancer Staging Manual. 7th ed. New York, NY; Springer-New York;2012. http://www.cancerstaging.org/staging/index.html.

24. http://www.johnshopkinshealthalerts.com/alerts/prostate_disorders/prostate-cancer-imaging-studies_5862-1.html Imaging studies for prostate cancer 2012.

25. Dahut W. Prostate Cancer Research at the National Institutes of Health, Department of Health & Human Services; 2010. http://www.hhs.gov/asl/testify/2010/03/t20100304k.html.

26. Alvarado LC. Total testosterone in young men is more closely associated than free testosterone with prostate cancer disparities. Ther Adv Urol. 2011;3(3):99-106.

27. Humphrey PA. Gleason grading and prognostic factors in carcinoma of the prostate. Modern Path. 2004;17:292-306.

28. Lecouvet et al. MRI or Bone scan or both for staging of prostate cancer? JCO. 2007;25(36):5837-38.

29. http://www.mskcc.org/cancer-care/adult/prostate Prostate cacner Memorial Sloan-Kettering Cancer Center 2012.

30. Rosenthal SA, Sandler HM. Treatment Strategies for high risk locally advanced prostate cancer; 2011. http://www.medscape.org/viewarticle/714549.

31. Akduman B, Crawford DE. Treatment of Localized Prostate Cancer. Rev Urol 2006;8(suppl 2):S15-21.

32. Tossoian JJ, Trock BJ, Landis P, et al. Active surveillance program for prostate cancer: an update of the John Hopkins experience. JCO 2011;29(16):2185-90.

33. http://www.nlm.nih.gov/medlineplus/ency/article/007300.htm 2012.

34. Alibhai SM, Leach M, Tomlinson G, et al. 30-day mortality and major complications after radical prostatectomy: influence of age and comorbidity. J Natl Cancer Inst 2005;97(20):1525-32.

35. Marsh DW, Lepor H. Predicting continence following radical prostatectomy. Curr Urolo Rep. 2001;2(3):248-252.

36. https://www.mayoclinic.com/health/cryotherapy-for-prostate-cancer/MY01634 2012.

37. Kumar M, Denham JW. Value of combined androgen blockade in the neoadjuvant treatment of localized prostate cancer: The jury must remain out. JCO 2010;29(25):445-46.

38. Scmitz M. Side effects of External Beam Radiation therapy for prostate cancer; 2009. http://prostatecancer.about.com/od/treatment/a/ebrtsideffects.htm.

39. Simon S. Study supports intensity modulated radiation therapy for prostate cancer; 2012. http://www.cancer.org/Cancer/news/study-supports-intensity-modulated-radiation-therapy-for-prostate-cancer.

40. Theodorescu D. Brachytherapy (Radioactive Seed Implantation Therapy) in Prostate Cancer. Drugs, Diseases & Procedures 2012. http://emedicine.medscape.com/article/453349-overview.

41. http://www.upmccancercenters.com/cancer/prostate/hormoneorchtherapy.html 2012.

42. Akaza H. Combined androgen blockade for prostate cancer: Review of efficacy, safety and cost effectiveness. Cancer Sci. 2011;102(1):51-56.

43. Suzuki K, Nukui A, Hara Y, Morita T. Glucose intolerance during hormonal therapy for prostate cancer. Pros Ca and Pros Dis. 2007;10:384-87.

44. http://www.prostate-cancer.com/prostate-cancer-glossary/chemical-castration.html 2012.

45. McLeod DG. Tolerability to nonsteroidal antiandrogens in the treatment of advanced prostate cancer. The Oncol 1997;2(1):18-27.

46. http://www.cancer.org/Cancer/ProstateCancer/DetailedGuide/prostate-cancer-treating-hormone-therapy 2012.

47. Scmitz M. Chemotherapy for Prostate Cancer; what you should know about prostate cancer chemotherapy, 2011.

http://prostatecancer.about.com/od/treatment/a/chem otherapy.htm.

48. Brawer MK. New treatments for castration resistant prostate cancer highlights form the 44th annual meeting of the American Society of Clinical Oncology, May 30-June 3, 2008, Chicago, IL Rev Urol 2008;10(4):294-96.

49. Gato DI, Carsten T, Vesterlund M, et al. Androgen independent effects of Serenoa repens extract (Prostasan) on prostatic epithelial cell proliferation and inflammation. Phytotherapy Res. 2012;26(2):259-64.

50. Takahashi T, et al. 2004. Isoliquiritigenin, a flavonoid from licorice, reduces prostaglandin E2 and nitric oxide, causes apoptosis and suppresses aberrant crypt foci development. Cancer Science. 95(5):448-63.

51. Kiemer AK, Hartung T, Huber C, Vollmar AM. 2003. Phyllanthus amarus has anti-inflammatory potential by inhibition of iNOS, COX-2, and cytokines via the NF-kappaB pathway. J Hepatol. 38:289-97.

52. Frondoza CG, Sohrabi A, Polotsky A, Phan PV, Hungerford DS, Lindmark L. An in vitro screening assay for inhibitors of proinflammatory mediators in herbal extracts using human synoviocyte cultures. In Vitro Cell Dev Biol Anim. 2004 Mar-Apr;40(3- 4):95-101.

53. Capodice, JL, Bemis, DL, Buttyan, R., Katz, AE. Zyflamend, a unique herbal preparation inhibits arachidonic acid metabolism and suppresses prostate cancer cells, in vitro. New York, NY: Columbia University Medical Center, 2004.

54. Zhang DY, Wu J, Ye F, et al. Inhibition of cancer cell proliferation and prostaglandin E2 synthesis by Scutellaria baicalensis. Cancer Res. 2003;63: 4037-43.

55. Cole WC, Prasad N. Contrasting effects of vitamins as modulators of apoptosis in cancer cells and normal cells: a review. Nutr Cancer. 1997;29(2):97-103.

56. Bach, SP, SE Williams, ST O'Dwyer, CS Potten, AJM Watson. 2006. Regional localization of p53-independent apoptosis determines toxicity of 5-fluoroouracil and pyrrolidinedithiocarbanate in the murine gut. British Journal of Cancer; 95:35-41.

57. Radhakrishna, PG., AS Srivastava, TI Hassanein, DP Chauhan, and E. Carrier. 2004. Induction of apoptosis in human lung cancer cells by curcumin. Cancer Lett. May 28;208(2):171-78.

58. Tyagi A, C Agarwal C, et al. Silibinin causes cell cycle arrest and apoptosis in human bladder transitional cell carcinoma cells by regulating CDKI-CDK-cyclin cascade, and caspase 3 and PARP cleavage. Carcinogeneisis. 2004 Sept;25(9):1711-20.

59. Lee LT, YT Huang, JJ Hwang, PP Lee, FC Ke, MP Nair, C Kanadaswam, Lee. Blockade of the epidermal growth factor receptor tyrosine kinase activity by quercitin and leteolin leads to growth inhibition and apoptosis of pancreatic tumor cells. Anticancer Res. 2002;May-June;22(3):1615-27.

60. Hostanska K, T. Nisslein, J. Freudenstein, J. Reichiling, and R. Saller. Cimicifuga racemosa extract inhibits proliferation of estrogen receptor positive and negative human breast carcinoma cell lines by induction of apoptosis. Breast Cancer Res Treat. 2004 Mar;84(2):151-60.

61. Lee YK, ND Bone, AK Stege, TD Shanafelt, DF Jelinek and NE Kay. VEGF receptor phosphorylation status and apoptosis is modulated by a green tea component, epigallocatechin-3-gallate (EGCG), in B-cell chronic lymphocytic leukemia. Blood. 2004 August 1; 104(3):788-94.

62. Li, YC., YS Tyan, HM Kuo, WC Chang, TC Hsia, and JG Chung. Baicalein induced in vitro apoptosis undergo caspases activity in human promyleoctyic leukemia HL-60 cells. Food and Chemical Toxicology. 2004;42:37-43.

63. Dinkova-Kostova A, Talalay P. 1999. Relation of structure of curcumin analogs to their potencies as inducers of Phase 2 detoxification enzymes. Carcinogenesis. 1999; 20(5), 911-14.

64. Chendil D, Ranga RS, et al.Curcumin confers radiosensitizing effect in prostate cancer cell line PC-3. Oncogene. 2004;Feb.26;23(8):1599-607.

65. Dorai T, Dutcher JP, Dempster DW, et al. Therapeutic potential of curcumin in prostate cancer-V: Interference with the osteomimetic properties of hormone refractory C4-2B prostate cancer cells. Prostate. 2004 Jun 15;60(1):1-17.

66. Manson MM, Farmer PB, Gescher A, Steward WP. Innovative agents in cancer prevention. Recent Results Cancer Res. 2005;166:257-75.

67. Klein EA, Thompson IM, Tangen CM, et al. Vitamin E and the risk of prostate cancer. The Selenium and Vitamin E Cancer Prevention Trial (SELECT). JAMA. 2011;306(14):1549-56.

68. Bowen P, Chen L, Stacewicz-Sapuntzakis M, et al. Tomato sauce supplementation and prostate cancer: lycopene accumulation and modulation of biomarkers of carcinogenesis. Exp Biol Med (Maywood). 2002 Nov;227(10):886-93.

69. Kucuk O, et al. Lycopene in the treatment of prostate cancer. Pure Appl. Chem. 2002;74(8):1443-50.

70. Beer T, Lemmon D, Lowe B, Henner W. High-dose weekly oral calcitriol in patients with a rising PSA after prostatectomy or radiation for prostate carcinoma. Cancer. 2003 Mar 1;97(5):1217-24.

71. Trump DL, Potter DM, Muindi J, Brufsky A, Johnson CS. Phase II trial of high-dose, intermittent calcitriol (1,25 dihydroxyvitamin D3) and dexamethasone in androgen-independent prostate cancer. Cancer. 2006 May 15;106(10):2136-42.

72. Chen, TC and MF Holick. 2003. Vitamin D and prostate cancer prevention and treatment. Trends Endocrinol Metab. Nov;14(9):423-30.

73. Helzlsouer KJ, et al. 2000. Association between alpha-tocopherol, gamma-tocopherol, selenium, and subsequent prostate cancer. J Natl Cancer Inst. 2000 Dec 20;92(24):2018-23.

74. Rose AT, McFadden DW. Alpha-tocopherol succinate inhibits growth of gastric cancer cells in vitro. J Surg Res. 2001 Jan;95(1):19-22.

75. Neuzil, J. et al. Induction of cancer cell apoptosis by a-tocopheryl succinate: molecular pathways and structural requirements. Faseb Jour . 2001;15(2);403-15.

76. Lippman, SM et al. Effect of selenium and vitamin E on risk of prostate cancer and other cancers: the selenium and vitamin E cancer prevention trial (SELECT). JAMA. 2009 Jan 7;301(1):39-51. Epub 2008 Dec 9.

77. Ebata J, Fukagai N, Furukawa H. Mechanisms of antimutagenesis by catechins towards N-nitrosodimethylamine. Environ Mutagen Res. 1998;20:45-50.

78. Klaunig JE, Xu Y, Han C, et al. The effect of tea consumption on oxidative stress in smokers and nonsmokers. PSEBM 1999;220(4):249-54.

79. Kuroda Y, Hara Y. Antimutagenic and anticarcinogenic activity of tea polyphenols. Mutat. Res. 1999; 436: 69-97.

80. Weisburger JH, Hara Y, Dolan L, Luo F-Q, Pittman B, Zang E. Tea polyphenols as inhibitors of mutagenicity of major classes of carcinogens. Mutation Res. 1996; 371: 57-63.

81. Seely D, Mills EJ, Wu P, Verma S, Guyatt GH. The effects of green tea consumption on incidence of breast cancer and recurrence of breast cancer: a systematic review and meta-analysis. Integr Cancer Ther. 2005 Jun; 4(2):144-55.

82. Lawenda BD, Smith D, et al. Dietary Antioxidant Supplementation During Radiation Therapy: Potential for Radiation Protection of Tumors. Department of Radiation Oncology, Naval Medical Center, San Diego, CA;2004.

83. Sarkar FH, Li Y. Soy isoflavones and cancer prevention. Cancer Invest. 2003;21(5):744-57.

84. Bemis, DL, Capodice, JL, Buttyan, R., Katz, AE. Botanicals in the Treatment of Prostate Cancer: Pre-clinical research. New York, NY: Columbia University Medical Center, NY;2004.

85. Bemis DL, Capodice JL, Desai M, Buttyan R, Katz AE. A concentrated aglycone isoflavone preparation (GCP) that demonstrates potent anti-prostate canceractivity in vitro and in vivo. Clin Cancer Res. 2004;10:5282-92.

86. Kumar NB.The Specific Role of Isoflavones in Reducing Prostate Cancer Risk. H. Lee Moffitt Cancer Center and Res. Inst., Tampa, FL;2004.

87. Nagata Y, Sonoda T, Mori M, et al. Dietary isoflavones may protect against prostate cancer in Japanese men. J Nutr. 2007;137(8):1947-79.

88. Adams BK, Ferstl EM, Davis MC, et al. Synthesis and biological evaluation of novel curcumin analogs as anti-cancer and anti-angiogenesis agents. Bioorg Med Chem. 2004 Jul 15;12(14):3871-83.

89. Adams BK, Cai J, Armstrong J, et al. EF24, a novel synthetic curcumin analog, induces apoptosis in cancer cells via a redox-dependent mechanism. Anticancer Drugs. 2005 Mar;16(3):263-75.

90. Bach, SP, SE Williams, ST O'Dwyer, CS Potten and AJM Watson. Regional localization of p53-independent apoptosis determines toxicity of 5-fluoroouracil and pyrrolidinedithiocarbanate in the murine gut. British Journal of Cancer. 2006; 95:35-41.

91. Barnard RJ, Aronson WJ. Preclinical models relevant to diet, exercise, and cancer risk. Recent results Cancer Res. 2005;166:47-61.

92. Bhatia N, Zhao J, Wolf DM, Agarwal R. Inhibition of human carcinoma cell growth and DNA synthesis by silibinin, an active constituent of milk thistle: comparison with silymarin. Cancer Lett. 1999 Dec 1;147(1-2):77-84.

93. Corpet DE, Point PF. From animal models to prevention of colon cancer. Systematic review of chemoprevention in min mice and choice of the model system. Cancer Epidemiol Biomarkers Prev. 2003 May;12(5):391-400.

94. Deeb D, Xu YX, Jiang H, et al. Curcumin (diferuloylmethane) enhances tumor necrosis factor-related apoptosis-inducing ligand-induced apoptosis in LNCaP prostate cancer cells. Mol Cancer Ther. 2003 Jan;2(1):95-103.

95. Deeb D, Jiang H, Gao X, et al. Curcumin sensitizes prostate cancer cells to tumor necrosis factor-related apoptosis-inducing ligand/Apo2L by inhibiting nuclear factor-kappaB through suppression of IkappaBalpha phosphorylation. Mol Cancer Ther. 2004 Jul;3(7):803-12.

96. Dhanalakshmi, Sivanandhan, G.U. Mallikarjuna, Rana P. Singh and Rajesh Agarwal. 2004. Silibinin prevents ultraviolet radiation-caused skin damages in SKH-1 hairless mice via a decrease in thymine dimer positive cells and an up-regulation of p53-p21/Cip1 in epidermis Carcinogenesis 25(8):1459-65.

97. Dorai T, Dutcher JP, Dempster DW, et al. Therapeutic potential of curcumin in prostate cancer-V: Interference with the osteomimetic properties of hormone refractory C4-2B prostate cancer cells. Prostate. 2004 Jun 15;60(1):1-17.

98. Helzlsouer KJ, et al. Association Between alpha-Tocopherol, gamma-Tocopherol, Selenium, and Subsequent Prostate Cancer. J Natl Cancer Inst. 2000 Dec 20;92(24):2018-23.

99. Inano Hiroshi, Makoto Onoda, et al. Chemoprevention by curcumin during the promotion stage of tumorigenesis of mammary gland in rats irradiated with -rays . Carcinogenesis. 1999; 20(6):1011-18.

100. Jee SH, Shen SC, Tseng CR, Chiu HC, Kuo ML. Curcumin induces a p53-dependent apoptosis in human basal cell carcinoma cells J Invest Dermatol. 19998 Oct;111(4):656-61.

101. Jo EH, Hong HD, et al. Modulations of the Bcl-2/Bax family were involved in the chemopreventive effects of licorice root (Glycyrrhiza uralensis Fisch) in MCF-7 human breast cancer cell. J Agric Food Chem. 2004 Mar 24;52(6):1715-19.

102. Li, YC., YS Tyan, et al. Baicalein induced in vitro apoptosis undergo caspases activity in human promyleoctyic leukemia HL-60 cells. Food and Chemical Toxicology. 2004;42:37-43.

103. Pathak A, et al. Potentiation of the effect of Paclitaxel and Carboplatin by antioxidant mixture on human lung cancer H520 cells. Journal of the American College of Nutrition. 2002;21(5): 416-21.

104. Prasad KN. Multiple dietary antioxidants enhance the efficacy of standard and experimental cancer therapies and

decrease their toxicity. Integrative Cancer Therapies. 2004;3(4):310-22.

105. Prasad, KN, A Kumar, V Kochupillia, WC Cole. High doses of multiple antioxidant vitamins: essential ingredients in improving the efficacy of standard cancer therapy. Journal of the American College of Nutrition, 1999;18(1):13-35.

106. Radhakrishna PG, et al. Induction of apoptosis in human lung cancer cells by curcumin. Cancer Lett. 2004 May 28;208(2):171-78.

107. Saada Helen N, Azab Khaled S. Role of lycopene in recovery of radiation induced injury to mammalian cellular organelles Pharmazie. 2001 Mar;56(3):239-41.

108. Sah JF, Balasubramanian S, Eckert RL, Rorke EA. Epigallocatechin-3-gallate inhibits epidermal growth factor receptor signaling pathway: evidence for direct inhibition of ERK1/2 and AKT kinases. J Biol Chem. 2004;279:12755-62.

109. Sarkar FH, Li Y. Soy isoflavones and cancer prevention. Cancer Invest. 2003;21(5):744-57.

110. Scambia G, De Vincenzo R, et al. Antiproliferative effect of silybin on gynaecological malignancies: synergism with cisplatin and doxorubicin Eur J Cancer. 1996 May;32A(5):877-82 (Cell Culture Study).

111. Upadhyay S, Neburi M, et al. Differential sensitivity of normal and malignant breast epithelial cells to genistein is partly mediated by p21(WAF1). Clin Cancer Res. 2001 Jun;7(6):1782-89.

112. Virgili F, Acconcia F, et al.Nutritional flavonoids modulate estrogen receptor alpha signaling. IUBMB Life. 2004 Mar;56(3):145-51.

113. Yi Ching Hsieh, Ross C, et al. Estrogenic effects of genistein on the growth of estrogen receptor-positive human breast cancer (MCF-7) cells in vitro and in vivo. Cancer Research. 1998;58, 3833-38.

114. Zhao KS, Mancini C, Doria G. 1990. Enhancement of immune response in mice by Astragalus membranaceus extracts. Immunopharmacolgy 20: 225-34

PART 5: NATUROPATHIC BEST PRACTICES CASE STUDIES

Case

BREAST CANCER

41-year-old female: pT1cN0, gravida 0, para 0

Dx: The initial lesion was found in the right breast in the right outer quadrant at 10:00; follow up with mammography and ultrasound guided biopsy revealed positive adenocarcinoma of the breast. Surgical excision with pathology revealed a 1.2 cm x 0.8 cm tumor without clean surgical margins; DCIS and invasive/inflammatory cell line with necrotic center and microcalcifications with invasive ductal cancer stage 2 without lymphovascular invasion; four sentinel lymph nodes all negative; and ER+, PR+, Her-2/neu- (by FISH), BRCA ½ -, BIRAD 6. An additional lump was found in left breast; biopsy revealed atypical hyperplasia.

+FMHx: Positive for breast cancer: maternal grandmother, maternal grandfather's sisters all died from breast cancer. Mother is currently in remission. PT has been having mammograms annually since she was 34 yo due to her family history and her large and fibrous breast tissue. With follow-up mammography, her breast cancer was detected early. The patient is feeling considerable stress and anxiety because of her diagnosis and her family history.

Tx: First oncologist opinion suggested chemotherapy following surgery with cyclophosphomide and Taxotere, infusion every 3 weeks for 4 rounds, followed by radiation for 5 weeks, with 5 days on 2 days off, with a 2 week booster at the end of the radiation sequence, followed by 5 years of oral Tamoxifen.

Second oncologist opinion suggested that because her BRCA ½ was negative, chemotherapy is not recommended. Oncotype Dx showed only an 11 for recurrence score of genetic typing of cancer. Suggested that only radiation is needed for 5 weeks with treatment for 5 days on 2 days off and then a 2 week booster at the end of the sequence, for a total of 7 weeks. PT decided to take this route, supplemented with oral Tamoxifen, to start with radiation treatment. The radiation application was IMRT. She was tattooed for accurate treatment fields.

NATUROPATHIC INTEGRATIVE TX:

The patient was established in my care prior to diagnosis so naturopathic best practices could be applied as soon as a suspicious lesion was found. The following management plan was implemented.

Before biopsy

All supplements were discontinued 3 days to 1 week prior and homeopathic pre- and post -surgery protocols were initiated.

Pre-surgery
- Homeopathics:
- Arnica: 1M one hour before surgery and in recovery, followed with Arnica 30c 1-3 pellets SL PO tid for 3-6 weeks
- Staphysagria: 6x 1-3 pellets SL PO tid for 3-6 weeks
- Thiosianmus 6x 1-3 pellets SL PO tid for 3-6 weeks
- Pectasol C™ (modified citrus pectin): 2 scoops qd
- CoQ10 (Vitaline): 200-400 mg qd

Post-surgery

After surgery when the patient was discharged and eating, eliminating, and sleeping normally, naturopathic integrative medicine was used aggressively while she awaited her first and second opinions from medical oncologists.
- CoQ10: 300 mg bid
- Pectasol C: 1 scoop bid
- Indole-3-Carbinol (MetaI3C Metagenics): 2 bid
- Calcium-D-glucarate: 1000 mg bid – tid
- Melatonin (Vital Nutrients): 20 mg qhs
- Minimal and Essential Vital Nutrients: 1 bid CC (a multivitamin without iron, calcium, magnesium, phosphorus, iodine, thus safe to use with chemo/radio therapies)
- Omega 3 fish oil (dose to EPA): 2-3 g qdin divided doses with food
- Protein: 100 g qd divided in 3 meals and 3 snacks with a protein snack before bedtime

Once the patient decided her medical oncology treatment course of action, L-Glutamine powder was added to the protocol at a dose of 10 g tid, swish and swallow, while the CoQ10 was discontinued 1 week prior to the radiation IMRT start date.

During radiation

Once the patient started radiation treatment:
- Oral Tamoxifen was administered
- Calcium-D-glucarate and MI3C were discontinued
- Green tea caps with 50%-85% polyphenols: 100-150 mg 2 bid
- Probiotics Theracomplete™ (Klaire Labs)

Post- radiation:

- Glutamine powder 4-6 weeks post radiation therapy discontinued
- Patient reported no effects of mucositis, stomatitis, nausea, diarrhea, fatigue, or leucopenia during treatment sequence and worked full time throughout her treatment
- 3 months after the completion of the radiation therapy and the start of oral Tamoxifen menopausal symptoms began. PT reported still having full bleeds and vaginal bleeds after intercourse
- Pelvic ultrasound WNL.
- Patient reports starting Zoloft for hot flashes, night sweats, irritability, mood swings and a general depression. She states that this started while she was in radiation therapy. 3 months after this date, her medical oncologist discontinued her Zoloft, thinking that it could interfere with the Tamoxifen, and switched her to Effexor. 3 months after this medication change, she stopped her menstrual cycle for the first time.

6. Outcomes

Depression: Patient reports that with cessation of menses she has more menopausal symptoms and with the family history of cancer recurrence, she feels more depression. Nevertheless, the patient has been enjoying her life, snowboarding with her partner and communing with her friends and family. She is very positive and active socially, but the depression was overwhelming for her until her Effexor medication was increased. She was then much more able to cope and enjoy life.

Hormone Balance: The next month we looked at her estrogen excretion with a Estronex™ (MetaMetrix) urine test. It was found that she was still dominated in both her 16-αOH-E1and 4-OH-E1, even on Tamox-

ifen. She started DiiM 600 mg b.i.d. to augment estrogen clearance toward the 2-OH-E1and2 pathway.

Stress: Her mother's cancer recurred, requiring her to move to a hospice for total care. This has increased her stress and anxiety, with associated depression. PT was started on:
- Seriphos™ (Interplexus) 2-4 prn and qhs
- L-Theanine 200-400 mg qd- tid
- Calmes Forte™ (Hyland): 1-3 pellets prn SL PO in conjunction with her current Effexor prescription

Long-Term: Her mother died. PT reports that for the following year she has had monthly cycles with PMS while still taking her Tamoxifen, Effexor, and naturopathic protocol.
- Repeated Estronex test and adjusted protocol to accommodate results of high 4-OH-E1 and low 2-OH-E1and2 in ratio to high 16-_OH-E1.
- Patient states she has not been taking her DiiM. DiiM restored to the protocol along with ground flax seeds (not oil!) 2 tbsp qd
- Omega 3 EPA: 3 g qd in divided doses with meals
- CoQ10: 200 mg qd
- Vitamin D-3: 5000 IU qd

Within 3 months of protocol change, PT reports that bleeding has stopped. During the course of follow-up visits signs were negative for recurrence and now she is nearing the completion of her Tamoxifen prescription. We will recheck her estrogen clearance and continue to monitor her progression, but now she is cancer free and enjoying life to the fullest.

CASE MANAGEMENT SKILLS

This patient had specific needs, both clinical and spiritual. Clinically, the patient wanted to explore the best treatment options for the best outcomes. The long-term treatment goals, which include enhancement of the conventional treatment strategy of using Tamoxifen for 5 years; can be managed with functional medicine tests that explore the success of the prescribed strategy. A whole patient- centered approach allows for the individuality needed to manage and improve this patients' treatment effect. This attention to clinical strategies and spiritual support is a characteristic of naturopathic integrative medical practice.

Case

COLORECTAL CANCER

62-year-old male, pT3N0Mx

PT contacted the clinic due to anxiety, insomnia, and a persistent rash that started on his scalp and spread to cover his entire body. PT was working with a local ND to help with his rash, unsuccessfully, and was referred to me as a specialist consult. The rash presented as a macular, popular, erythematous, edematous, pruritic rash that spread concentrically to cover his entire body. It was extremely inflammatory.

Hx: Protocols for topical relief given by his local ND, including topical abx ointment, topical vitamin E, and shea butter with mixed herbs, all exacerbated the condition and increased the burning sensation. The local ND ran stool tests, and I recommended a salivary hormone assay for his stress about his wife's ill health. He was sent to a dermatologist for a work up, and a biopsy of several sites gave a diagnosis as spongiosus dermatitis. The dermatologist gave a prescription of topical hydrocodone cream.

The stool test returned as a O&Px2 and showed a 3+fungi, 2+cocci bacteria and a +KOH. The salivary tests returned with only slight abnormalities. The local ND put the patient on antibiotic clindamycin 450 mg Q 6hrs for 10 days along with probiotics. The patient put himself on TCHM herbs CalmEZ, which he stated is an herbal prednisone. Within 7 days he reported to his local ND rectal bleeding, suspecting hemorrhoids, as he has had them in the past. He reported that his stress is tremendous because his wife has to have back surgery and he is her only care giver. She is bedridden and he has to take her to rehabilitation therapy post surgery.

The dermatologist changed his topical prescription to betamethasone 0.5% bid, which improved his topical rash globally. The patient reported that he still had remnants of the rash on his torso, but it was less pruritic and inflamed.

Suspecting something more serious than spongiosus dermatitis, I suggested that he get a colonoscopy due to his persistent rectal bleeding. At the age of 50, he had never had a baseline colonoscopy. I related to him the experiences I have had with other patients where persistent rectal bleed was not due to hemorrhoids but were symptoms of other conditions, such as systemic candidiasis and colorectal cancer. Patients with these symptoms and the associated inflammatory dermatitis, chronically high stress with insomnia, and

other lifestyle issues all led to my recommendation for a colonoscopy. Sometimes experience and expertise ignites your medical intuition.

About 3 months later he followed up with his local ND, still without a colonoscopy. His rectal bleeding was persistent as was his rash. He completed treatments for systemic candidiasis and dysbiosis without any resolution. The local ND (without visual inspection) gave him an astringent rectal suppository protocol for his hemorrhoids, using Collinsonia and Hammelis herbal rectal implants. Probiotics, anti-inflammatory herbals, biotin, vitamin A, and liver supporting herbs were also given to him by his local ND at that time.

Two days after his visit to his local ND, the patient and I had a telephone follow up. He reported to me that his skin patches were drying with decreased incidence while using the betamethasone ointment, but his skin was thinning with the repeated use of betamethasone. He reported that the local ND treatment of the candidiasis did help with his skin symptoms but did not resolve them. When he had to go on the antibiotics, the skin symptoms flared up without resolution and the rectal bleed increased. He did contact a gastroenterologist to set up his colonoscopy. An incidental chest x-ray was done as preparation for the colonoscopy and it was within normal limits.

Dx: One month later, PT had a colonoscopy, which revealed that he had rectal adenocarcinoma, specifically clinical stage IIA adenocarcinoma of the rectum, 1-2 cm from anus. Diagnostic colonoscopy for pathology found 5 polyps that were suspicious. They were removed.

Pathology revealed adenocarcinoma of the rectum, clinical stage IIA, CEA 21. CT scans showed positive on staging.

NATUROPATHIC INTEGRATIVE TX

All supplements had been discontinued prior to the colonoscopy. While a conventional treatment plan was being determined, PT was started on a naturopathic integrative oncological protocol.

- L-glutamine: 10 g tid, swish and swallow
- MCP: 1 scoop bid
- Melatonin: 20 mg qhs
- Meriva™ (Thorne phytosomal activated curcumin): 500-1000 mg bid-tid
- Vitamin D-3: 5000 IU qd
- Minimal and Essential™ Vital Nutrients: 1 bid CC
- Theracomplete™ (Klaire Labs) probiotics: 1 bid IC

Within 3 weeks, the patient met with his radiation oncologist, and it was decided that neoadjuvant chemotherapy with radiation therapy followed by a surgical resection could cure the cancer and leave him without a permanent colostomy.

The sensitizing chemotherapeutic was Xeloda, used neoadjuvantly with radiation applied for 5 days on, 2 days off for 8 weeks, followed in 4-6 weeks with surgery.

During neoadjuvant chemoradiation, the Meriva was discontinued, but all other supplements were continued until 1 week prior to surgery.

Outcomes

Stress: Note about the psychoneuroimmunology of the patient – he has had a lifetime of stress and unhappiness. It is not until his relocation and marriage to his wife that he has been happy. He stated frankly to me that he is worried about his health, but more about his wife and who would take care of her if he got treatment for his cancer. We had a long discussion about using his care team of friends to help: establishing someone to come and clean his house, do their laundry and cook meals and freeze them while he is in radiation treatment. We discussed how this gives his friends and loved ones something 'to do' to help him as well as take some of the burden off of him during his treatment course. This seemed to relieve some of his stress and make it all seem more possible for him.

CASE MANAGEMENT SKILLS

A primary management principle seen in this case is to not relent when diagnosing an apparently chronic superficial disease like candidiasis. In this case, chronic candida infection was a cofactor in colorectal cancer but this was misdiagnosed. This type of misdiagnosis can be lethal, in that the earlier detection and diagnosis of colorectal cancer leads to a greater cure rate, while late stage diagnosis is often incurable.

Likewise, a condition like idiopathic dermatitis may be a cofactor that leads to a diagnosis of cancer. A head-to-toe spongiotic dermatitis of unknown origin is definitely related to a systemic IgE response, and by what we know about inflammation, TH2 and IgE and stress are directly related.

Long-term stress creates the mileu or hot bed for cancer cells to mutate into creation, changing protooncogene to oncogene. Stress arising from an oppressive childhood with physical, sexual, and psychological abuse can lead to an adulthood of substance abuse and depression.

Foremost of all case management principles is simple: chronic rectal bleeding must always be diagnosed!

Case

LEUKEMIA

64-year-old female: myelodysplastic anemia syndrome cancer of the bone marrow that turned into AML Stage IV

PT presented with mild thrombocytopenia and neutropenia and anemia, extreme anxiety attacks, and chronic B-12 deficiency with above normal serum folate.

Hx: PT was diagnosed with MDS 10 years prior to her leukemia diagnosis. She started hormone replacement therapy around the same time as she started to have symptoms of fatigue. Biopsy at the time revealed hypercellular marrow with relative erythroid hyperplasia and some dysplastic megakaryocytes. She was given injections of procrit for her low RBC and vitamin B-12 for her megaloblastic anemia. She was followed for a decade and considered to be without symptoms, except with the continuation of fatigue that was extreme by the end of the day. Her chief complaints were chronic anxiety and depression due to a traumatic past.

She sought out integrative naturopathic therapies to help with her chronic fatigue, anxiety, and depression. She was interested in testing for heavy metals because her long-time exposure to toxins in her profession. She also had questions regarding the value of taking CoQ10, curcumin, and other supplements. PT had solicited several second opinions from different cancer centers and now wanted to work with her local cancer clinic. A full autoimmune work up with MD was negative.

NATUROPATHIC INTEGRATIVE TX

Initial protocol

For her symptoms, we initiated a naturopathic integrative protocol:

- Seriphos: 2-4 qhs and prn for anxiety and PTSD
- IgGDF 2000: 1 scoop bid
- CoQ10: 200-300 mg bid
- Mushroom extracts: reishi, maitake, shitake, tid

Within a month, a repeat bone marrow test revealed M6 AML, with a blast count of 22, which was considered a sequelae of her long-standing MDS. It was recommended that she start chemotherapy: daunorubincin with 7 days of ara-C and a consideration of decitabine.

During Gemcitabine chemotherapy

Her protocol was upgraded to:

- Minimal and Essential: 1 bid CC (Vital Nutrients)
- Omega 3 (dose to EPA): 2-3 g CC
- L-glutamine: 10 g tid, swish and swallow
- CoQ10 was discontinued
- Melatonin was contraindicated

After chemotherapy

PT reported that after chemotherapy she was able to visit with her grandchildren who lived in a different state. One of her goals had been to be healthy enough to visit with her grandchildren due to her leucopenia. It had previously been contraindicated. She was very happy to have met this goal and it gave her hope to continue with treatment.

Outcomes

Bone marrow transplant: The Gemcitabine did not work that well, but she underwent a successful bone marrow transplant with cord blood. This positive effect lasted for about a year, although she was hospitalized most of this time and in isolation due to her very low leucopenia. Doxirubicin became the chemotherapy of choice after the bone marrow transplant failed. It was administered as an IV infusion every 4 weeks, which resulted in a slight increase in WBC to a low normal of 3.0.

Adverse reactions: 3 weeks after starting the new chemotherapy, there were some adverse reactions to the chemo with systemic purpurea edema on her tibial shins. One week later there was a 10% increase in AML cells, and one week after that, a 45% increase in AML cells. PT was given 4 weeks to live at that time.

After prognosis

Despite this prognosis, an aggressive naturopathic integrative protocol was started for AML and cachexia:
- Minimal and Essential (Vital Nutrients): 1 bid CC
- IgGDF 2000: 1 tbsp bid
- CoQ10: 300 mg bid
- L-glutamine: 10 g tid, swish and swallow
- Curcumin (activated): 2 tid
- Stametes7: 2 bid-tid
- Turkey tails: 2 bid-tid
- Biovegetarian™: 2 tid prn
- Protein supplementation: New Zealand whey protein as meal replacement bid
- Seriphos: 2-4 qhs and prn

While following this protocol, PT reported that she had a purpurea rash and that her energy had improved. She did not feel so overwhelmed and felt more capable. She had started to get her final affairs in order and felt that her self esteem had improved. She is now able to have visitors. One of her daughters has moved in to help her. She is looking forward to a visit from her children and grandchildren, as well as finding adoptive homes for her horses and other pets. She is receiving blood transfusions of packed red blood cells as needed. She is getting vitamins B-12 1 cc IM weekly from a hospice and a transfusion about every 2 weeks. WBC and RBC all WNL, and she reports feeling better every week. Four weeks after she was told she had only 4 weeks to live, she had just a little fatigue and had gained 4 lbs. Here rash had resolved and she continued with weekly transfusions and labs.

Infection: PT reported an infection that was triggered by infusion, with high fever. She was using abx prescriptions. At one month follow up, she was great spirits. She was taking platelet transfusions every 3 weeks and packed RBC transfusion every 3 weeks on different weeks than the platelet transfusion. PT was placed on low daily dose of prednisone to decrease reactions to transfusions. The blood infection was resolved, and with the help of the naturopathic integrative protocol, she was able to fight off a cold with a sore throat within 3 days. The medicinal mushroom protocol was changed to Cordyceps, Grifola, and Trametes as leukemia specific treatment.

Pain: At the next month follow up, PT had some edema and weight loss. The hospice had told her that her liver was no longer able to accept the transfusions. She was suffering from some secondary infections of HSVI and II. These infections caused excruciating pain and decreased her will to live. She asked her medical oncologist to change her pain medication. It was changed to a fentanyl transdermal patch with a secondary pain medication if the fentanyl was not controlling the pain.

To give further comfort, an HSV naturopathic protocol was initiated, including:
- NAC: 600 mg tid
- HSV nosode (professional health formulations) :10 gtt tid SL PO
- Topical licorice gel with added lysine (500-1000 mg): applied topically to lesions

Longevity and quality of life: PT died from her disease within 6 weeks of these herpetic infective events. It should be noted that after the patient was sent home from a cancer treatment center of excellence and told she had 4 weeks to live, she lived an additional 4 months with a high quality of life while following a naturopathic integrative protocol. The patient was extremely happy to be home and to be able to take care of her pets and farm animals, set her affairs in order, live with her daughter and boyfriend, and see her family and friends, all in those 4 months. The patient had another chance to see her grandchildren and when she told me how much that meant to her she had tears in her eyes. These are the things life is for!

CASE MANAGEMENT SKILLS

Promoting quality of life, establishing plans for meeting the end of life, and exploring the spirituality of dying - these are characteristic naturopathic integrative medical practice. This involves not just looking at the patient as an object of diagnosis and treatment but as an individual. This is what I call the family standard. If you treat your patients as you would one of your family members or someone whom you love, you will raise that standard of care for that patient and include that patient in the formative decisions about their own end of life process. This is the care we must give our patients, centered on their concerns and needs.

Case

LUNG CANCER

45-year-old male: NSCLC Stage IV adenocarcinoma

PT presented after he noticed some dyspnea while singing in the navy choir. The dyspnea was then noted with exertion, but because of a large GI bleed that required 2 transfusions and left him with an ileus, the dyspnea was forgotten. After a chest CT showed positive for pleural effusion, thoracentesis was performed but was non diagnostic. A second thoracentesis was unsuccessful.

Dx: One year later the patient noticed again that the dyspnea was worsening and had a CT scan, revealing a positive recurrent and chronic right pleural effusion with thickened pleura and nodularity in the right lung. Bronchoscopy for pathologic biopsy with right thorascope and right thoracotomy with 3 wedge resections and pleural decortications revealed nodularity of pearly white nodules implanted along the lung surface. Pathology reported a Stage IV adenocarcinoma of the right lower lung lobe as well as the chest wall lining, with positive mets to 3 lymph nodes and chronic pleural effusion.

Tx: Chemotherapy was initiated with Cisplatin and Pemetrexed IV infusions and the patient sought naturopathic integrative oncology therapies.

NATUROPATHIC INTEGRATIVE TX

The following protocol was integrated with the chemotherapy regimen:
- L-Glutamine: 10 g tid, swish and swallow
- Pectasol-C: 1 scoop bid
- Melatonin: 20 mg qhs
- Probiotics Theracomplete 1 bid IC
- Minimal and Essential (Vital Nutrients): 1 qd-bid
- Omega 3 dose to EPA: 2-3g CC in divided doses

Glutamine gave instant help with mucositis diarrhea and led to more muscle strength and energy. Repeat CT scan after 2 rounds of chemotherapy revealed some interval improvement with residual FDG avid disease at the right supra-clavicale, upper paratracheal, and retrocrural regions. On genetic testing, the cancer cell had a positive EML4-alk translocation, which indicated that the cancer could possibly be treated more effectively with an alk inhibitor.

One more round of the Cisplatin with Pemetrexed was given and the patient reported extreme fatigue and lower ADLs, with an increase in pleural pain. His medical oncologist discontinued the Cisplatin and gave only the Pemetrexed infusion.

Outcomes

Stress: During this transitional time the patient reported that his father had died due to esophageal cancer. This was a very stressful time for him as he was unable to care for himself with his extreme fatigue and reduced ADLs. The patient expressed for the first time some emotion over his diagnosis and the longevity of his life and his wanting to be there for his children and wife.

Clinical trial: After two rounds of the Pemetrexed, it was decided he would be a good candidate for a clinical trial because of the alk infusion gene mutation and a PET/CT scan showing progressive disease with the reduced infusion. The trial involved Crizonitib, otherwise known as 1066 or PF-02341066 in a clinical study in advanced stage NSCLC patients with EML4-alk fusion gene mutation (echinoderm microtubule-associated protein-like 4 anaplastic lymphoma kinase). Patients with this gene mutation have NSCLC without a history of smoking cigarettes and do not have an EGFR mutation (epidermal growth factor receptor gene) or a Kras gene mutation. Only 4% of patients with NSCLC that have these specific criteria.

PT wanted to be in this trial; it gave him hope for his future.

While waiting for the trial to begin, he followed a naturopathic integrative protocol.

- CoQ10: 300 mg tid
- Meriva: 500 mg bid-tid
- Stametes7: 2 bid-tid

30 days after the discontinuance of Cisplatin, all GI complaints were resolved as long as he continued the naturopathic integrative protocol. His ADL functions were all restored to normal.

Second Line Tx

Crizonitib was initiated as a second line therapy due to the EML4-alk translocation with IV infusion every 3 weeks. Patient reported that dyspnea has improved, hoarseness was stable, and pain in his right chest wall pleura had also improved. His ADLs were normal as well as his energy, with a mild interval decrease noted in his disease. PT was excited, animated, and hopeful. He is to be restaged after 4 cycles with follow up scans. He remains on his integrative naturopathic protocol with the discontinuance of the CoQ10 and Meriva with the trial, but all other supplements allowed in the protocol.

CASE MANAGEMENT SKILLS

How we "meet" our patients is the naturopathic integrative principle at work here. This patient is a very conventional conservative man who never had naturopathic care of any kind. He came to naturopathy for integrative care and hope. The improvement of his side effects with integrative protocols enabled him to improve his health status as well as allow him to enhance his cancer treatment.

Case

NON HODGKIN LYMPHOMA

52-year-old male: diffuse large B cell NHL

Hx: PT was first diagnosed at 47 yo with diffuse large B cell NHL, initially with CD30+, CD20+, BCL-2+, BCL-6+, Alk-1 negative. He had a flu infective event that did not resolve until after about a month. Several months later he had another bout of this flu and went to the ER for evaluation. CT of pelvis and abdomen was done and showed extensive peraortic adenopathy. PT has a history of beta thalassemia trait and has been on folate treatment during his adult life.

Dx: A retroperitoneal CT guided biopsy revealed a B cell lymphoma, large cell type. Follow up CT scan revealed progressive disease below the diaphragm and compression of the IAC. Pathology revealed a high risk lymphoma with both CD20 and 30 positivity. Labs revealed WBC WNL, Hgb low at 9.2, Hct low at 30.1, ESR elevated at 90, and LDH elevated at 1018.

Tx: CHOP/Rituxan chemotherapy was started at high dose, followed by autologous stem cell rescue after chemotherapy. Therapy was successful and the lymphoma was in remission for several years.

Recurrence: Approximately 2 years later, a recurrence of the NHL was found in the left thigh. RICE chemotherapy was started since the recurrence showed a pathology of CD30 negative large B cell lymphoma. Two rounds of the RICE therapy was followed by a peripheral stem cell transplant with BEAM chemotherapy. This treatment gave an excellent post transplant response and was determined successful. PET/CT showed no progressive disease

NATUROPATHIC INTEGRATIVE TX

PT requested naturopathic integrative therapies to lower risk of recurrence.

- CoQ10: 200-300 mg bid-tid
- Minimal and Essential: 1 bid CC (Vital Nutrients)
- Vitamin D-3: 2000-5000 IU qd
- L-glutamine: 10 g qd-tid, swish and swallow
- Omega 3 dose to EPA: 2-3 g qd CC in divided doses
- Green tea caps with 50-85% polyphenols tid
- Dietary proteins: 100 g qd with 3 meals and 3 snacks

Vaccination therapy: Upon annual follow up with CT scan, there was no evidence of disease progression, but blood labs found more cytopenia. The medical oncologist suggested a 12 month vaccine therapy with tetanus and diphtheria/hemophillus, to be followed by a 12 month vaccination protocol with tetanus and a 14 month vaccination protocol with diphtheria/hemophillus. After 24 months of the vaccine therapy, PET/CT scan showed no progressive disease, WBC low at 3.2, ANC 1.4, Hgb low at 10.4, Platelet at 193, MCV 69. He remained on his naturopathic integrative protocol. At his 4 month follow up, labs showed WBC back to normal, Hgb stable, and platelet count stable. A quantatative immunoglobulin study was ordered and showed WNL. PET/CT revealed new localized activity at the left axillary, which was suspected to be recurrent lymphoma. The anomaly was found to be the site where his vaccination therapy was administered 48 hours previous to the PET/CT scan.

Lifestyle change: PT changed his life completely upon initial diagnosis of NHL. He retired from his high powered cooperate job and began studying meditation and yoga while practicing the ancient exchange of "giving the light," an energetic use of chakra light energy to heal and balance. Currently, the patient is considered to be in complete NHL remission 2 years after his last treatment. He has continued to use his alternative lifestyle, spirituality, and philosophy to remain healthy and cancer free. His current labs reveal low levels of vitamin D-3 and slight cardiomyopathy secondary to his extensive chemotherapeutics.

PT continues to follow a naturopathic integrative protocol:

- CoQ10: 200-300 mg qd-bid
- Minimal and Essential: 1 bid CC
- Vitamin D-3: 2000-5000 IU qd
- Omega 3 dose to EPA: 2-3 g qd in divided doses CC
- Green tea: 5-6 cups qd
- Stametes7: 2 bid
- Meriva: 500 mg bid
- By his own self prescription he has added in Essiac tea, yogi tea and flaxseed oil

CASE MANAGEMENT SKILLS

In this case, we see how the patient's investment in his own health has an exceptional effect on his ability to heal himself. This patient changed his life. He had the means to quit working and began studying a spiritual life and a healing practice. As he worked on healing himself, he recognized the importance of sharing that healing energy with others. This is the most important lesson anyone can learn – and the very special gift cancer patients give to their doctors....a life lesson of unconventional love.

Case

OVARIAN CANCER

67-year-old female: pT3cN4M2 adenocarcenoma

Dx: Gravid 3, para 3, diagnosed with the initial suspicion arising after a post menopausal bleed after 10 years without a menstrual cycle. Upon GYN pelvic examination, leiomyoma was suspected, but upon ultrasonography, it was found to be a large 10 cm diameter ovarian growth on the left ovary. The right ovary had multiple smaller growths.

Her history and her family history were negative for cancer. CT/MRI examinations revealed multiple sites of lymphadenopathy within the abdominal and pelvic lymphatics. Tumor markers were positive with elevated CA125, HcG and LDH. PT was complaining of shortness of breath at the time of diagnosis and abdominal ascites was found pathologic upon thorancentesis.

Tx: It was decided that neoadjuvant chemotherapy would be used prior to surgical intervention. Taxol and carboplatin were chosen as the neoadjuvant protocol to be administered weekly for 3-4 weeks prior to surgery.

PT was diagnosed at a known cancer treatment center of excellence and was admitted to an integrative hospital system. She received patient centered care with naturopathic integrative treatments, physical therapy, psychotherapy, and pastoral care, all at the time of diagnosis. The integrative protocol was to be inclusive of both her 'IN' hospital patient status and her 'OUT' of hospital patient status. All departments met with the patient individually and then with each other to establish the best patient specific patient-centered approach possible. The patient was able to receive her neoadjuvant chemotherapy as an outpatient and commute locally from home.

NATUROPATHIC INTEGRATIVE TX:

All supplements to be discontinued one week prior to surgery. Homeopathic Pre and Post surgery protocol to be administered at that time.

- Minimal and Essential (Vital Nutrients): 1 bid CC
- Omega 3 dose to EPA: 2-3 g qd in divided doses CC
- Vitamin D-3: 2000 IU qd
- Pectasol-C: 1 scoop bid
- L-glutamine: 10 g tid, swish and swallow
- Calcium-d-glucarate 1000 mg tid
- Rhizinate: dgl, prn, suck or chew for xerostoma
- Cal Appatite Forte™ (Metagenics): 3 qhs
- Protein: 100 g protein
- Colorful fruits and veggies in small frequent meals throughout the day

Outcomes

Rehabilitation fitted her for a prosthetic wig due to the side effect of alopecia from her chemotherapy. Physical rehab with acupuncture for post surgery was recommended, and massage once the surgical site had healed. PhD psychologist to have ongoing meetings with the patient and her husband when they are here for infusions to help with processing the diagnosis and the anger and disbelief both of them are feeling.

Pastoral care: Pastoral care was determined by patient to be better served by the pastor at her local church, which she attends weekly. She describes herself as a deeply religious and faith-based person, who is hopeful and has a lot to do before she is ready to die.

Surgery: After the patient's neoadjuvant therapy was complete, the tumor had successfully shrunk and oncological surgery was determined to be appropriate. Surgery involved an extensive full bilateral oopherectomy and radical hysterectomy, as well as an infrolic omenectomy and a peritoneal scrapping and wash. It was determined that there were up to 7 possible sentinel lymph nodes that were removed from the pelvis and lower abdominal regions. Pathology revealed that only 4 out of those 7 were positive for her disease. Adenocarcinoma of the ovaries had metastasized to the peritoneal cavity, at the greater omentum and inguinal lymph nodes. Genetic testing showed BRCA1/2 negative. The surgeon was a skilled oncological surgeon and for almost 5 hours 'peeled' the cancer off her perotineal cavity. This decreased the overall tumor burden significantly.

Chemotherapy: Her care team and the patient determined that staging and grading of her cancer indicated Gemcitabine IV infusion every 3 weeks for 6 rounds as her post surgical protocol. The patient was positive and hopeful, wanting to go home as soon as possible and see her family: her granddaughter in particular was of elementary school age and lived with her grandparents half of the time. The patient's surgical recovery was swift and within a few days she was at home with her family.

During the next year the patient was treated successfully with the gemcitabine infusion with CT negative follow ups and CA 125 WNL and very little side effects while on the integrative protocol. Approximately 1 ½ years into the chemotherapy, adjuvant therapy ceased to work. Her CA 125 marker began to rise, and a metastasis to her liver was found. Her chemotherapy was changed to Adriamycin and Taxotere, to be administered as an IV infusion every 2 weeks if tolerated. The patient had many more side effects to this protocol, with neutropenia, frank leucopenia, and anemia requiring neupagen and procrit injections to be administered with infusions. The patient complained of fatigue, anxiety, and a sense of dread with the new chemotherapeutics. After two rounds,it was determined that the protocol was not successful by her continual elevation of CA 125 tumor marker.

The patient was then placed on a tertiary oral chemotherapy, Tarceva 100 mg qd, and sent home to return in a one week follow up. Upon return she was complaining of difficulty breathing, and it was observed that she had abdominal ascites. Thorancentsis was administered and it was confirmed to be pathologic ascites. It was discussed at that time that thorancentesis could be administered weekly to biweekly as needed for the comfort of the patient. The patient stated that she did not want to be hospitalized and would rather be at home with her family, friends, and loved ones. Her WBC/RBC counts were good enough for her to be at home with hospice care.

PT succumbed to her disease 6 months from being discharged to her home with hospice. The patient had several end-of-life goals. When she came to the cancer treatment center of excellence her first oncology opinion gave her only 4-6 months to live. In her second choice of treatment with the integrative approach, she lived for 2 years post diagnosis and most of those months she was well and in full functioning capacity. She was extremely happy for the extra time with her husband and family, and it allowed her to heal and have closure with her nuclear family and set her own heart and affairs in order.

CASE MANAGEMENT SKILLS

This patient's faith in her systems of care enabled her to go through grueling treatment with minimal side effects. The elderly often have fewer reactions to and tolerate better the challenges of chemotherapy and radiotherapy. In younger women, these same treatments cause increased side effects, but in women in their sixties or older these same doses produce minimal side effects.

Case

PANCREATIC CANCER

69-year-old female Stage IV adenocarcinoma

Dx: Pancreatic cancer was diagnosed after a non-descriptive, left-sided pain 'under the rib cage' progressively worsened. It progressed to a sharper left-sided epigratic pain during the winter without any other GI, GU, pulmonary, or cardiac complaints. But CT scan was positive in the spring for a tumor 3.5 cm x 2.6 cm in the tail of the pancreas and multiple liver lesions: right liver lobe with 6 small lesions; and left lobe with a 3.2 cm x 2.4 cm tumor with some ductal dilatation distally. Pathologic biopsy, ultrasound guided, revealed pancreatic adenocarcinoma, CK19+, HepPar-1 negative, CA19-9 at 41.6 and elevated CEA at the time of diagnosis.

Tx: A second oncologist at a known cancer center of excellence agreed with her local oncologist to start with oral Tarceva, in conjunction with an IV infusion of Gemcitabine Q 3 weeks. The patient does have concomitant Mediterranean thalassemia anemia, HTN, and hyperlipidemia. FOLFOX was the other therapy suggested, but only if the combination therapy failed. She started oral Tarceva and Gemcitabine infusions. Almost immediately she had a positive response to the Tarceva by having a "rash response." The Tarceva rash is an erythematous, macular rash that has raised, dry lesions, dime size. It is highly pruritic. Neutropenia and an increase to her anemia occurred within 3 weeks of the start of chemotherapy. This became so fulminant that the next infusion she was scheduled for had to be postponed.

NATUROPATHIC INTEGRATIVE TX

PT began to follow a naturopathic integrative protocol soon after diagnosis.

1. After diagnosis

- CoQ10: 300 mg bid-tid
- L-Glutamine: 10 g tid, swish and swallow
- Omeg 3 dose to EPA: 2-3g in divided doses qd CC
- Minimal and Essential multivitamin™: 1 bid CC
- Pectasol-C™: 1 scoop bid
- Pancreatic digestive enzymes, including HCL and ox bile acid with food
- Probiotic, Theracomplete™:1 bid IC
- Protein: 100 g daily with 3 meals and 3 snacks
- Organic, whole foods and organic meats and dairy only.

2. During chemotherapy

Added to her integrative naturopathic protocol:

- Stametes7™: 2 bid-tid fungi perfecti
- Turkey Tails™: 1-2 bid-tid fungi perfecti
- EGCG as 50-85% polyphenols: 125-200 mg bid-tid
- Tace minerals as LDA Mineral™ (Klaire Labs): qd
- Iron complex™: 100 mg ferrous gluconate qd CC in divided doses

PT was able to resume her chemotherapy, and her WBC and RBC have become stable. It was suggested that she use the neulasta/neupagen protocol with her oncologist so that her treatment cycles will not be interrupted again. She has used these interventions before but has severe leg cramps, pain and flu-like symptoms with each use and cannot tolerate the adverse effects. Ashwagandha (BanYan company) was used to enhance the mushroom protocol, and she was bumped up to all three interventions at top doses of 2 each tid. The WBC responded quite favorably. IgGDF2000 and bone marrow soup stocks were added to her protocol. The cancer center of excellence also had her on acupuncture for mucositis, but that was discontinued due to her low WBC leucopenia and the threat of cellulitis. A substitute was cranial & sacral therapy if she wanted it.

PT reported that with the addition of ashwagandha her energy has improved, and she is getting more exercise and social activity. This woman is highly supported by her family. Her first office visit included her husband and two adult daughters. She is well supported and loved by her family and it shows in her outlook on life. She is social, happy, and very tied to her family and friends. Her outlook has always been that of a positive cancer fighter, that moves forward with the love and help of her family, friends, and community.

For 1 year she continued on this chemotherapeutic regimen with minimal side effects of a little diarrhea the first few days after infusion. Re-evaluative scans showed that her liver lesions were reduced and pancreatic lesions stable. After about one year, CT scan showed a slight increase in the size of the original pancreatic tumor, and in response the chemotherapy regimen was changed to Oxaliplatin, Irinotecan and 5FU (FOLFOX) IV infusion every 3 weeks.

Naturopathic Integrative Protocol:
PT wanted to discontinue several supplements but her medical oncologist told her not to change anything she was doing because it is working for her. However, her naturopathic doctor recommended:

- Castor oil (hexane free) applied topically to

palms of hands and soles of feet bilaterally as prophylactic to hand foot syndrome. (PPE)

- Sublingual vitamin B-2, B-6 and FA
- Catnep tea for nausea and vomiting
- Medical marijuana: for low appetite and neuralgia a discussion of medical marijuana was had by both her naturopathic and medical oncology doctors.

Sleep intrusion, anxiety, and extreme leucopenia ensued right after the new chemotherapy was started, CA 19-9 @ 96. She received a neupagen shot and added to her protocol:

- Stamets7: 2 tid fungi perfecti
- Turkey tails: 2 tid fungi perfecti
- Ashwagandha: 2 tid
- IgGDF 2000: 1 tbsp bid
- Iron complex: 2 bid CC
- Seriphos™ (phosphorylated serine) 2-4 qhs

Within 2 months, CT scans showed improved tumor shrinkage, and 5 more rounds of FOLFOX were ordered. No hand foot syndrome was reported, and the patient was active, happy, and highly functioning. She did lose all of her hair, but got a fabulous wig and kept on going!

Two months later her CA 19-9 was reduced to 25, and CT scans showed stable disease in the liver and pancreas, while others lesions in these organs had shrunk. The FOLFOX was given every 2 weeks at this point, with the only side effect being slight peripheral neuropathy manifesting as tingling in hands, which cold to touch objects make worse. PT reports that she discontinued the glutamine herself for no reason and will put herself back on the protocol. The patient's medical oncologist was so pleased with her results that she decided to take out the Oxaliplatin and do the infusions every 3 weeks. This was done for 3 months with good results of a low CA 19-9 to 11, which is normal!

A block in the colon required the chemotherapy to be discontinued, but CT with colonoscopy revealed no mass or cancerous growth in the colon. The blockage may have been due to swollen tissue from inflammation, and a surgical diversion of the small bowel with a temporary colostomy bag is currently scheduled. There was no chemotherapy one month prior to this operation. Homeopathic surgery protocol was initiated pending surgery.

Continual blockage led to further exploration and PT underwent exploratory surgery. Surgery revealed that she had multiple metastases on the outside of the colon, which had created a compression on the colon

due to the size and amount of the lesions. Partial removal of the colon and a colostomy bag was placed at the time of this surgery. While the CT scans showed a remission status the metastatic cancer was actually growing in another area at a rapid rate. It was therefore regarded as chemorefractory at this point. The patient eventually was released to home with hospice aid and the aid of her daughters and husband. She became cachexic while hospitalized and weighed around 89 lbs. at the time of discharge. The integrative team was to try to increase her body weight and then reassess for treatment options. However, the patient succumbed to her disease, surrounded by her family at home after living almost 2 years beyond her initial cancer prognosis at the time of diagnosis.

CASE MANAGEMENT SKILLS

Cancer patients die, which is disturbing to the family and the physician. This patient had far outlived her expected outcomes and lived with a high quality of life until the last 6 weeks of her life. She was able to live her life to full capacity and was in Florida on vacation when she took a turn for the worst. Her time on this Earth was enhanced, and she enjoyed her family and friends This is the *Vis* in action.

Case

PROSTATE CANCER

74- year-old male adenocarcinoma

Hx: PT was diagnosed with prostate cancer in 1991 after attending a local health fair and discovering that his PSA screening was elevated. He followed up with his medical doctor and had a prostate biopsy that showed 5 out of 5 core samples positive for adenocarcinoma of the prostate gland. The patient underwent a radical prostatectomy within 1 year of the health fair screening. Watchful Waiting therapy ensued for the next decade.

Metastasis: Approximately 10 years post radical prostatetectomy, metastatic disease was found in the left hip and sacrum when his PSA was found to be elevated. PT started Lupron and Casodex orally, and the PSA levels went down to undetectable limits. He reports that about this time he became a vegan as a complete dietary change from the high fat, processed non organic foods diet he had previously. The patient has cofactorial disease: obesity, NIDDM, HTN, and hyperlipidemia. His vegan diet change led to weight loss of 100+ lbs.

Zometa IV infusion for bone density was started and continued throughout care. One month after starting lupron and casodex therapies, they were discontinued due to side effects of 2+ pitting independent edema. The Lupron was continued and did control the PSA for almost three years in conjunction with the patient's organic vegan diet.

Orchiectomy: At this time the PSA began to rise and the patient was offered a switch to a different GnRH agonist, the patient declined. Instead the patient opted to have a bilateral orchiectomy with his investigation of hormone blockade and orchiectomy. The orchiectomy was successful in decreasing the PSA to neglible limits .

NATUROPATHIC INTEGRATIVE TX

After surgery, PT sought integrative naturopathic therapies.

Initial protocol:

- CoQ10: 400 mg qd-tid
- Calcium-D-glucarate: 1000 mg tid
- Zyflamend™ (New Chapter):1-2 bid
- Vitamin D-3: 2000-5000 IU qd
- Omega 3 dose to EPA: 2-3 g qd CC
- Minimal and Essential (Vital Nutrients): 1 bid CC
- Saw Palmetto complex with 85% betasitosterols, including Nettle root, Pumpkin seeds, Pygeum,
- Zinc picolinate 30-60 mcg bid

Outcome

Lifestyle: For 3 years he continued on this protocol, along with his upgraded protein addition to his vegan diet with more soy proteins, legumes and whole grains. Naturopathic best practices continued to work on his ongoing metabolic syndrome, creating better glucose tolerance and decreasing his need for oral glucophage use. Diet and lifestyle changes regulated his hypertension, and herbal therapies for HTN were successful in controlling his BP without allopathic medication.

PT is a very spiritual person with positive and sunny personality. He and his wife are 'snowbirds' and usually spend the winters in Florida with family members. Allowing for his spirit-mind-body connection this was strongly encouraged. The PSA remained undetectable, the boney mets to the hip and sacrum remained stable and non progressive, and he remained highly functioning.

Stress: Several high stress incidents occurred during these three years, including a job loss and an inability to find another, his wife's health deterioration, and

financial stressors from the economic devastation of his retirement investments. PSA levels jumped sharply and his medical oncologist put him back on the Casodex. PSA levels continued to rise while on Casodex and it was discontinued. Within a year, boney mets spread to the left calvarium, left proximal femur, and thoracic spine, as well as the left hip. Sacrum mets increased. These metastases caused pain with ambulation, such that he could not get up and down his stairs in his home.

PT went to Florida, where his local oncologist applied spot external beam radiation therapy with good results. This resulted in much improved ADLs and mobility without prosthesis. Upon return in the spring, it was found that his PSA was rising, and a follow-up bone scan showed new boney mets the to left clavicle, scapulae bilaterally, the skull, right femur, and the sternum. He was started on Ketaconazole and hydrocortisone with a PSA at that time of 45. He rapidly developed dyspnea, orthopnea, muscle weakness, extreme fatigue, and bradycardia. Ketaconazole was discontinued, and an emergency pacemaker was placed due to a complete heart block.

Stem Cell Transplant Tx: PT changed his medical oncologist because of a failure to explain the side effects of ketoconazole. His new medical oncologist suggested autologous stem cell transplant therapy called Provenge as his next best intervention. His integrative naturopathic protocol was changed to accommodate that protocol, which causes extreme leucopenia and anemia as a side effect. Treatment was for 3 rounds, and it was suggested that Taxotere or Abiraterone be used post treatment as the next chemotherapeutic intervention.

- Stametes7™ (Fungi Perfecti): Medicinal mycelia of 7 mushrooms, 2 bid
- Melatonin: 20 mg qhs (Vital Nutrients)
- IgGDF2000™ (Xymogen) immunoglobulin IgG dairy and colostrums free: 1-2 g qd
- Turkey Tails™ (Fungi Perfecti): 1-2 tid
- Vitamin D-3: 10 k qd for 30 Days (by Medical Doctor)

The Provenge treatment was completed with severe anemia and neutropenia remaining 4-6 weeks after completion. Naturopathic integrative strategies continued to work to increase WBC/RBC formation, and it was suggested that the patient add some organic wild red meats in the diet. Sublingual vitamin B-12 and folate was previously added as well as ferrous gluconate supplementation to hold back anemia. PT did comply and noted that his energy was improved. At the next visit it was suggested that he consider some organic local poultry and immune tonic soups: boiling the bones of an organic chicken to make a thick chicken stock to use to make a soup adding in vegetables and medicinal mushrooms of shitake, maitake and reishi as well as super foods of garlic and onions. It was also suggested that he contact a local organic meat grower and get some large stew bones with marrow and create another soup stock for stews out of the marrow bones. In addition to this diet change, L-glutamine 10 g tid, swish and swallow, was added to the naturopathic integrative protocol, while calcium-D-glucarate, saw palmetto complex, CoQ10, and Zyflamend were discontinued with the start of chemotherapy.

Unfortunately, the patient had a metastatic lesion growing behind his right eye. He was placed in rehabilitation after having the lesion surgical resected. The patient was weakened because status he also had metastatic disease in his bones. The surgery was successful for a craniotomy that scraped the cancer from behind his eye and off the periphery of the frontal lobe of his brain. The patient was released to hospice and home care and has recovered remarkably. He is now ambulatory with only a walking cane, has some vision restoration in the right eye, has had a successful reverse colostomy, and continues to thrive and enjoy his life to this day. He continues to take his supplements as well as a tertiary chemotherapy regimen and is being managed successfully in a collaborative fashion with the patient the center of the focus and healing.

ADDENDUM: The patient's faith never wavered, although his spirits 'dipped' at times as he described it. His Vis and the support of church, family, and friends has kept his spirit strong during this challenging time of his life. He continues to be an inspiration to his patients and colleagues a great healer.

CASE MANAGEMENT SKILLS
The threat at this time is that the patient's faith and spirit will be brought down due to these setbacks. His ability to always look at the glass as half full has served him in his fight against cancer. My concern is that he will begin to fail in his fight. The challenge is to encourage the *Vis* in his constitution – his ability to heal. Surrounded by his family and friends he has responded well to being home and rehabilitating. His community church has provided rides, meals and support.